Diagnosing history

MANCHESTER
1824

Manchester University Press

Diagnosing history

Medicine in television period drama

Edited by Katherine Byrne, Julie Anne Taddeo and James Leggott

MANCHESTER UNIVERSITY PRESS

Published by Manchester University Press
Oxford Road, Manchester M13 9PL

www.manchesteruniversitypress.co.uk

British Library Cataloguing-in-Publication Data

A catalogue record for this book is available from the British Library

ISBN 978 1 5261 6328 8 hardback

First published 2022

Typeset by Deanta Global Publishing Services,
Chennai, India

This book is dedicated to all the physicians, nurses, and researchers, past and present, whose hard work has changed our lives for the better.

Contents

Figures

Contributors

Gordon R. Alley-Young, PhD, is a Communication Studies Professor at Kingsborough Community College – CUNY. His study 'Co-opting Voice and Cultivating Fantasy: Contextualizing and Critiquing the *A Gay Girl in Damascus* Hoax Blog' appears in the book *Ethics, Ethnocentrism and Social Science Research* (Routledge, 2020). His research focus includes critical cultural studies of teachers/students, politics, and intersectional identities in popular media.

Marie Allitt is an Early Career Teaching and Research Fellow in Twentieth Century Literature at the University of Edinburgh. Prior to this role, she was Humanities and Healthcare Fellow at the University of Oxford, involved in integrating humanities and professionalism teaching in the medical school. Her research focuses on literary medical humanities, medical life writing, the senses, spaces, environments, and architectures of medicine and health, and medical education. She is the author of the forthcoming *Medical Caregiving Narratives of the First World War: Geographies of Care* (Edinburgh University Press, 2022).

Jacqueline D. Antonovich is an Assistant Professor in History at Muhlenberg College in Allentown, Pennsylvania, where she specialises in the history of medicine and politics in the United States. Her current research focuses on women physicians and medical imperialism in the American West. She is the creator, co-founder, and executive editor of Nursing Clio, a peer-reviewed collaborative blog project that ties historical scholarship to present-day issues related to gender, health, and medicine.

Kristin Brig is a PhD candidate in the history of medicine at Johns Hopkins. She is broadly interested in the history of public health in nineteenth-century British Africa. She is currently working on her dissertation, which examines how municipal and resident water management strategies reacted to and co-existed with one another in nineteenth-century Cape Colony and Natal port cities.

Katherine Byrne is a lecturer in English at Ulster University. She is the author of *Tuberculosis and the Victorian Literary Imagination* (Cambridge University Press, 2011) and *Edwardians on Screen: From Downton Abbey to Parade's End* (Palgrave, 2015). She is one of the editors of *Conflicting Masculinities: Men in Television Period Drama* (IB Tauris, 2018) and co-author (with Julie Anne Taddeo) of a book on rape in period drama television.

Emily J. Clark is a PhD Candidate in the History of Medicine at Johns Hopkins University. She specialises in the study of reproduction and sexuality in the seventeenth- and eighteenth-century Atlantic World, with a particular focus on issues of gender, class, and race. Her dissertation, titled 'Laboring Bodies: Dispossessed Women and Reproduction in Colonial New England', argues that gender and racial norms were shaped in reaction to the productive and reproductive labours of enslaved, servant, and poor working women.

Sarah E. Fanning is the Director of Drama and Lecturer in English at Mount Allison University. She is the editor of the journal *Brontë Studies* and co-editor with Dr Claire O'Callaghan (Loughborough University) of the forthcoming edited collection *Serial Killing on Screen: Adaptation, True Crime and Popular Culture* (Palgrave, 2022). Her research interests include the Brontës, adaptation, the Victorians, period drama, mental health, and true crime.

Jennifer M. Fogel is an Associate Professor of Broadcasting and Mass Communication at SUNY-Oswego. Her research examines contemporary popular culture, particularly the way that gender is represented on television. Her previous work has analysed the gendered marketing of *Star Wars* toys, the commodification of Carrie Fisher's image as Princess Leia in *Star Wars*, cognitive dissonance in fandom, and articulations of family life in twenty-first-century television series.

Guillermo González-Donoso is a Historian from the Pontificia Universidad Católica de Chile. He received his Diploma in Art History from the Adolfo Ibáñez University and is pursuing his MPhil at Bath Spa University (UK), specialising in Early Modern History, historiography, and theory of history. He is the Content Director of the Chilean NGO Red Cultural website.

James Leggott is an Associate Professor in Film and Television at Northumbria University. He is the author of *In Fading Light: The Films of the Amber Collective* (Berghahn, 2020) and *The Representation of North East England in Film and Television* (Palgrave, 2021). He has published on various aspects of British film and television history and culture, including contemporary British cinema, comedy, and period drama. He has co-edited collections on historical drama, cult comedy, and British science fiction film and television.

Kevin McQueeney (PhD, Georgetown University) is an Assistant Professor of History at Nicholls State University. He specialises in African American health and healthcare history. The University of North Carolina Press will publish his first manuscript, *A City Without Care: Racialized Health Care, Racial Health Disparities, and Black Health Activism in New Orleans 1718–2018*, in autumn 2022. In 2019, he received the Richard Harrison Shryock Medal from the American Association for the History of Medicine.

Jessica Meyer is an Associate Professor of Modern British History at the University of Leeds. Her research interests lie at the intersection of the histories of gender, war, medicine, and popular culture. Her most recent publication is *An Equal Burden: The Men of the Royal Army Medical Corps in the First World War* (Oxford University Press, 2019).

Claire O'Callaghan is a Lecturer in English at Loughborough University. Her research interests include the lives and works of the Brontës, Sarah Waters, and the representation of gender and sexuality across neo-Victorian media. Claire is the author of *Sarah Waters: Gender and Sexual Politics* (Bloomsbury, 2017) and *Emily Brontë Reappraised* (Saraband, 2018). Her work has appeared in *Victorians: A Journal of Literature and Culture*; *Brontë Studies*; *Women: A Cultural Review*; *Victoriographies*; *Critique: Studies in Contemporary Fiction*; *Contemporary Women's Writing*; and *Neo-Victorian Studies*.

Patricia Palma is an Assistant Professor in the Department of Historical and Geographic Sciences at the Universidad de Tarapacá, Chile. She is a specialist in the history of medicine in Latin America, and her current project studies the Chinese diaspora in Peru and Chile.

José Ragas is an Assistant Professor at the Instituto de Historia in Pontificia Universidad Católica de Chile. His main research focus is the transnational history of science and technology, and he is currently examining the transition from natural ice to artificial cold in South America in the late nineteenth century.

Barbara Sadler is a Senior Lecturer and programme leader for Film and Media at the University of Sunderland, UK. She attained her PhD from the University of Lincoln, UK, as part of the AHRC-funded 'Televising History' project. Her research involved a production and reception study of regional television history programming and a history of ITV from the regional perspective. This work included analysis of television station identifiers (and other interstitials) as historical artefacts.

Aeleah Soine is an Associate Professor of History at Saint Mary's College of California. Her research interests include nursing, gender, transnational movements, and citizenship in the nineteenth and twentieth centuries, and her most recent work can be found in *Gender & History*, the *Journal of Women's History*, *German Studies Review*, and *Media History*. She is also the project director of a National Endowment for the Humanities (NEH) grant to introduce community-based public (and popular) history to the undergraduate curriculum.

Serenity Sutherland is an Assistant Professor of Broadcasting and Mass Communication at SUNY-Oswego. Her research intersects American women's history, science and technology studies, digital humanities, and media studies. Her dissertation was a biography of MIT chemist Ellen Swallow Richards who became a leader in the early twentieth-century home economics movement.

Julie Anne Taddeo is a Research Professor in Modern British History at the University of Maryland, USA. She is the author of *Lytton Strachey and the Search for Modern Sexual Identity* (Haworth, 2002). She has edited and co-edited the following collections: *Conflicting Masculinities: Men in Television Period Drama* (with Katherine Byrne and James Leggott, Bloomsbury, 2018); *Upstairs and Downstairs: British Costume Drama Television from* The Forsyte Saga *to* Downton Abbey (with James Leggott, Rowman and Littlefield, 2014); *Steaming into a Victorian Future: A Steampunk Anthology* (with Cynthia J. Miller, Rowman and Littlefield, 2012); *Catherine Cookson Country: On the Borders of Legitimacy, Fiction and History* (Routledge, 2012); *The Tube Has Spoken: Reality TV & History* (with Ken Dvorak, University Press of Kentucky, 2009). Her current projects include a book co-authored with Katherine Byrne on rape in TV period dramas and an edited collection (with Jo Parnell) on Australian period drama TV and film.

Dan Ward is a lecturer in Media and Cultural Studies at the University of Sunderland. His PhD focused on masculinity and violence in contemporary US crime drama, and he has published on a range of topics including *Game of Thrones*, sports documentaries, and Cold War films. His most recent research explores celebrity branding in the age of social media, with particular emphasis on notions of authenticity.

Andrea Wright is a senior lecturer in Film Studies at Edge Hill University. Fantasy/fairy tales, New Zealand cinema, and television costume drama are central to her research interests. She has written on production design, landscape, gender representation, and national identity. Recent publications include essays on the British television series *Downton Abbey* and the films of New Zealand director Taika Waititi.

Acknowledgements

The three of us have now worked on multiple projects together, both as co-contributors and as co-editors, and from the start, our collaborations consistently have been labours of love, not just because we get to write about a genre we personally have enjoyed since our childhoods, but because working together often feels effortless and so very pleasurable.

Immediately after our last edited collection, *Conflicting Masculinities* (IB Tauris, 2018), went to press, we realised we still had so much to explore about period drama television, not only because new TV series are constantly gracing our screens, but because these programmes continue to engage with so many pressing historical and contemporary issues and resonate with audiences worldwide. Much of this book was completed before we went into lockdown in March 2020, but the COVID-19 pandemic added a sense of urgency to our work, prompting us to reassess some of the dramas and re-examine them from the vantage point of our current moment of crisis.

We want to thank our contributors who have had to cope with the additional burdens of teaching online while worrying about the health and safety of their loved ones as well as themselves. Thanks very much to Giuliana Monteverde for her brilliant help preparing the manuscript and to Dr Frank Ferguson and the Research Recovery Fund at Ulster University for their much-appreciated support. The entire production team at Manchester University Press has been fantastic, steering us through the process from start to finish, and under increasingly difficult conditions. Neal Street Productions have been incredibly generous in granting us permission for our cover image from *Call the Midwife*. And, once again, our families deserve endless praise for supporting our pressing need to watch so much television for our work.

Introduction

Katherine Byrne, Julie Anne Taddeo, and James Leggott

The idea for this collection came about as a result of noticing that many of our favourite period dramas shared a common theme: medicine. Diseases of various kinds, and their treatment, seemed to be an important part of the shows we enjoyed watching on television, and we were interested in exploring that further. We had no idea at that point that during the writing of this book a global pandemic was going to change all our lives, and that infection, vaccines, hygiene, and hospitals were no longer just plotlines, but would soon become things we discussed, watched, and worried about every day, all the time. Medicine was, for us, initially a way of accessing or expressing important anxieties about our world, but now it has become the bedrock of that world, the fundamental part that decides how and where we can function. Doctors and nurses are no longer complex and at times problematic professionals, often in conflict with themselves and others; they have become, in recent months, the most important and heroic members of our society, people who risk their own lives and on whom our collective hopes are pinned. Of course, all these things were always true, but we were often able to ignore them, to ignore ill health and those who work with it until we were personally confronted with illness, even to enjoy the plot opportunities it offered on television. Now, of course, it is very different. We feel, however, that this book is more timely than ever, for it reminds us how important it is to understand and learn from the pathologies, experimentations, and breakthroughs of the past, as they become an ever greater part of our shared future. And of course, at this time of anxiety and confinement, the need for escapism via the small screen is greater than ever; so much of our culture has come to a temporary halt as we write this, but we are thankful television endures, to inform, distract, and entertain.

Our screen may be full of the news of the pandemic at present, but it has long been filled with and fascinated by many aspects of public health. As Joseph Turow notes, 'medicine as a profession is very much in style on television' (2010: 1). This is not a recent phenomenon; there has been a long relationship between medicine and the small screen, and many of TV's most popular shows, on both sides of the Atlantic, have been medical in focus. These range from hospital-set dramas like *ER* (1994–2009) to reality TV shows and docudramas like *One Born Every Minute* (2010–) and the long-running *Your Life in Their Hands* (1958–1964). This fascination with doctors, hospitals, and bodies is also shared by period drama on television, but scholarship has paid little attention to this intersection. Recent period series including *The Knick* (2014–2016), *Mercy Street* (2016–2017), and *Charité* (2017), for example, use the hospital setting familiar from older shows like *Bramwell* (1995–1998) to address larger themes about the professionalisation of medicine, medical innovations and failures, and the gender politics that surround the profession. Dramas like *Call the Midwife* (2012–) document the progress of the NHS and female reproductive health while also engaging in contemporary debates about contraception, abortion, and disability. In addition, medical-driven narratives abound in almost every period drama on our screens today: war-induced mental and physical trauma in *Peaky Blinders* (2013–); Spanish flu in *The Village* (2013–2014); gay conversion plotlines in *A Place to Call Home* (2013–2018); bodily and facial disfigurement in *Home Fires* (2015–2016); medical experimentation and monstrosity in *Penny Dreadful* (2014–2016) and *Frankenstein Chronicles* (2015–2017); nursing as a vehicle of female emancipation in *The Crimson Field* (2014) and *Morocco: Love in Times of War* (2017); and all of the above and many more in *Downton Abbey* (2010–2015), whose most famous plotlines, from Lady Sybil's death in childbirth to the war-induced injuries and deaths experienced by the men of the Abbey (upstairs and downstairs), are medical in nature. Such a preoccupation with medical plots and settings across such a range of period shows implies that, for the contemporary viewer, illness, healing, and the medical profession are fundamental ways of accessing and understanding the past – even, perhaps, that history is most fascinating or most relatable when placed in focus by the diseased or suffering body. The popularity of the topic is also surprising because these are the aspects of history the modern viewer is least likely to feel nostalgic for; these pre-antibiotic, pre-anaesthetic, often unsanitary pasts are not places most of us would want to be a patient in. Yet revisit them, in all their primitive and often gruesome limitations, these dramas frequently do. In doing so they chart and explore the gender and class politics that surrounded patient care, the moral and philosophical implications of scientific advances and experimentation, and the changing nature of the increasingly powerful medical profession.

These dramas do not only reveal much about how we view our corporeal past, however. All these issues are still pertinent today, and frequently they also function as a commentary on, and often a critique of, the issues surrounding medicine in the present day. Even without the shadow of COVID-19 hanging over the writing and reading of this collection, there are so many contemporary issues that these dramas tackle: in particular, debates around public health provision, the politics of reproduction, and genetic testing and research. For example, shows like *Call the Midwife* firmly locate the NHS as an essential part of British 'heritage', while others, like *Downton*, hint that its creation is an irrelevance – a view which even the harshest conservative critics of the NHS have since retracted. *The Frankenstein Chronicles* is as anxious about the ethics of medical experimentation as its source text, while *The Knick* pursues knowledge and progress as a holy grail. And like our current crisis, *La Peste*'s (2018–) recreation of the plague in sixteenth-century Spain reveals how some are more vulnerable than others to the devastating effects of pandemics. This collection considers these key issues, alongside the appeal and popularity of the medical plot, and the way medicine has become 'heritage' due to its inclusion in period drama.

Scope of the collection

We begin with period dramas set in the early modern period of European, British, and American history, a time when medicine as a profession was coming into its own, as trained experts tried to push out those they considered 'quacks' and experimented with new techniques, drugs, and therapies. From the plague to syphilis, disease, often compounded by superstition and prejudice, ravaged the lives of millions as medical and lay practitioners struggled to assert their own authority. As we see especially in the TV series set during – and, in the case of time-travelling *Outlander* (2014–), after – the eighteenth century, efforts to modernise and professionalise medicine were accompanied by the marginalisation of women who had long worked in their communities as midwives and healers and who, despite the exclusionary practices being put in place, continued to treat members of their community, primarily poor women.

Our first chapter examines the Spanish TV series *La Peste*, which, although it was released in 2018 to mark the centennial of the 1918 influenza pandemic, has felt appropriately and frighteningly relevant now amidst the ongoing ravages of COVID-19. Ragas, Palma, and González-Donoso recall the clever social media campaign to promote the series (including the placement of giant golden rats around Seville) but more significant still is their discussion of how this period drama unveils the multiple yet contradictory ways people from various social groups and backgrounds reacted to and were impacted by the plague. The series depicts characters who wish to protect their own lives, to procure a cure for others, or just to profit from the sanitary crisis, and how economic concerns struggle with protecting public health. Although the plague is intended as the backdrop to a murder mystery, *La Peste* ultimately puts health and disease at the centre of the narrative – one of the reasons, perhaps, for the series' enduring international commercial success.

Just as social class dictates how disease spreads and is treated in *La Peste*, gender dominates the medical narratives in Diana Gabaldon's time-travelling book series *Outlander* (1991–) and its current television adaptation. Claire Randall Fraser practices medicine in backdrops where women fought for recognition as bona fide practitioners, as shown in Fogel and Sutherland's chapter. In settings such as eighteenth-century Jacobin Scotland, pre-Revolutionary France, colonial America, World War II European battlefronts, and 1950s–1960s Harvard University, Claire's medical acumen proves she is a talented healer despite the frequent scepticism and disapproval of those around her. The ways in which Claire utilises her medical skill – both holistically and scientifically – serve as an avenue of agency and survival. Overall, *Outlander* allows for a fictional exchange of ideas about medicine and gender across the centuries that serves as a commentary on women's access to medicine off-screen, particularly in the episodes in which Claire dispenses advice about contraception and abortion. The show's presentation of gender politics across three centuries reminds historians of the back and forth shifts women have made as practitioners in medicine and science.

By season five of *Outlander*, Claire has set up her own clinic and even attempts to make penicillin as her husband entangles himself in the conflict between the Crown and colonists that will result in the Revolutionary War. It is that same war in which the Cornish hero of *Poldark* (2015–2019) finds himself fighting in the opening episode of the series, and (as we learn in a later episode) in which Dr Dwight Enys will not only save Poldark's life but experiment with surgical techniques that he will later apply to the mining community of Cornwall. Sadler's chapter on this second television adaptation of Winston Graham's *Poldark* novels (the first was made in the 1970s) focuses on Enys and the quiet battles he fights with his medical colleagues as he resists the class prejudices of their profession. Whether he is experimenting with dissection, resuscitating drowning victims, or treating mental illness with kindness rather than punishment, Enys reflects actual changes and debates that marked the end of the eighteenth century. Sadler further shows how *Poldark*'s portrayal of the ideal doctor – empathetic (especially in his treatment of women's bodies and minds) and constantly inquisitive – reflect modern viewers' expectations of medical care within the larger political debates surrounding Britain's National Health Service (a theme which runs through many of the British series under discussion in this collection).

The one disease Enys never encounters – despite some characters in *Poldark* frequenting bawdy houses – is syphilis, even though the disease infected one out of five Georgian Londoners by their mid-thirties. During the eighteenth century, as London grew, so did the number of women working as prostitutes, who were at risk of contracting and spreading the disease, and who are the subject of *Harlots*' (2017–) second episode discussed by Brig and Clark. Prostitutes typically feature as minor characters in period drama TV, which is what sets this drama apart, especially from its co-producer, ITV's, more conservative Sunday evening fare like *Downton Abbey* and *Victoria* (2016–). In this particular episode, it is the women's roles as lay healers and mourners, not prostitutes, that take centre stage. Brig and Clark offer a detailed discussion of the illness, death, and funeral preparations of the character Mary Cooper to highlight the spaces in which early modern English prostitution and illness took place, the different perspectives early modern Londoners had on the 'French Pox' and the kinds of domestic medical practices employed to help Mary in her suffering. *Harlots*, they conclude, inverts the traditional Western medical narrative and prompts viewers to reconsider their preconceptions of where, how, and why medicine took place.

Our second section revisits a familiar trope of period television: the medical practitioner as pioneer and hero but sometimes villain. The series under discussion here showcase doctors, nurses, and midwives at the forefront of modernising their professions, sometimes risking their own lives to save others. Some of the dramas covered in this section complicate the narrative by humanising their heroes with such flaws as addiction or the espousal of racist views as they work with colleagues and provide services to patients often marginalised by their respective societies (and historically ignored by period television). These series help us rethink the work performed not just by medical professionals but by nostalgia; viewers certainly do not miss the diseases that can now be defeated by vaccines, surgeries, and antibiotics, but the attractiveness of the leads and their romantic entanglements helps us to forget or forgive some of the less pleasant historical realities of the past under consideration.

Although most of the series under discussion in this book were (and some still are) filmed in the last two decades, we have deliberately included in this section two (*Dr. Quinn, Medicine Woman* and *Bramwell*) from the late twentieth century that suggest a marked change in depictions of women in medicine – namely, how the 'lady physician' has disappeared from the twenty-first-century period drama. Antonovich's chapter on *Dr. Quinn, Medicine Woman* (1993–1998) explores how women in 1867 America had to carefully balance their professional ambitions with the demands and expectations of femininity. Unlike the 'grittier' medical dramas produced in the last decade, this 1990s series was marketed as 'family friendly' fare. Significantly, as Antonovich shows, its hero, Dr Quinn, is just one of a long line of fictionalised female physicians in American popular culture. The 'lady physician' on the frontier became an archetypical character in nineteenth- and twentieth-century fiction and film for examining shifting ideological debates over gender, sex, race, and politics. Likewise, Dr Quinn embodied the goals of first-wave feminism, while also embracing a distinct 1990s multiculturalism that elided the very troubling racial politics and eugenicist beliefs of actual women physicians that populated the American West at the turn of the century.

As a 'civilising' force on the frontier, Dr Quinn helps her community overcome racial prejudice, but as we see in the five series (*M*A*S*H* [1972–1983], *Mercy Street*, *The Knick*, *Copper* [2012–2013], and *Masters of Sex* [2013–2016]) surveyed in McQueeney's chapter, the history of American medicine cannot be so easily untangled from racism. The characters in these seemingly different period series are based either directly on historical figures or are representative of a composite of Black physicians. The most common story arcs detail the struggles of Black doctors in gaining acceptance from white patients and peers, with *The Knick* and *Mercy Street* refusing to sugarcoat the realities of lynchings and mob violence. But, while period TV has the potential to restore these marginalised voices, McQueeney is concerned that the narrative focus on violent oppression has also led to the erasure of Black women as nurses and doctors as well as the more uplifting history of political activism of Black medical professionals. Furthermore, McQueeney notes how American period dramas have fallen behind their British counterparts, which in recent years have showcased doctors, nurses, and midwives of colour as the main, not secondary, characters.

Women in general have not been cast in the roles of doctors in medical period dramas produced in the last decade, a surprising change given the popular success not only of *Dr. Quinn* but also the British series *Bramwell* of the 1990s (discussed in Taddeo's chapter). Instead, the depiction of women in medicine has typically centred on their more traditionally designated roles as nurses. Since the 1979 BBC's adaptation of Vera Britain's World War I nursing memoir, *Testament of Youth* (1933), wartime nurses have remained a common fixture in British period drama. More recent dramas, however, represent a transnational cohort of nurse-centred dramas, from Spain's *Morocco: Love in Times of War* to Germany's *Charité*, but as Soine's chapter argues, these dramas, when read together, promote heteronormative, racialised, and class-based assumptions that nurses in particular represent women in general. Unlike the myriad of other women's medical roles that might be (but only occasionally have been) featured in period drama series, nursing narratives offer a celebration of women's intellect, independence, and adventure without uncomfortably challenging mainstream viewers' assumptions about their embodied femininity, whiteness, or respectability.

On the surface, *Call the Midwife* also seems to reaffirm such assumptions as we watch the midwives in their sensible cardigans, dispensing advice and services to the working-class residents of London's East End in the early 1960s. But during the course of its nine-season (and continuing) run, *Call the Midwife* has been hailed as the grittier, feminist alternative to period fare like *Downton Abbey*, as it prioritises women's bodies, vocations, and friendships. As Byrne demonstrates, midwives have always been engaged in power struggles, as male doctors tried to push them out of practising obstetrics in the nineteenth century. What is so unusual in the case of *Call the Midwife* is how it has actively been used as a recruitment tool for the midwifery profession, and more problematically, has been embraced by proponents of 'natural' birth. Reflecting the debates and policy changes that have dogged midwifery in Britain over the last few years, while looking back nostalgically to a time when birth followed the 'social' rather than 'medical' model, this drama displays just how political, and influential, period TV can be.

While *Call the Midwife* is primarily centred on female medical professionals, Dr Patrick Turner (Stephen McGann) presents viewers with a staunch champion of the National Health Service as well as the type of doctor we all wish for: compassionate, caring, and tireless in his care for the women and children of the East End. James Leggott's chapter takes us back to the pre-NHS days in *When the Boat Comes In* (1976–81), about working-class life and aspiration in working-class Tyneside in the period between the world wars. As with *Poldark*, the show weaves medical plots and ideas about progressive health care practices into its sweeping saga of romance and industry in a far-flung corner of the British Isles. Although for many viewers, the obvious focal point of the programme was the character of Jack Ford, played by James Bolam as a scheming, venal, yet oddly honourable social climber, Leggott turns his attention to the character who is in many ways the antithesis of Jack. As *When the Boat Comes In* progresses, it gives increasing attention to the character of Billy Seaton, a young doctor and staunch socialist, who eschews the possible wealth and privileges of the profession and instead makes a philanthropic commitment to treating, without any hope of remuneration, only the very poorest of his tough, working-class town. The series captures something of the tensions at work in the pre-NHS landscape of UK health care, but it also seems to take an ambivalent stance on whether its earnest doctor is, as another character wonders, a 'saint or an idiot'.

A darker, sometimes criminal, side of medicine features in the third section of our collection as we examine neo-gothic period dramas that present doctors as either 'mad' or so power-hungry that they are willing to do the unspeakable to advance their research. Series like *Penny Dreadful*, *The*

Frankenstein Chronicles, and *The Alienist* (2018–) borrow from familiar nineteenth-century literary texts and real-life figures, mashing them together for intertextual commentaries on the successes and pitfalls of scientific investigation. As Wright demonstrates, *The Frankenstein Chronicles* uses the history of anatomy and dissection as a backdrop for a re-imagining of Mary Shelley's story and the series' narrative is littered with historical figures including the author, members of her circle, and William Blake, while *The Alienist* speaks to Victorians' (and our own) fascination with serial killers and the evolution of policing based on pathological investigation and evidence-based forensic science. Taddeo's chapter on *Penny Dreadful* further builds on the neo-gothic obsession with dissection (and the female anatomy) as well as the asylum as an institution of terror, not cure. Focusing on the story arcs of its two main female characters whose encounters with doctors involve attempts to 'tame' and re-fashion them into 'ideal women', Taddeo interprets the neo-gothic series as a feminist intervention (albeit a flawed one) in the history of Victorian medicine.

Allitt's chapter on representations of surgery in period drama further complicates the portrayal of the doctor-as-villain embodied in *Penny Dreadful*'s Victor Frankenstein, who boasts that he's not afraid to 'pierc[e] the tissue that separates life from death'. Allitt discusses *Casualty 1900s* (2009) and *The Knick*, which she argues consciously encourage viewers to reflect on their own relationship with medicine, in turn destroying any nostalgic impulse one might assume from a period drama. Nevertheless, we are given an up-close look at early twentieth-century medical, clinical, and technological innovations that radically influenced surgical practice and from which we all benefit today. Similar to Byrne's chapter on *Call the Midwife*, Allitt's observes how *Casualty 1900s* frames itself in relation to the NHS, on the one hand showing its British audience that they have it so much better than before, while also showing what they risk without it – a risk that underpins the New York City charitable institution featured in *The Knick*, whose American viewers are still debating universal health care.

The final section of the book pays particular attention to period drama's depiction of mental illness, theories, and treatments, and the doctor–patient power dynamic – themes touched on throughout the book but which merit closer analysis here. While Taddeo notes how mental illness in Victorian-themed period drama is typically depicted as 'a female malady', O'Callaghan and Fanning's chapter on the miniseries *To Walk Invisible* (2016) about the Brontë siblings showcases a rare dramatic example of the male sufferer. However, as they detail, this series distorted Victorian discourses on alcoholism and male insanity to present a moralistic view of Branwell Brontë, blaming him for his illness. While the series empowers the sisters' narrative in very modern ways through a feminocentric focus on their plights and achievements in a world hostile to women's intellectual pursuits, it fails to understand Branwell's illness in relation to how it affected *him*.

Representing male mental illness within the context of and result of military service is the subject of Dan Ward's chapter on the work of screenwriter Stephen Knight. Although separated by a century, the backstories of the male characters in Knight's *Taboo* (2017–) and *Peaky Blinders* (service in the East India Company army and on the Western Front, respectively) allow for an exploration of how men cope with trauma through addiction and violence. Ultimately, as Ward notes, Knight uses the genre to not only elucidate contemporary concerns through a period lens, but to draw attention to the aspects of our culture (namely attitudes about mental illness and masculinity) which appear stubbornly resistant to change over time.

The final chapter of the collection by Alley-Young looks at one such aspect that has been particularly resistant to change: the designation of homosexuality as a medical and moral pathology in need of a 'cure'. *A Place to Call Home* has been called 'the Australian *Downton Abbey*' for its soap opera treatment of class interactions in the post–World War II era, but the series' inclusion of previously marginalised characters (an Aborigine veteran, for example) and its storylines around rape and gay conversion therapy have marked it as more progressive than *Downton*, which also dealt with such topics (in the cases of Anna Bates and Thomas Barrow respectively). Alley-Young provides a detailed analysis of how James Bligh's homosexuality is medically pathologised and treated within the larger media, moral, medical/scientific, and socio-cultural discourses of the era (1950s–1980s). The series aired its episodes on James's gay conversion therapy as debates about marriage equality dominated Australian headlines and thus suggests, yet again, the power of period drama to use the past to reflect on the present and even help change the future of its audience.

We have tried to cover here what we felt were the key topics and issues surrounding the televisual representation of the history of medicine, largely in the West. However, as the last few pages have indicated, there is a huge wealth of material to choose from, and what we have here is not exhaustive. Indeed, so popular are medical storylines in period drama that this collection could have been twice the length and still not included them all. Moreover, we expect that medicine will be an even more popular topic for period series in the wake of the COVID-19 pandemic and that many more shows will explore these issues over the next few years. Far from being confined to the past, illness and public health are, it seems, sadly and unavoidably part of our shared future. As the dramas explored here show, period television has a unique ability to allow us to use the past to understand the present. At the same time, of course, it offers the reassurance that our society has long had to cope with terrible diseases, and yet has always learnt from, endured, and survived them.

Reference

Turow, J. (2010). *Playing Doctor: Television, Storytelling, and Medical Power*. University of Michigan Press.

Part I

Early modern professions and disease

1

Golden rats and sick empires: portraying medicine, poverty, and the bubonic plague in *La Peste*[1]

José Ragas, Patricia Palma, and Guillermo González-Donoso

Introduction

Since the COVID-19 epidemic arrived in our countries, it has managed to transform our everyday lives, disrupting our established routines and introducing new habits. During the mandatory confinement enforced by national governments, television and online streaming platforms gained sudden prominence and installed binge-watching as a regular activity. In a similar manner to readers who turned frantically to Giovanni Boccacio's *Decameron* (c. 1351) and Albert Camus's *The Plague* (1947) to find solace during these anxious times, viewers looked for answers in online movies and series (Esteban, 2020). Not surprisingly, movies such as *Outbreak* (1995), *Contagion* (2011), *World War Z* (2013), and Netflix's *Pandemic* (2020) rapidly jumped to the top of the most viewed worldwide. For instance, in Hong Kong *Contagion* remained in the top ten for several weeks while *Plague Inc.* was one of the most popular mobile phone games, allowing players to control a deadly pathogen (*The Economic Times*, 2020). As the journalist Heather Kelly (2020) observed, 'the compulsion to watch these fictionalized, sometimes graphic versions of things that are unfolding in the real world can be a way of making sense of what's happening when we are faced with uncertainty'.

The compulsory search for both films and TV series with an epidemic background has not been limited to the Global North. The lethal and dramatic impact of the epidemic in Spain and Latin America was accompanied by an increasing interest in science fiction and how diseases had affected the region in the past. Although it was released two years before the arrival of COVID-19 to Europe and the Americas, the TV series *La Peste* (2018–2020) portrayed a grim overview of a society ravaged by an epidemic in the sixteenth century. The series, like the movies mentioned above, enabled current viewers to observe and learn about diseases within the safe environment of their own households. Viewers were then exposed to topics such as quarantines, anti-science sentiments, the lack of vaccines, the role of physicians, and the harsh debate between the protection of the local economy versus the protection of human lives without knowing that a few months later they would be experiencing those issues in real life. Heather Kerry points out that the fascination with these types of movies and TV series confers on viewers a certain tranquillity even when they portray the worst scenarios, reassuring them that even lethal epidemics like the plague in *La Peste* will eventually disappear.

La Peste combines historical accuracy and fictional drama of the bubonic plague that affected Spain in the late sixteenth century, portraying everyday life during the pandemic. This chapter analyses how *La Peste* marks a milestone for Spanish television, as a series that accounts for global disasters in local settings with high doses of realism. The series portrays how political and medical authorities, and especially the larger population, tried to escape or overcome the consequences of the epidemic. *La Peste*'s release coincided with the centennial of the epidemic, commonly known as the Spanish flu, that killed twenty to fifty million people around the globe (Spinney, 2018). Like its twentieth-century counterpart, the early modern plague inflicted significant damage on Spanish society during the peak of Spanish dominance in the Atlantic World. The show presents a dark and sombre portrayal of how the disease corroded the social tissue of Seville and its residents. In placing a massive epidemic like the bubonic plague at the core of the narrative, *La Peste* unveils the multiple yet contradictory ways people from various social groups and backgrounds reacted to the pandemic, whether to save their own lives, to procure a cure for others, or just to profit from the sanitary crisis. Such complex scenarios of power, economic growth, and personal dilemmas are the ones chosen by the creators of *La Peste*, the most expensive and successful show produced by Spanish television to date (Arroyo, 2018).

In its first season, *La Peste* follows Mateo Núñez's efforts to fulfil a promise made to his old friend Germán Larrea, a veteran from the Eighty Years War, to find his son in Seville, a city infested by the plague. The series shows a variety of distinct forces including a powerful merchant guild, transnational commerce to the New World, and the everyday poverty and dirtiness that made the inhabitants of Seville and Europe generally vulnerable to epidemics. The main storyline follows Mateo risking his life to return to Seville, the city he abandoned after being accused by the Holy Office of printing banned books, to find Larrea's son, Valerio. Once Mateo manages to find Valerio, who makes a living by selling clothing from the victims of the plague, he is betrayed by the latter and delivered to the authorities. Celso de Guevara, the Grand Inquisitor, offers Mateo an official pardon in exchange for finding a serial killer who has committed several crimes in the city. While the murder mystery plotline is the centre of the series, the plague is used as a historical backdrop and as a metaphor for the corrupt city. As

Mateo chases the clues left by the murderer, the epidemic threatens the city and its inhabitants. In this way, we can see various social actors – such as civil authorities, merchants, and the impoverished – living with the plague.

In this chapter, we aim to highlight what makes *La Peste* a relevant case study for those interested in the history of medicine and the analysis of popular culture through the lens of a television series. As a result of a carefully designed campaign to promote the release of the show, *La Peste* constitutes a fascinating example of the possibilities offered by TV shows as vehicles for disseminating historical medical knowledge to a vast audience. Rather than just adding to nostalgia for a time when Spain dominated the globe, the show confronts viewers with the picture of an emergent empire coexisting with the daily misery lived on the streets and on every corner of urban spaces (Martínez Shaw, 2019). To assess how an early modern epidemic provided the major backdrop to such an ambitious production, we start by placing the medical narrative in the genealogy of Spanish TV dramas and note the early influence of American medical shows that aired before Spanish producers developed their own medical productions. We then turn to the story of the epidemic, its dissemination, and the end of the disease. We also present the tension between fiction and reality that the show aims to resolve by examining the character of Monardes, an actual physician who lived in sixteenth-century Seville. In the final section, we analyse the strategies deployed by producers to build an audience through its interaction with historical content and an unexpected character: rats.

La Peste and the Spanish (television) Golden Age

With a budget of €10 million, 130 locations, and with 400 extras on set, *La Peste*'s first season is a six-episode TV show produced by the Spanish communication conglomerate Movistar. It became the most ambitious production in Spanish television and an overnight sensation among viewers and critics (Martínez, 2018). Yet, *La Peste*'s success did not occur in a vacuum, nor was it a sudden phenomenon.[2] It was the result of a combined effort on the part of producers, broadcasters, and the audience that supported ambitious projects during the transition from conventional TV shows to global digital platforms. Within the constellation of TV series, medical TV shows occupy a special place in the genealogy of Spanish TV. We can relate the origins of medical series to the spread of television since the mid-twentieth century. Spain was not absent from this phenomenon. Avid watchers of American and European series, Spaniards closely followed productions where medical drama was the dominant plotline. Due to the global expansion of Spanish TV as a result of the collective work of producers, digital platforms, and screenwriters in addition to the rise of digital television, Spanish series themselves started to incorporate medical topics within the last decade.

Translation into different languages along with subtitled versions contributed to the further expansion and prestige of medical TV shows outside the English-speaking audience. Besides cable and local stations, TV shows were consumed by a growing audience through illegal cable connections, online pirate platforms, and locally manufactured DVDs (Aunión, 2019; Rivas Moreno, 2018). Televisión Española (TVE), the Spanish broadcasting station created in 1956, started to broadcast American medical series in the 1960s and 1970s when the country was still under the authoritarian regime of General Francisco Franco. In the following decades, private stations got exclusive rights to popular shows, making people familiar with this particular genre. In the 1990s, pharmacists, doctors, and nurses gained prominence in local series productions. However, it would not be until the 2000s that the first regional productions such as *Hospital Central* (2000–2012) and *MIR* (2007–2009) positioned medical dramas among Spanish series. Inspired by the American medical drama *ER* (1994–2009), *Hospital Central* is one of the most successful shows in the history of Spanish television with 6.5 million viewers across its eight seasons ('Record de audiencia', 2005).

As American, British, and Spanish medical shows garnered more viewers, concerns surrounding the potential negative effects of (hyper)realistic narratives on audiences loomed among professional medical organisations. Attempting to increase their audiences while trying to obtain approval from the medical community, TV producers did not hesitate to stress realism in episodes by including actual physicians on their production teams. In turn, medical organisations urged Spanish medical TV shows to disseminate positive health habits to increase disease prevention.

In 2008, the Spanish Medical Colleges Organization (*Organización Médica Colegial de España*), the national entity responsible for organising and regulating the medical profession in the country, published a report which warned of the 'risk' of misinformation that the public may receive by watching these series. Some of the outcomes from such exposure were already taking shape in hospitals and health centres, where doctors reported that the number of people attending medical consultations had suddenly increased, with patients demanding unnecessary treatments, searching for experimental therapies, and harbouring ideas of unrealistic recoveries (Lacalle, 2008). In a particular incident, several women rushed to health centres requesting breast cancer tests after the Venezuelan soap opera *Cristal* (1985–1986) aired an episode where the main character, Inocencia, was diagnosed with the illness.[3] Despite numerous recommendations to be cautious, the audience continued to grow, creating a direct and problematic pipeline from living rooms – where people gathered to watch these TV shows – to hospitals. Producers are caught between keeping realistic medical representations and increasing drama by distorting medical procedures (and recoveries) that usually take weeks and months in order to format them for television. 'If TV shows depict exactly what happens in a hospital, they will be extremely boring', said Juan Algarra, a physician and screenwriter for *Hospital Central* (Benito, 2008).

The advent of digital platforms like Netflix and Movistar+ provided the necessary boost to reach a global audience for Spanish TV shows rather than just importing foreign medical series or limiting their national productions to local viewers. Both digital platforms invested in producing and financing historical series, where doctors and diseases played an important role. In 2015, TVE premiered *El Ministerio del Tiempo* (2015–2020), which is currently broadcast in more than 190 countries. The series follows the activities of a secret Spanish Ministry in charge of guarding several doors that provide access to various eras of Spanish history to keep the past as it is and to prevent any disruption of the present. During the first two seasons, the patrol responsible for carrying out secret missions in the past was formed by Alonso de Entrerríos (Nacho Fresneda), a sixteenth-century soldier and a veteran of the Eighty Years War; Amelia Foch (Aura Garrido), one of the first Spanish women to attend university at the end of the nineteenth century; and Julián Martínez (Rodolfo Sancho), a paramedic from the present who accidentally discovers the gates while rescuing a person from a burning building and is invited to join the Ministry.

In some cases, the disease was the main protagonist of the drama. For instance, in the episode 'Un virus de otro tiempo' ('A virus from another time') the show revolves around the early twentieth-century Spanish flu epidemic, two years before the centennial of the pandemic that claimed the lives of millions of people around the world. During a mission in 1918 to witness the birth of the famous Spanish Flamenco dancer (*bailaora*) Carmen Amaya, a member of the 'time patrol' (Irene Larra) catches the flu and develops its first symptoms. Against the protocol, the newly appointed sub-secretary orders Irene back to the twenty-first century to cure her. In doing so, the flu rapidly spreads throughout the Ministry, provoking the contagion and subsequent death of its personnel.

In a similar manner to *El Ministerio del Tiempo*, *La Peste* was a remarkable television success. *La Peste* has had considerable diffusion throughout Latin America through the Movistar+ platform, and in the coming months of writing this chapter, due to its popularity, the series will reach the English-speaking world with the purchase of the transmission rights by the BBC. Although this deal with the BBC was made in 2018, the pandemic has since only increased viewer interest in TV series about contagious diseases. In the next section, we will analyse the historical context in which the series *La Peste* takes place, highlighting the authorities' management of the epidemic, the impact of its spread throughout the city, and the prominent role of the doctor Nicolás Monardes and his urban and intellectual environment.

Between fiction and reality

La Peste constitutes a disturbing recreation of underground Spanish Golden Age society. Producers conjured both a digital reconstruction of the urban landscape as well as taking account of historical information to recreate the living conditions in which the plague took place.[4] Producers and the director focused on showcasing 'Seville dirty, poor, and infested with rats where people died of contagion' (Bermejo, 2018). As we watch the episodes, the plague corrodes and distorts everything. Its manifestations are visible, with deformed bodies and corpses rapidly buried in mass graves. But it is also an invisible but permanent menace that affects everyone. 'The plague is an excuse to talk about an extreme situation', explains Alberto Rodríguez, one of the creators of the show. *La Peste* turns viewers into helpless witnesses of how their ancestors faced diseases before the development of modern vaccines and antibiotics.

With its magnificent palaces, booming population, diversity of languages, and endless source of wealth, Seville became one of the most vibrant cosmopolitan places in the early modern world. The city was, above all, the gate from and to the New World.[5] It was also a broad market, bringing affluence to many other sites in the kingdom and elsewhere (Hamilton, 1934; González Mariscal, 2015). Occupying a place that nowadays belongs to New York, Singapore, or Shanghai, the Spanish port was undoubtedly an impressive accomplishment for a place that just a few decades before could not distinguish itself from other small ports or towns along the Mediterranean maritime space (Abulafia, 2011). As one of the critical early modern European hubs, it was a place of transit for travellers as well as those who participated in Iberian globalisation. It is also important to note that Seville was embedded in the European Renaissance. This robust cultural platform favoured curiosity and the expansion of knowledge through routes that connected the New World with convention centres in the Italian Peninsula and elsewhere. Furthermore, Andalusia was an attractive place for intellectuals willing to work with and prosper economically from the new ideas that were reformulating the world. Along with the magnificent infrastructure and the new 1 per cent that took advantage of the currency flow, there was an underworld populated by underdogs who lived side by side with imperial and religious authorities and who struggled to survive in a hostile environment.

The reconstruction of the city in *La Peste* is consistent with the image of narrow, unhygienic streets, crowded with passionate people, who practised an intense spirituality that made their existence bearable during the disease (Martínez, 2018). Producers pulled every available resource to recreate the dense environment of early modern cities like Seville. 'We had to create everything', said Pepe Domínguez del Olmo, *La Peste*'s art director (Bermejo, 2018). The team generated organic trash to use on set. Patricia López Arnaiz, who played Teresa Pinelo, a fierce entrepreneurial widow on the show, said, 'it smelled like fish, there were rats and rotten vegetables everywhere'. Producers concentrated their efforts on filming outdoors, which posed several challenges. Visual effects played a significant part in bringing Seville and its inhabitants back to life. Art director Iñigo Rotaetxe worked for nearly ten months with experts and art historians to recreate even the smallest details in terms of not only material culture but also social behaviour and urban planning (Failes, 2018). The outcome holds a high degree of accuracy which allows viewers to confidently interpret the overt contradictions of the Spanish Renaissance.

The spiritual universe permeates the episodes and determines not only the Sevillians' mental horizons but the framework in which the epidemic is contested and understood. In general terms, the epoch was marked by the dominance of the Catholic Church, which considered itself a pillar of the Spanish global monarchy. The hegemony of the Catholic Church set the contours of intellectual freedom and religious reform. In the series, the Holy Office, represented by Inquisitor Celso de Guevara, supports and manipulates Mateo's investigation to discover a hidden network of local and dominant Protestants, who will be burned alive for conspiring against the Church. This storyline portrays the cultural tensions that occurred in sixteenth-century Andalusia where religious persecutions took place side by side with a rich body of unorthodox ideas and intellectual traditions, such as the former Muslim occupation of the region, the cults formed by African slaves, grassroots Catholicism, Protestants, surviving crypto-Jewish traditions, and other faiths harboured by the maritime nature of the city. For the General Inquisitor Celso de Guevara, the suspicion and further arrest of prominent heretics is a testimony to how Andalusia was both a space of cultural and religious pluralism and an important site of large Protestant groups and heretical subversives.

The core narrative of this season revolves around one major issue that echoes in pandemics throughout history: the dilemma between maintaining the economy and protecting public health. Current viewers of the show will likely relate to this particular dilemma which for almost two years has pervaded the public debate on how to manage the current pandemic crisis: should we prioritise the economy or people's health? As policy makers and authorities enforced quarantine and social distancing to prevent the spread of the coronavirus, some commentators raised the alarm about the economic repercussions of such pre-emptive measures. Likewise, in the TV series, the merchants' guild – represented by Luis de Zúñiga (Francisco León Barrios) – attempts desperately to silence any news or rumour about the presence of the plague in the city. As soon as he learns about the first outbreak in a *chabela* (slum), he manages to contain the plague within the area by placing it under military quarantine, with 'an armed man every two hundred meters'. Morata, a member of the local council and an associate of Zúñiga, appeals to the other members of the council (the Veinticuatro) by invoking the prestige of the city and a feud with another major Spanish port (Cádiz) as a reason to withhold information about the plague: 'If we make this information public, we will have to close the city. And if that happens, we will for sure lose the monopoly of the trade with the New World.' When his proposal is defeated, Zúñiga tries to bribe the other member who opposed Morata. In the end, Zúñiga will obtain his vote by blackmailing him.

For merchants, receiving silver and goods coming from the New World was a matter of life and death. To accomplish this goal, and to preserve the status of the port as the main gate from and to the Americas, Zúñiga does not hesitate to sacrifice the lives of Sevillians, in particular of its most vulnerable group, orphaned children. As Morata claims in his address to the local council, 'this city has never been so close to becoming the capital of the kingdom like now. We should not miss this opportunity.' In order to execute his plan of imposing a military quarantine in those places with an outbreak, Zúñiga suggests that children should be in charge of feeding the people in quarantine. The reference to orphaned children as disposable emanates from the early modern literary genre known as *picaresca* (or picaresque in English). With the *pícaro* (rogue or rascal) as the central character of this genre, writers such as Miguel de Cervantes and artists like Bartolomé Esteban Murillo sought to convey the misadventures of these orphans who lived in urban areas and tried to survive by using their skills. The series depicts orphans like Valerio and Leandra as a floating population that provides cheap labour to the city (Figure 1.1).

In the end, the efforts deployed by Zúñiga to establish a sanitary belt around the slums prove to be unrealistic. The main reason behind this failure is the profound inequality that runs through the Sevillian population. While Zúñiga and the upper class can take all the required measures to avoid being infected by the plague, lower socioeconomic groups risk exposing themselves to contagion by continuing to work in adverse conditions. Regardless of their status or economic background, every inhabitant of Seville is touched by the plague. An impoverished woman who works trading used clothes – sometimes those from victims of the epidemic – will be

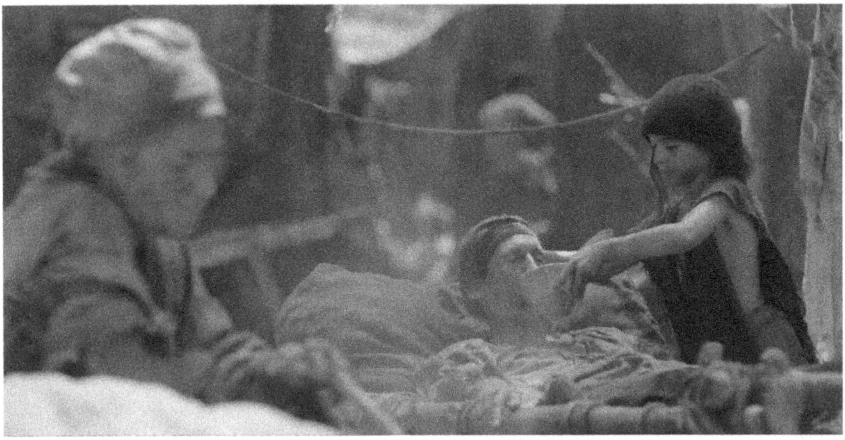

Figure 1.1 An orphan child provides assistance to sick people (*La Peste*, S1E1)

ultimately responsible for introducing the plague to Seville. When one of the guards attempts to register her, she offers him a piece of soap to look the other way. As the camera follows her entrance to the city pulling the cart with the infected clothes, the viewer anticipates the dire consequences of that action.

Once the disease enters the city, chaos is inevitable. The series rapidly removes any sign of hope that the epidemic could be brought under control and shows even less hope for finding a cure. It also shows that the disease does not distinguish between social groups, although medical care does depend on the financial resources of patients. The epidemic also exacerbates the weak social tissue, expanding the gap between the rich and the needy. While the vast majority try to find room in crowded hospices, the rich can enjoy benefits that provide them comfort in their agony. One of the more brutal scenes is when Mateo and Valerio enter the lazaretto looking for a patient. Sick people crowd the doors trying to get in, but there is no more space, and the guards violently prevent them from entering by throwing them out onto the street. 'It is very easy to get out from here, the difficult thing is to get in', says one of the physicians, while in the background piles of bodies are being thrown into carts to be burned or buried in mass graves. As Mateo points out to Valerio, 'you don't have to die to go to hell. Here you have it. Sickness is hell' (see Figure 1.2).

The series also portrays the ineffectiveness of the medical treatments of the time to save patients. At the same time, it shows the reluctance of doctors and authorities to adopt new healing knowledge, especially from the New World, with one notable exception. The flux of both traditional and new medical knowledge in such an adverse setting is elegantly embodied by

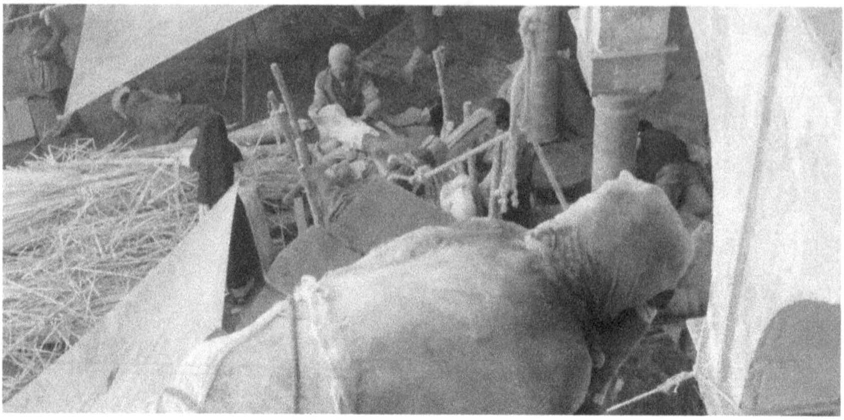

Figure 1.2 Bodies piled in the hospital awaiting burial in a mass grave (*La Peste*, S1E4)

Monardes, played by Tomás del Estal. The character is based on an actual physician named Nicolás Monardes Alfaro (1493–1588) who resided in Seville and cultivated one of the first medical, botanical gardens in the city.[6] Throughout the episodes, Monardes looms as both an erudite but also a moral character amid the rapid decline of ethical paradigms as the epidemic expands. For instance, in his first appearance in the show, he refuses to accept money from merchants in exchange for keeping their silence regarding the expected spread of the plague in the city. The interpretation of Tomás del Estal presents Monardes as a character who conjures wisdom, is confident in his medical knowledge, and demonstrates perpetual curiosity, but also as a character who is extremely cautious to not break any laws such as performing simple medical procedures like an autopsy. A careful observer himself, Monardes is one of the first to consider the relationship between the epidemic and whether or not the rats are the actual carriers of the disease.

The Monardes' household in *La Peste* is many things at the same time: a medical facility, a recovery place, a laboratory, and a medical garden. The city of Seville later recognised the real-life Monardes as a pioneer in treating and diagnosing diseases with plants and herbs brought from the New World with a plaque outside his first household that reads: 'Universal Sevillian and introducer of medical knowledge from the Americas into Europe'. In a scene where he is attempting to save Valerio's romantic interest, *La Peste*'s Monardes mentions pineapples as a plant 'used by Indians to treat wounds and clean the blood'. The real-life Monardes increased his collection with the specimens brought by ships to observe their full vital cycle: from planting them in the soil to applying them on patients for different forms of treatment. The possession of a botanical garden also suggests the complex acclimatisation of exotic items and their further preservation: 'With half of what you see here, I might cure more than one hundred diseases. Yet I have to hide myself [from the Inquisition]', says a disappointed Monardes while he looks at his garden in another scene.

Heterodoxy, spirituality, power, freedom, and persecution are the elements that coexisted in the Seville reconstructed by the production crew.[7] *La Peste* developed the capacity to bring to life the vibrant urban landscape and its actors in a decisive moment. In doing so, producers were able to convey the social and cultural tensions that are embedded during an epidemic, and how epidemics and society mutually interact with each other. The plague itself operates as a background that permeates every human action, and exploits every social and political fracture to secure its transmission and spread throughout the city. As we explain in the next section, the series had to come up with novel ways to transmit the emotions and personal experiences from five centuries ago to a new generation of viewers.

Breaking the fourth wall

In an increasingly competitive and global market, Spanish TV shows have had to adopt innovative strategies to capture the attention of viewers and gain momentum. Developing a robust audience is important not only during the screening of a show but also to create the necessary dose of expectation to extend the show for another season. Many Spanish producers take advantage of social media to share advanced content and gain followers. The case of *La Casa de Papel* (*Money Heist*, 2017), for example, utilised elements from popular culture such as anti-fascist chants ('La Bella Ciao') from World War II or the masks from Spanish surrealist artist Salvador Dalí as a strategy to reach new audiences beyond Spain and the Spanish language (Locard, 2019). In general, the development of a new and different repertoire of strategies is a constant concern among Spanish producers and broadcasters during the current transformation of television and its products.

La Peste therefore represents a hallmark of how Spanish TV shows sought to engage new audiences. Its producers appealed to the public sphere and digital platforms to develop a narrative available to various groups. Mostly, there were three campaign strategies deployed by the TV show, carefully crafted to generate a reaction from the public. The first strategy was the incorporation of the public sphere. Overnight, dozens if not hundreds of mid-sized golden rats appeared throughout Seville. In the TV show, rats are the most essential non-human character. They spread everywhere in the city without anyone knowing that they were carrying the epidemic. Valerio makes rat-hunting an unusual way of living. Armed with a big stick, he enters sites under quarantine to kill them and sell the dead bodies to a local officer. To make these animals the centre of attention, there were three different kinds of rat used during the shooting: trained, street, and digital rats. According to José 'Pepe' Domínguez, the artistic director of the series, 'some rats have more hours of experience on stage than myself'. Having well-trained animals also posed an unexpected problem. In a scene where rats viciously attacked one of the characters, the trained ones did not respond to the command. Producers had to replace them with the street ones (Machuca, 2018). In giving such rodents a prominent place within the storyline, producers aimed to equate rats with the marginal people inhabiting the city. As a plaque placed by the production team explained later, the display of artificial rats was a tribute to those 'uncomfortable people of Seville': 'These golden figures are a tribute to the people who, for living and thinking on their terms, were uncomfortable, feared, persecuted, forced to hide themselves and yet, they spread these streets with their golden freedom.'

The ubiquitous presence of mock rodents on the streets generated particular reactions from bystanders and viewers. The production team strategically placed them in key historical locations where residents and tourists frequently walked, such as La Cárcel Real, the Imprenta Cromberger, Barrio Triana, Casa Monardes, the Mint House, and the University of Seville (R. V., 2018). Rats served as markers to historical locations, and bystanders could access information about these sites through a QR code placed on a plaque next to the designated location. People welcomed golden rats and uploaded pictures of them to social media. Some enthusiasts posed with them, and one person even took a picture kissing one. In the days before the release, the actors posed with golden rats to promote the show. Over the past few centuries, people have turned rats into the universal archetypes of urban filth and imminent epidemics.[8] However, the campaign turned the image of the rodents into something more acceptable and mock rats were soon embraced and 'domesticated' by bystanders, who found them harmless. Perhaps because the spread of modern epidemics is now attributed to agents like mosquitoes (or even bats) rather than rats, their presence was more approachable for bystanders.[9]

A second strategy pursued by producers was a dynamic presence on social media. They took advantage of the multiplying effect of social media and the ongoing global audience to introduce the show and its content beyond Spain. The show displayed information on major sites, where it reached a significant number of followers. For instance, on Instagram, it reached 3,758 followers, and on Facebook, it had 4,169 followers. Every one of the platforms permitted sharing and disseminating different information and material related to the show, fostering interaction with other platforms or physical spaces where the production team was promoting it. The official Instagram account received and shared art created by fans who saw their pieces posted and liked by other members of the virtual community. It also allowed followers to leave their impressions and comments on the show or other elements related to the show.

The third and final strategy developed to engage audiences was an interactive website launched simultaneously with the TV show. The website allowed visitors to easily navigate its content, and it helped update audiences with news about the series. A wiki platform designed exclusively for the show by its fans in December 2017 provided the 'most possible information' about the characters, the actors, the locations, and its historical background. One of the mini-sites was precisely devoted to explaining 'the plague' as a historical phenomenon, based on information from the World Health Organization. It plainly and succinctly explains the various types of plagues as well as their symptoms, how they were spread, the existing methods to cure them, and how to prevent their dissemination. An interactive itinerary hosted on the official website named 'The Route of The Plague' highlighted the historical sites in Seville and the prime locations seen on the show. There were eleven sites placed along the river Guadalquivir, including the publishing house, the red-light district, the jail, the Cathedral, and the garden, among other locations. The website suggests two different routes to follow on the site: a shorter one, which lasts an hour and a half, and a longer route that encompasses all the locations. The Hospital of the Cinco Llagas is one of the chosen places along the way. The building is now the Parlamento de Andalucía, but for centuries, it was 'a landmark of public health for the city'. As the website mentions, 'in the event of an epidemic, hospitals served more to isolate infected people than to cure them'. The hospital is depicted as a detested place where patients crowded outside the building without any hope of being properly treated. They spent their last days and hours in poor conditions, and they were divided according to their social status. One of the characters appears wearing the iconic bird-like mask used by physicians to combat the plague in Europe in the mid-seventeenth century.

Conclusion

With a second season released in November 2019 and an agreement to broadcast the show in the United Kingdom through the BBC, *La Peste* is one of the most famous TV shows in the Spanish language. It is also a historical drama where health and disease are at the centre of the narrative and serve as a compelling background to the six episodes of the show. Through the story of a political and religious conspiracy accidentally unveiled by veteran Mateo Núñez, we experience the adverse living conditions of both the rich and the poor in one of the megacities of the Spanish Empire during the epidemic of the bubonic plague. The thorough reconstruction of the urban milieu does allow viewers to become immersed in the strategies and (limited) possibilities encountered by urban dwellers to combat the disease. The vivid recreation of such personal experiences, from hopeless patients to prominent physicians such as Monardes, highlights the effects and human reactions of an epidemic that took place nearly five centuries ago.

Although *La Peste* was aired two years prior to the global outbreak of COVID-19, viewers may find disturbing similarities between the fate of the fictional characters during the Spanish Golden Age and their own experience during the current pandemic. As a fictional narrative with a medical background at its core, *La Peste* provides valuable lessons for scholars, viewers, and even policy makers and health specialists: pandemics are not just 'medical' events. They are complex social, political, and economic phenomena. The visual and narrative foci of the producers of the show is a testament to how pandemics penetrate and exploit our social fractures, whether in the past or the present, by using them as vehicles to spread and rapidly erode institutions, scientific certainties, and moral bonds.

Notes

1 We would like to express our gratitude to Kenia Munguia and Giselle Gibbons for their proofreading of previous versions of this chapter.
2 On the complicated characterisation of the TV 'Golden Age', see Wilson (2019).
3 On how health issues are portrayed among female TV characters in Spanish TV, see Lacalle and Gómez Morales (2018).
4 A recent paper by Parrilla Valero (2019) examines the impact of the Black Death on the Crown of Aragon.
5 For a detailed vision of sixteenth-century Seville, see Wilson (2013).
6 A brief critical bibliography about the life of Dr Monardes includes: Diaz-Delgado Penas (2015); López Pinero and López Terrada (1997); Olmedilla and Puig (1897); and Rodriguez Marin (1925). Our major reference for this chapter is Pardo Tomás (2002). See also Sheaves (2015) and González Donoso (2019).
7 On the relationship between Monardes and heterodox movements, see Díaz-Delgado Peñas (2015: 16–17).
8 See 'The Global War Against the Rat and the Epistemic Emergence of Zoonosis' website project, developed by Dr Christos Lynteris and hosted by the University of St Andrews. Accessed 4 October 2021. https://wwrat.wp.st-andrews.ac.uk/.
9 On how mosquitoes are the most lethal agents in history, see Winegard (2019).

References

Abulafia, D. (2011). *The Great Sea. A Human History of the Mediterranean.* (London: Oxford University Press).

Arroyo, A. (2018). 'La serie española de los 10 millones de euros', *Estrella* (10 January). Accessed 21 July 2020. www.estrelladigital.es/articulo/television/serie-espanola-10-millones-euros/20180110183310339133.html

Aunión, J.A. (2019). 'El auge de las plataformas contribuye a la caída en picado de la piratería cultural', *El País* (30 September). Accessed 21 July 2020. https://elpais.com/cultura/2019/09/30/actualidad/1569839007_661135.html?ssm=TW_CM

Benito, E. de (2008). 'Los médicos no se reconocen en la serie de médicos', *El País* (19 January). Accessed 21 July 2020. https://elpais.com/diario/2008/01/19/radiotv/1200697204_850215.html

Bermejo, A. G. (2018). 'La Peste: miedo y asco en Sevilla', *Cinemanía* (18 January). Accessed 21 July 2020. https://cinemania.20minutos.es/series/la-peste-miedo-asco-sevilla/?platform=hootsuite

Diaz-Delgado Peñas, I. (2015). *Estudio Crítico de Nicolás Monardes Alfaro* (Madrid: Fundacion Ignacio Larramendi).

Esteban, I. (2020). 'Los lectores se contagian del poder de *La peste*', *El Correo* (14 March). Accesed 21 July 2020. www.elcorreo.com/culturas/libros/lectores-contagian-poder-20200314140533-ntrc.html

Failes, I. (2018). 'VFX takes audience back to 16th century Spain in *The Plague*', *VFX. The Magazine of the Visual Effects Society* (30 May). Accessed 21 July 2020. http://vfxvoice.com/vfx-takes-audiences-back-to-16th-century-spain-in-the-plague/

González Donoso, G. (2019). 'El sevillano galeno y las simples americanas. Posibilidades epistemológicas de un tratado de medicina del siglo XVI', in *Seminario Simon Collier 2019* (Santiago: Instituto de Historia, Pontificia Universidad Católica de Chile), 107–136.

González Mariscal, M. (2015). 'Inflación y niveles de vida en Sevilla durante la revolución de los precios', *Revista de Historia Económica. Journal of Iberian and Latin American Economic History*, 33:3, 353–386.

Hamilton, E. (1934). *American Treasure and the Price Revolution in Spain, 1501–1650* (Cambridge, MA: Harvard University Press).

Karpf, A. (1988). *Doctoring the Media. The Reporting of Health and Medicine* (London: Routledge).

Lacalle, C. (2008). 'Los médicos en la ficción televisiva', *Quaderns del CAC*, 30 (January–June): 55–65.

Lacalle, C. and B. Gómez Morales (2018). 'Educar entreteniendo: los problemas de salud de los personajes femeninos en la ficción TV española'. *Signo y Pensamiento*, 37.73. https://doi.org/10.11144/Javeriana.syp37-73.eeps.

Locard, M. (2019). 'Pourquoi "La Casa de Papel" nous rend aussi across', *Le Nouvel Observateur* (18 July). Accessed 21 July 2020. www.nouvelobs.com/culture/20190718.OBS16116/pourquoi-la-casa-de-papel-nous-rend-aussi-accros.html

López P., José M. and M. L. L. Terrada (1997). *La influencia española en la introducción en Europa de las plantas americanas (1493–1623)* (Valencia: Universitàt de Valencia & CSIC).

Machuca, F. (2018). 'Las ratas acabaron con la Sevilla llena de luz y de magia, valiente y emprendedora', *ABC* (5 February). Accessed 21 July 2020. https://sevilla.abc.es/play/series/sevi-ratas-acabaron-sevilla-llena-y-magia-valiente-y-emprendedora-201802051049_noticia.html.

Martínez, B. (2018). 'Alberto Rodríguez: Queríamos que *La Peste* fuera una experiencia inmersiva', *Revista GQ* (11 January). Accessed 21 July 2020. www.revistagq.com/noticias/cultura/articulos/alberto-rodriguez-entrevista-la-peste/27771

Martínez, M. (2018). 'El pasado inacabado. Sobre *La Peste*', *Revista Contexto* 152 (17 January). Accessed 21 July 2020. https://ctxt.es/es/20180117/Culturas/17378/La-peste-serie-tv-Sevilla-historia-trama.htm

Martínez Shaw, C. (2019). 'Contra el triunfo de la confusión', *El País* (27 July). Accessed 21 July 2020. https://elpais.com/cultura/2019/06/20/babelia/1561046875_735107.html

Olmedilla y Puig, J. (1897). *Estudio histórico de la vida y escritos del sabio y medico español Nicolás Monardes* (Madrid: Imprenta de los hijos de M. G. Hernández).

Pardo Tomás, J. (2002). *El tesoro natural de América. Colonialismo y ciencia en el siglo XVI* (Madrid: Nivola Libros y Ediciones).

Parrilla Valero, F. (2019). 'La Peste Negra del 1348 a la Corona d'Aragó. Una revolución social, econòmica i salubrista', *Gimbernat. Revista d'Història de la Medici*na i de les Ciències de la Salut, 71 (2019): 13–22.

'Record de audiencia de *Hospital Central*', *El Periódico* (27 January 27). Accessed 21 July 2020. https://web.archive.org/web/20090122025749/http://www.elperiodicoextremadura.com/noticias/noticia.asp?pkid=154173

Rivas Moreno, S. (2018). 'El ocaso de la televisión tradicional', *El País. Retina* (5 January). Accessed 12 October 2019. https://retina.elpais.com/retina/2017/12/28/tendencias/1514477436_454556.html

R. V. (2018). 'Sevilla, llena de ratas por la peste', *ABC* (6 February). Accessed 21 July 2020. https://sevilla.abc.es/play/series/sevi-sevilla-llena-ratas-peste-201802060928_noticia.html

Sheaves, M. (2015). 'Notes from the field: Retracing sixteenth-century steps in Seville', *Not Even Past* (8 April). Accessed 21 July 2020. https://notevenpast.org/notes-from-the-field-retracing-steps-in-sixteenth-century-seville/

Spinney, L. (2018). *Pale Rider. The Spanish Flu of 1918 and How It Changed the World* (London: Vintage).

The Economic Times (2020). '"Contagion", "Pandemic", "Plague Inc": Demand for disease-themed movies, games at an all-time high amidst coronavirus outbreak', *The Economic Times* (February 21). Accessed 21 July 2020. https://economictimes.indiatimes.com/magazines/panache/contagion-pandemic-plague-inc-demand-for-disease-themed-movies-games-at-an-all-time-high/articleshow/74241416.cms

Wilson, A. (2019). 'Good Bad Bad Good. What was the Golden Age of TV?', *Harpers Magazine* (11 October). Accessed 21 July 2020. https://harpers.org/archive/2019/10/good-bad-bad-good-golden-age-of-television/

Wilson, K. (2013). *Plague and Public Health in Early Modern Seville. Rochester Studies in Medical History* (Rochester, NY: University of Rochester Press).

Winegard, T. C. (2019). 'The mosquitoes are coming for us', *The New York Times* (27 July). Accessed 21 July 2020. www.nytimes.com/2019/07/27/opinion/sunday/mosquitoes-malaria-zika-history.html?fbclid=IwAR1wkGhXj-lhUpd-ah5UApL4IEszw7ALnpesUHkwEt2efq6N0nZUNTHryt0

2

Wellness, womanhood, and witchcraft in *Outlander*: televised historical portrayals of women's shifting roles in medicine

Jennifer M. Fogel and Serenity Sutherland

Claire Randall Fraser (Caitriona Balfe), the heroine in Diana Gabaldon's time-travelling book series *Outlander* and its television adaptation, practises as a nurse, healer, and physician in backdrops where women have historically struggled for recognition as bona fide medical practitioners. In settings such as eighteenth-century Jacobin Scotland, pre-Revolutionary France, colonial America, World War II European battlefronts, and 1950s–1960s Harvard University, Claire's medical acumen proves she is a talented healer despite the frequent scepticism and disapproval of those around her. In all time periods Claire finds herself, she must negotiate the gender politics and cultural expectations of women's gendered roles, which often results in her taking a stand to defend her medical expertise. Unlike contemporary television medical dramas that offer a more egalitarian perspective on women's abilities to practise medicine – although still marred by conflict between a woman's personal happiness and professional success – *Outlander* portrays a woman pitched through time with only her knowledge of medicine and future events to find her footing.

While Claire's story is fictional, her experience of inclusion and exclusion in the male-dominated world of medicine from the mid-eighteenth century to the 1970s echoes much of the historiography of women's experiences in medicine. Londa Schiebinger reminds us in *Has Feminism Changed Science?* (1999) that women's access to scientific opportunities is full of ebbs and flows, never totally exclusionary but never completely inclusive, either. In Britain and the Americas, women's involvement as practitioners of medicine has undulated since the 1700s, throughout which time medical knowledge provided women positions of both power and danger within their wider communities. In eighteenth-century Scotland, it is Claire's medical knowledge that offers access to clan Mackenzie when she sets Jamie Fraser's dislocated shoulder and treats Colum Mackenzie's Toulouse-Lautrec Syndrome, a degenerative disease that renders his legs immobile. This does not mean Claire's expertise is taken wholesale, however. Men and women within the clan treat Claire with a fragile mix of suspicion and grudging respect, even accusing her of witchcraft.

This chapter examines the ways in which Claire utilises her medical skills – holistically and scientifically – as an avenue of agency and survival. The show's presentation of gender politics across three centuries reminds historians of the back and forth shifts women have made as practitioners in medicine and science. To fully explore the ways in which *Outlander*, and Claire specifically, acts as a fictional historical narrative of a medical pioneer, this chapter will focus on three areas: first, Claire's status as 'Sassenach' not only labels her as an outsider in Scotland but also alludes to her isolation as a female healer. Second, we examine the domestication of medicine within *Outlander* and the ways Claire (and other female 'healers' in the series) navigate accusations of witchcraft. Last, we assess the ways in which *Outlander* utilises communitarian ideology to service Claire's modern-day progressivism and romanticise the historical narrative. Throughout this chapter, Claire's experience is situated within the historical record and scholarship on the history of women in medicine to assess the television series' portrayal of women's role in medicine and professionalisation and to interrogate whether Claire's story can be read as a feminist narrative that is true to the historical context.

The televised medical drama as a genre

The adaptation of Gabaldon's *Outlander* series premiered on Starz in August 2014. Like the novels on which it is based, the television series is a complex mix of genres: a dramatic romance with a historical bent. While popularised as a breath-taking love story between Claire Beauchamp Randall and Jamie Fraser (Sam Heughan), *Outlander* in its first five seasons envelops their romance within some of the most contentious moments of Scottish and American history. But it also offers a twist on contemporary medical dramas. Today's medical dramas like *Grey's Anatomy* (2005–), *Chicago Med* (2015–), and *The Resident* (2018–) often offer harrowing 'disease of the week' narratives peppered with sub-storylines focused on the complex and lively personal stories of young doctors.

Although media critics are more likely to accurately comment on the lack of racial diversity and invisible discussion of the health care system writ large, women in these television series still wrestle with hegemonic gender norms in what was, and in many ways continues to be, a male-dominated profession. Media effects scholar Emily Moyer-Gusé (2008) notes that medical dramas can act as entertainment-education to influence and persuade viewers' attitudes and behaviours towards health-related issues. Similarly, medical dramas can shape viewers' perceptions of medical professionals (Chory-Assad and Tamborini, 2003). What distinguishes the impact of entertainment narratives from more traditional health campaigns is the unique aspect of transportation into the fictionalised story and, more importantly, identification with the drama's characters (Cohen, 2001; Green and Brock, 2001). Relationally, if viewers' attitudes and behaviours can be affected by medical dramas, it stands to reason that the portrayal of gender in these same series can also perpetuate and influence gender norms within the medical profession.

A content analysis by Parul Jain and Michael D. Slater (2013: 717) found that 'Women are portrayed as doctors at proportions similar to or exceeding their representation in the physician population'. However, medical dramas 'disproportionately focused on their sexuality and romantic relationships as opposed to their professional role' (2013: 717). Furthermore, even though many current medical dramas feature female leads and an equal presence of women in the hospital hierarchy, these series quite often highlight the continued work–life imbalance of female physicians and nurses. As noted in the *New York Times*, 'The structure of medical training has changed little since the 1960s ... nor has the division of domestic labour shifted to reflect the rise of women in the medical work force' (Khullar, 2017). Thus, women characters in medical series still confront a historical gender bias but one that is now less defined by lack of access and rather a confrontation of competing poles of maternalism and careerism.

Medical dramas set in a historicised past, on the other hand, are more soundly centred on emerging practices in the medical field, and too often marginalise the interrogation of gender roles. The last decade has seen an uptick in historical medical dramas – many of which are mentioned in this book – that take a decidedly similar path, with women struggling to make their mark in the medical profession as nurses or midwives (e.g., *Call the Midwife*, 2012–; *Mercy Street*, 2016–2018) whereas men are depicted on the brink of pioneering medical innovations (e.g., *The Knick*, 2014; *The Alienist*, 2018–2020; *Charité* 2017–). *Outlander* defies this trend by constructing the female lead as an outsider within the interleaving patriarchal cultures of medicine and history. In this way, it is quite similar to another popular television series (also discussed in this volume), *Dr. Quinn, Medicine Woman* (1993–1998). Instead of the brutish Scottish Highlands of the eighteenth century, *Dr. Quinn* takes place in the post–Civil War frontier West with its title character unconventionally practising medicine in a setting ill-prepared to acknowledge a female doctor. In *Prime Time Feminism*, feminist media scholar Bonnie Dow (1996: 170) argues that the success of *Dr. Quinn* was tied to it strategically using the nostalgic frontier as a frame for a larger postfeminist discussion on contemporary (i.e. 1990s) gender anxieties. *Dr. Quinn* followed Dr Michaela 'Mike' Quinn putting up her shingle in frontier Colorado Springs, a town unwelcoming to both outsiders and a female doctor. Dow argues that *Dr. Quinn* was feminist within the context of its historical setting but clearly avoided larger political discussions of feminism in favour of Dr Mike drawing on her professional career to enact great domestic and community change, rather than enact a town-wide feminist revolution. According to Dow (1996: 178), the series reflects maternal feminism, a faction of feminism that recognises differences between the sexes, specifically linking maternalism within the domestic space and affirmation of motherhood in an egalitarian society. Despite earning backlash from obstinate neighbours for being a 'woman doctor' with liberal genteel ideals (learned from being raised in Boston), Dr Mike is immediately endowed with a trio of children, placing her ultimately as a mother, thereby softening her image as a single career woman.

Moreover, media scholar Mimi White (2000) argues that Dr Mike's professional successes and eventual respect from the town cannot, necessarily, be read as a win for traditional feminism. Played by the glamorous Jane Seymour, Dr Mike's fight against sexism 'is tempered, in particular by her extremely conventional femininity, evident not only in her physical appearance, but also in her tender and morally balanced mothering, and her artless romance behaviours' (White, 2000: 31). White characterises *Dr. Quinn* as 'communitarian postfeminism', where Dr Mike is at the centre of progressive reforms and historically interpolates a number of contemporary social concerns, but 'nevertheless conform[s] to conventional expectations of woman's place in culture' (White, 2000: 35). In fact, as Bonnie Dow (1996: 180–181) explains, 'Dr. Mike's expertise as a doctor is enhanced by her sensitivity and relationship skills as a woman and, in particular, as a mother'. Furthermore, Dr Mike's love interest, Sully (Joe Lando), is a thoroughly idealised romantic partner awash in an intriguing mixture of liberal male feminist and hypermasculine mountain man. Still, the series ultimately romanticises Dr Mike's independence, masking much of her professional success through personal familial attainment, particularly once she is deemed an asset to the townspeople.

In many ways, *Outlander* similarly expresses a muted feminist message of a female outsider within a thoroughly patriarchal society. Claire Fraser continually asserts her independence in two disparate time periods locked within a burgeoning social revolution. But unlike *Dr. Quinn*, Claire's choices are more consciously rooted in survival and cleverness than maternalism and cultural change. While Claire's beauty, too, is similarly remarked upon by numerous characters, she becomes equally renowned for her medical abilities. Her skills are not meant to be an agent of female independence, but they do serve to give her more agency than other women in the *Outlander* series. The idealised romantic hero, Jamie, whose liberal views on gender and racial equality are masked underneath a hypermasculine Highlander exterior, aids Claire throughout the narrative. The partnership between the couple is not only critical to the popularisation of this romantic narrative, but also affords Claire a front-row seat on the historical events permeating the novels – many of which Claire and Jamie desperately try to intercede in and effect change. Importantly, it is Claire's *general* knowledge of the past that drives the narrative forward with her agency as a 'healer' providing access to numerous historical scenes and figures. Thus, not only is the character of Claire Fraser a manifestation of a pseudo-historian of Scottish and American history reminiscent of time-travelling science fiction series, but also the personification of chronicling developments in the medical field itself – a role typically reserved for male physicians in historical medical dramas.

Female physician as Sassenach

In the stifling patriarchy of Highland Scotland, Claire is granted agency few of her gender could earn. Her medical expertise – initially cursory nursing knowledge from the battlefronts of WWII and herbal remedies – vaults her to the title of 'Beaton' within clan MacKenzie and earns the respect of many of the men, although she is still considered a prisoner of the clan's chieftain Colum MacKenzie (Gary Lewis). The Beaton was a type of cunning folk, or wise women and men in late medieval and modern Europe, possessing a set of special skills relating to healing and specialist knowledge passed down through generations (de Blecourt, 1994). Claire fits this model with her healing knowledge, and her possession of seemingly insider information minimises her outsider status. Author Sarah Stegall notes (2016: 98), 'The title and respect of a "Beaton" allow Claire to make decisions and to act in ways that would not have been permitted even to a woman born into the clan, let alone an outsider.' Claire's education, traversing the world with her archaeologist uncle during childhood, and training as a nurse all fuse together to offer her a privileged status that empowers her within the clan's male power structure (Stegall, 2016). Nevertheless, Claire is the consummate outsider, a Sassenach both as a female healer and Englishwoman in Scotland.

An outsider both to the clan and the eighteenth-century time period, Claire often fails to disguise her contempt for the political and cultural injustices she observes. The laws regulating eighteenth-century Highland life, including those that posited women as property of men, continually thwart her agency and ability to practise medicine. Although Claire believes that caring for the people of clan MacKenzie will afford her eventual release, she understands that she will have to 'find a way to apply twentieth-century medicine using only the methods and equipment of the eighteenth century'

('The Way Out', S1E3). But Claire's reliance on scientific methods runs contrary not only to the hegemonic gender norms of the time period, but also the dogma of the Church relying on religious faith to heal the sick as well as the supernatural mysticism of Scottish folklore. In the season one episode 'The Way Out', Claire discovers that two boys who were playing in the ruins of a Benedictine monastery have become ill, and one has already died. The clanspeople tell Claire that demons roam free inside the ruins and sickened the boys. Despite numerous warnings, Claire refuses to back down from helping the boy, earning the contempt of Father Bain (Tim McInnerny) when she contradicts his evaluation of the boy's illness as demonic possession. She skilfully discovers the boy had eaten poisonous flora and attempts to cure him, eliciting disdain from Father Bain when he labels Claire a blasphemer, refusing to listen to a woman. Eventually the boy's aunt courageously stands up to Father Bain allowing Claire to heal the boy. While seemingly a victory for Claire and her medical skills, the move earns her the abject scorn of Father Bain (and thus the Church). It also further ingratiates her to Colum MacKenzie, who views her as a worthy possession within his castle thereby decreasing her chances of release from his service.

As the narrative turns, Claire marries Jamie Fraser to avoid arrest by Black Jack Randall (Tobias Menzies), a type of protective custody through coverture. The marriage offers much more freedom for Claire, as Jamie – similar to Sully in *Dr. Quinn, Medicine Woman* – expresses more egalitarian notions of marriage as a partnership and supports her medical practice. Jamie also foresees the practicality of Claire's historical knowledge and medicinal skills to further the couple's survival amidst the bourgeoisie bluebloods of eighteenth-century France and the British compatriots of colonial America. Still, he baulks at Claire's desire to nurse the destitute denizens of France at the L'Hôpital des Anges run by the convent's Mother Hildegarde ('Useful Occupations and Deception', S2E3). At this point (in season two), Claire is pregnant with Jamie's child and the two work to infiltrate Prince Charles's inner circle in order to foil Jacobite efforts and halt the looming death knell of 1745's Battle of Culloden. But Claire takes the opportunity not only to trade courtly gossip with the women in her new circle of friends, but also further her medicinal skills through the mentorship of Mother Hildegarde (Frances de la Tour) and Master Raymond (a mystic apothecary played by Dominique Pinon) who both encourage her healing talents.

When their ministrations in France come to naught, Jamie and Claire return to Scotland to prepare for war and the impending doom of the Jacobite rebellion. Claire accompanies Jamie to the front lines and establishes a field hospital (and later clinic) to minister to soldiers and townsfolk. This, once more, establishes her unusual agency for the time period. While Jamie and his cohort train the farmers of the Highlands to fight as soldiers, it is Claire who organises the women in preparing medical supplies, remedies, and nourishment for the men ('Prestonpans', S2E10). In 'Je Suis Prest' (S2E9), the episode provides flashbacks to Claire's time with the Allied armies at a field hospital training soldiers in proper hygiene and nursing the injured, which parallels her current situation amongst the Highlanders. In seasons three and four, she brings this same steadfastness to situations ranging from treating typhoid fever as a ship's surgeon aboard the British man-of-war *Porpoise* ('Heaven and Earth', S3E10) to midwifery of slaves and immigrants of colonial America.

Although Claire's doctoring skills become essential to her survival in the past, they are also the cause for much of her isolation outside of her marriage to Jamie. Even having confessed to Jamie that she is a time traveller, Claire is still continually stifled by her historical knowledge of the past and rendered strange by her seemingly magical ability to heal the sick. Women, in particular, distrust her a great deal. Claire's status as Sassenach gives her an unusual position in the gendered hierarchy of clan life and identifies her as peculiar from the eighteenth-century norms of womanhood. Claire becomes even more isolated when she returns to the twentieth century. Season three begins with Claire's return to the 'future' and Frank Randall (also played by Tobias Menzies), pregnant with Jamie's child. Claire and Frank decide to move to the United States to start anew. But in 1950s Boston, Claire is bored by the domesticity she once craved with Frank (and Jamie) and – having grown accustomed to her wartime authority amongst eighteenth-century Scottish men – vexes Frank's male Harvard colleagues by freely offering her opinions on current events ('The Battle Joined', S3E1). After her daughter, Brianna, is born, Claire acknowledges that something is missing in her life and decides to enroll in medical school to once more be a part of something greater than herself ('Surrender', S3E2). But in doing so, she not only faces isolation as the only woman in her class, but also further separates herself from her marriage to Frank. The dissolution of their marriage is captured in a series of vignettes in 'All Debts Paid' (S3E3) as Claire becomes a surgeon, Frank participates in numerous 'discreet' affairs, and Brianna grows into a young woman with an emotionally strained relationship with her mother. Claire's advancing medical skills, once a measure of her survival in the eighteenth century, now cocoon her from the grief of lost love and an inability to move on from the past (see Figure 2.1).

While we are not privy to much of Claire's work as a practising surgeon in a 1960s Boston hospital, she evidently makes strides towards breaking the glass ceiling of the medical field, which reflects similar real-life accounts of women surgeons practising in a male-dominated sphere (Cassell, 1998; Conley, 1999). However, the male faculty and her peers initially marginalise Claire during medical school. Her only ally is the similarly dismissed

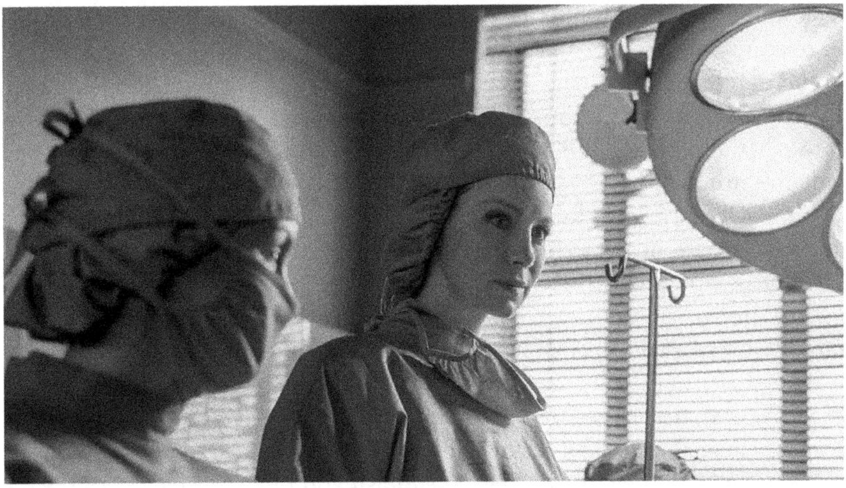

Figure 2.1 A circa-1960s Claire breaking the glass ceiling as a surgeon in a Boston hospital (*Outlander*)

African American colleague Joe Abernathy (Wil Johnson). Abernathy serves as a narrative foil illustrating the analogous types of isolation both characters experienced working in a male-dominated field, as well as the types of disrespect white men directed towards women and people of colour attempting to practise medicine. These sentiments are continually reinforced in *Outlander* as Claire is introduced to other 'healers' from various cultures (i.e., Haitian, Native American, Quaker, etc.) during her journey into the past. It is likely due to Claire's intimate familiarity with being dismissed by men (in multiple time periods) that causes her to form strong kinships with those relegated to 'outsider' status within the patriarchal hierarchy.

Furthermore, Claire's compassionate rigidity displayed in both Highland Scotland and WWII battlements is certainly set apart from the tempestuous personal and professional lives of women doctors in contemporary television medical dramas. We don't see Claire ruthlessly covet surgeries like the interns of *Grey's Anatomy* (2005–) or deal with administrative blowback for performing a costly experimental surgery like on *New Amsterdam* (2018–), but viewers witness the constant barrage of disbelief and derision Claire earns from many of the men (and women) as she struggles throughout the centuries to assert her medical expertise. For example, season four finds Claire and Jamie installed in pre–Revolutionary War North Carolina. Claire's attempts to offer medical advice to an ailing Edmund Fanning (a colonial administrator and friend of the governor, played by Samuel Collins) are snubbed, with the man deferring to his male physician ('Wilmington', S4E8). As the man lies dying, men in wigs and surcoats surround the makeshift operating table debating whether or not it is proper for Claire to operate on Fanning. Once Fanning's physician arrives and he sees Claire in the middle of emergency surgery he exclaims, 'What hath hell wrought. [...] You've butchered him, madam. All he needed was tobacco smoke up through the rear.' To which the governor responds, 'No need of you, the lady has it in hand.'

Similarly, in season five, although Claire is offered a position of power as Jamie's wife in rural North Carolina, she is often rendered powerless in implementing scientific medical care as the other women of her community prefer the quackery of medicinal elixirs and powders riddled with life-threatening poisons like mercury. In 'Between Two Fires' (S5E2), Claire listens as a group of women doing laundry discuss a remedy for healing a burn. At first, the suggestions are mere wives' tales that Claire explains have some medicinal truth, but then the women report that a local male physician condemned them as hackneyed rubbish and prescribed a fever powder used by the King. Even as Claire tries to reason with the women that the powder contains a poison, the women – though they acknowledge Claire is a 'fine healer' – prefer the advice of a 'learned physician'. Desperate to impart her knowledge of preventative twentieth-century health care to the settlers of North Carolina and realising the hindrance of her sex, Claire adopts the pseudonym of 'Doctor Rawlings' and pens a pamphlet on the proper use of domestic remedies. Unfortunately, Claire's efforts are seemingly for naught after a local newspaper accidentally publishes her pamphlet and the women of a neighbouring community simply mock the medical advice of 'Doctor Rawlings' ('The Company We Keep', S5E4). By the season finale, Claire's alias has been uncovered by Lionel Brown (played by Ned Dennehy). Already aggrieved by Claire's liberated medical advice and its effect on his marriage, as well as her overall lack of deference to men and Jamie's antagonism of the Brown family, Lionel kidnaps and eventually initiates a gang-rape of Claire.

'Answer me true ... are ye a witch?': witchcraft and wellness

Claire's fictional experiences offer a grounding in reality when compared to the real-life medical professions of colonial New England midwife Martha Ballard and 'lady' physician Elizabeth Blackwell, the first female physician in the United States, who graduated from Geneva Medical College in 1849. Many women followed Ballard and Blackwell into the profession throughout the nineteenth century. As historian Mary Roth Walsh documents (1977), women in medicine experienced a backlash in the early to mid-1900s. Other historians have acknowledged how women struggled to obtain training as professionals in medicine in America (Abrams, 1985; Luchetti, 1989; Moldow, 1987; Peitzman, 2000; Walsh, 1977) and Britain (Pringle, 1998), just as Claire struggled to do in 1950s Boston, with many, as one historian termed it, travelling to the ends of the earth (Bonner, 1992). Claire, it seems, travels not just to the ends of the earth, but to the limits of time. Claire's journey throughout time and space and the struggles she faces in every setting to practise medicine symbolises the great distances women in their time took to achieve medical education.

Historians have well documented women's role as caregivers during childbirth, with many noting the prevalence of female midwives until the turn of the nineteenth century when the presence of male physicians increasingly favoured a medical model that emphasised the educated male doctor and his birthing tools of forceps and the emerging science of obstetrics (Leavitt, 1986, 1999; Wertz and Wertz, 1977). This is most clearly represented in Laurel Thatcher Ulrich's *A Midwife's Tale: The Life of Martha Ballard, Based on Her Diary, 1785–1812* (1990), which traces the life of Martha Ballard, a midwife and healer living in New England. Ballard kept a diary in which she recorded all the babies she delivered, noting a variety of demographic information and any complications that may have arisen during the birth, and sometimes after. Increasingly towards the end of Ballard's life, male doctors became more common during delivery due to the 'era when old childbirth practices were being challenged in both England and America by a new "scientific" obstetrics promoted by male physicians' (Ulrich, 1990: 27; Leavitt, 1986). Ulrich argues, however, that in colonial New England male doctors could not do without female healers and often called in midwives to assist, although this disrupted the balance of who controlled the delivery significantly. In England as well, the 1858 Medical Act in Britain restricted who could practise medicine to men, thus restricting midwives and their practice (Roberts, 2009).

Claire performs midwifery throughout her time in the past, although the audience does not see her assist with a birth until 'The Watch' (S1E13) in season one when she helps her sister-in-law Jenny McMurray (Laura Donnelly) with delivering a daughter. In fact, Jenny is the first woman the show portrays as having been assisted by Claire's medical knowledge and this reinforces the misperception that the only medical attention women of the eighteenth century required was reproductive health. Typically Claire spends her healing efforts on the men of the show: setting Jamie Fraser's dislocated arm ('Sassenach', S1E1), easing Colum MacKenzie's pain from Toulouse-Lautrec Syndrome ('The Way Out', S1E3), and tending to a dying man on a boar hunt ('The Gathering', S1E4). The men, with the exception of Colum MacKenzie, seek treatment for wounds earned while hunting, raiding, war, and defence of the clan. There is no doubt that in the eighteenth century, childbirth could be just as dangerous as the predatory activities of men. In the 1740s, nearly 10 per cent of women died in childbirth (Marshall, 1983: 227). Blame fell on midwives for maternal casualties in the 1800s, according to historian Christine Théré (1999: 558). Yet women also required treatment for ailments beyond childbearing; however, the show provides only one type of medical narrative (reproductive health) for women within the first season.

The modern viewer might deem Claire's occupation as a female physician as 'out of time' for the period, but she is essentially practising the feminine domestic labour of 'caring for another's body' (Barclay, 2013: 4). Thus, as argued by Stegall (2016: 103), 'Gabaldon has deliberately chosen Claire's profession as one which will more or less fit into the mid-1700s'. In eighteenth-century Scotland, it was not uncommon for women to care for others as healers and midwives. At the same time, however, 'the ability to heal gave women more power than men were comfortable with' leading to accusations of witchcraft (Stegall, 2016: 102). Claire often experiences such recriminations, although she, at times, uses this to her advantage. She becomes La Dame Blanche ('The White Lady') among the French bourgeoisie and the Gaelic *ban-druidh* ('The White Witch') to the people of the Lallybroch estate. Gabaldon (1999: 195) herself comments, 'Given Claire's naturally pale complexion, her healing arts (and the ruthlessness which is a natural part of them), and her supernatural connections (both real and perceived), it seemed only reasonable to endow her with the title.' Both titles offer Claire a modicum of physical protection by warding off many seeking to harass her, but also emphasise her place as an outsider in league with the mysticism of medieval Scottish folk tales. Media scholar Valerie Estelle Frankel notes in *Symbolism and Sources of Outlander* (2015b: 186) that 'In French, Dutch, and Germanic folklore, White Ladies were a type of vicious fairy. […] La Dame Blanche makes a formidable friend or enemy and expects respect from the men who want her aid.' Many Scottish clansmen believe in Claire's preternatural abilities, thereby allowing her access and agency to assert her medical expertise, but, more often than not, the religiosity of the Church and its congregation is far warier of Claire's medicinal powers. Thus, the show plays with the tensions of how institutions viewed women healers throughout the centuries.

Can a feminist travel through time? *Outlander* and the communitarian ideal

Due to her time-travelling abilities, twentieth-century modern woman Claire serves as a type of surrogate for historians themselves, although

Claire actually lives in the past with her cultural assumptions, instead of analysing with the benefit of hindsight as historians do (Gaddis, 2002). Like the historian, Claire's modern perspective on issues such as women's rights, slavery, and colonialism cause a disconnect with eighteenth-century historical actors, such as the powerful men she encounters. Claire's exposure to 1950s and '60s Boston would have made her familiar with feminism and women's rights. This raises the question of whether or not Claire Fraser can be read as a feminist, both within the context and storyline of the show and as a comparative figure within the televised medical costume genre. Certainly compared against the backdrop of other televised medical women, such as Dr Mike, Claire is a much more progressive take on what a female healer set in the past can and should look like. Having said this, though, we read the show's treatment of Claire's power and autonomy through the role of a female healer as less an expression of modern-day feminism and more a validation of communitarianism, or the common good for all. Through this claim, we argue against *Buzzfeed*'s assertion that the show is cable television's 'feminist answer to *Game of Thrones*' and its intolerable treatment of its female heroines (Petersen, 2014).

The show's hesitancy to portray Claire as a feminist can be seen in how the narrative handles reproductive topics for women. Claire expresses progressive ideals about a woman's right to decide her own approach to reproductive health care, but never outright portrays herself as a feminist. Perhaps because in the eighteenth-century settings in which she finds herself, feminism, a term first widely used in the early 1900s (Cott, 1987: 3), is incredibly anachronistic – but this seems an odd strategy for a story that is all about twentieth-century viewpoints clashing with those of the eighteenth century. Claire's willingness to perform abortions – though we don't actually see her do so in the television series – functions as a panacea to the lack of reproductive health care for women in the eighteenth century and not necessarily as a women's rights issue, although she certainly expresses that it is a woman's choice ('The Deep Heart's Core', S4E10). In her examination of birth control in *Outlander*, Nicole M. duPlessis (2016: 86) argues that the series 'rather grudgingly accepts abortion, casting it as painful and desperate, but reserving it as an option primarily (though not exclusively) because the existing social structure forces women to consider it an option'. Although Claire offers Brianna (Sophie Skelton) the choice of an abortion when the paternity of her child is in question (either her lover Roger, played by Richard Rankin, or rapist Stephen Bonnet, played by Ed Speleers), Claire had two seasons earlier counselled Prince Charles Stuart's married mistress against aborting the foetus and instead assists her scheme to keep the child ('Untimely Resurrection', S2E5). Instead, *Outlander* is more politically feminist in discussions of birth control, with Claire continually promoting contraceptive techniques to women in both the eighteenth and twentieth centuries (duPlessis, 2016). For example, Claire learns of eighteenth-century birth control techniques from prostitutes in a brothel ('A. Malcolm', S3E6), which she later shares with her stepdaughter Marsali (Lauren Lyle) and daughter Brianna. Claire's motivations here seem to stem from maintaining the domestic relations of the community by preserving the health of its women more so than protecting a woman's right to choose, especially when the choice is abortion. It is important to note that communitarianism can exist alongside feminism and the two are not incompatible; however, the show's narrative defaults to communitarian explanations for issues of women's reproductive rights and gender issues, rather than presenting an unapologetically feminist argument.

Even beyond the scenes of conflict and resolution featuring issues of reproductive politics, communitarianism rather than liberal social justice efforts guide the narrative. For example, Claire plays a role in two physician-assisted suicides: the first is Colum MacKenzie who requires Claire's help to release him from his disabling and painful disease ('The Hail Mary', S2E12), and the second offers a peaceful release to a convicted slave in lieu of a painful execution by southern gentry ('Do No Harm', S4E2). Colum's death will pave the way for his son to become clan chieftain and fare better after the Jacobite 'Rising' when the British enforce harsh penalties on the Scottish clans. The death of Rufus (Jerome Holder), one of Jamie's aunt's slaves, is a bitter compromise that will both assuage the neighbouring landowners' vigilante justice and protect the plantation's other inhabitants. Thus, Claire's actions are less about liberal or reformist ideology, and more service to ameliorating the community and its demands, which is especially clear when Claire handles patients in an unbiased way – treating Redcoat, Jacobite, and slave alike. Communitarianism is particularly emphasised in season four as the Frasers discover and befriend the Native American Tuscarora tribe. Under the tutelage of various members, the Frasers begin to understand the importance of the ancient traditions established to keep the community thriving even amidst westward expansion. As noted by Valerie Estelle Frankel (2015a: 137), the Tuscarora 'believe everything around them is part of an infinite web'. This aligns with leadership scholar Craig E. Johnson's (2005) central premise of communitarianism as a society of intersecting communities.

Similarly, communitarianism is a large part of the narrative in season five, as Claire morphs a significant part of her home on Fraser's Ridge into a surgery. While Claire tends to the ailments of her patients, Jamie surreptitiously uses the promise of his wife's medical expertise to strengthen the Fraser's Ridge community. In 'The Fiery Cross' (S5E1), when a young Josiah Beardsley comes to the Ridge for a cure for his throat pain (diagnosed later as abscessed tonsils), Jamie implies that payment for treatment would be Josiah settling at the Ridge since he is an excellent hunter and would be an asset to the burgeoning community. Claire also struggles to enact some preternatural medicinal progress as the burden of future historical knowledge weighs on her shoulders. In 'Between Two Fires' (S5E2), she first recruits her daughter-in-law, Marsali, to become her surgical apprentice – even roguishly procuring a corpse to instruct her on anatomy. This serves a two-fold purpose: Claire is able to pass on her knowledge to a competent assistant, and an apprentice can be a 'healer' when she is absent from the Ridge. Second, Claire becomes determined to 'create' penicillin with mouldy bread – even though penicillin would not be used as an antibiotic until the twentieth century – in order to further treat more patients on the Ridge despite the impact it could have on the future. In fact, her experimentation comes to fruition when she uses the nascent drug to aid her in the tonsillectomies she performs on Josiah and his brother Keziah. Thus, Claire's occupation as a female physician and healer is not necessarily driven by second-wave feminist notions of equality, but rather communitarian resistance to the strictures of the eighteenth (and later twentieth) century.

Reading Claire's narrative as a type of biography offers a comparison of how the show portrays Claire's womanhood as a progressive communitarian ideal with how real women physicians viewed themselves within the gender politics of their societies. Claire's biographical foil within the show for the first three seasons is Geillis Duncan (Lotta Verbeek), also a time traveller and knowledgeable about herbs and healing. Unlike Claire, though, Geillis is an antiheroine: she is not motivated by the Hippocratic Oath in her practice of medicine. Geillis kills many male characters throughout the show: she poisons her eighteenth-century husband to be with her lover ('By the Pricking of My Thumbs', S1E10); she sacrifices her twentieth-century husband to travel back in time through the stones at Craigh Na Dunne ('Of Lost Things', S3E4); and she rapes and then murders many young boys in an attempt to harness their virginal power ('The Bakra', S3E12). Geillis's violence against the male body contrasts with Claire's, who out of a sense of moral obligation always tries to heal even those men, such as Colum MacKenzie and Captain Jack Randall, who would imprison or harm her. Furthermore, Geillis's practice of the healing arts is more malevolently spiritual than Claire's scientific rigidity. Blood sacrifices, communing naked in nature, poisons, charms, and abortive elixirs are the tools of her trade, whilst Claire utilises 'everyday, domestic objects, utensils, and kitchen herbs to heal' (Ty, 2016: 59). Geillis's medical motivations, then, are power, revenge, and social ascendency. Historical biographies of real women physicians show that a range of motivations and medical epistemologies exist for women in medical professions. Biographies also feature personal struggles and geographical distances women undertook to pursue advanced medical training (Bittel, 2009; Jensen, 2012; More, 1999; Tuchman, 2006; Wu, 2005). Claire's story in *Outlander*, traversing vast distances of time and space, mimics the biographical approach of recovering women's stories and featuring the voices of individual women. But here the show is limited as the individual woman's experience viewers always see is Claire's – a white, British woman from the mid-twentieth century.

Conclusion

As historical fiction, *Outlander* serves as an entertaining pathway to discovering the complicated evolution of gender roles – here, specifically within the medical field. Overall, the show allows for a fictional exchange of ideas about medicine and gender across the centuries that serves as a commentary on women's access to medicine off-screen. The presentation of gender politics undulating across three centuries reminds viewers of the back and forth shifts women have made as practitioners in medicine and science. While viewers may cast Claire's modern-day progressivism as feminist within the more patriarchal periods in which she finds herself, we argue that her idealism and quest for egalitarian gender roles are actually more connected to narrative tropes of the romance. From the perspective of a historical medical drama, Claire – as a woman doctor – constantly finds herself at odds with patriarchal rule. And yet, she manages to ultimately utilise her medical acumen to not only prove her usefulness to the powerful men she is surrounded by, but also provide a sympathetic heroine who drives the medical field to not only embrace the traditions and communitarianism of more natural remedies, but also accept women as capable scientific pioneers.

References

Abrams, R. (ed.) (1985). *'Send us a lady physician': Women doctors in America, 1835–1920*, W.W. Norton, New York.

Barclay, K. (ed.) (2013). *Women in eighteenth-century Scotland: Intimate, intellectual and private lives*, Ashgate, London.

Bittel, C. (2009). *Mary Putnam Jacobi and the politics of medicine in nineteenth-century America*, University of North Carolina Press, Chapel Hill, NC.

Bonner, T. N. (1992). *To the ends of the earth: Women's search for education in medicine*, Harvard University Press, Cambridge, MA.

Cassell, J. (1998). *The woman in the surgeon's body*, Harvard University Press, Cambridge, MA.

Chory-Assad, R. M. and Tamborini, R. (2003). 'Television exposure and the public's perceptions of physicians', *Journal of Broadcasting and Electronic Media*, vol. 47, pp. 197–215.

Cohen, J. (2001). 'Defining identification: A theoretical look at the identification of audiences with media characters', *Mass Communication & Society*, vol. 4, pp. 245–264.

Conley, F. (1999). *Walking out on the boys*, Firrar, Straus, and Giraux, New York.

Cott, N. (1987). *The grounding of modern Feminism*, Yale University Press, New Haven, CT.

de Blecourt, Willem (1994). 'Witch doctors, soothsayers and priests. On cunning folk in European historiography and tradition', *Social History*, vol. 19, pp. 285–303.

Dow, B. J. (1996). *Prime-time feminism: Television, media culture, and the women's movement since 1970*, University of Pennsylvania Press, Philadelphia, PA.

duPlessis, N. M. (2016). 'Men, women and birth control in the early *Outlander* books', in V. E. Frankel (ed.), *Outlander's Sassenachs: Essays on gender, race, orientation and the Other in the novels and television series*, McFarland, Jefferson, NC, pp. 82–96.

Frankel, V. E. (2015a). *Scots, Sassenachs, and spankings: Feminism and gender roles in Outlander*, LitCrit Press, Middletown, DE.

Frankel, V. E. (2015b). *The symbolism and sources of Outlander: The Scottish fairies, folklore, ballads, magic and meanings that inspired the series*, McFarland, Jefferson, NC.

Gabaldon, D. (1999). *The Outlandish companion*. Delacorte Press, New York.

Gaddis, J. L. (2002). *The landscape of history: How historians map the past*, Oxford University Press, Oxford, pp. 17–34.

Green, M. C. and Brock, T. C. (2000). 'The role of transportation in the persuasiveness of public narratives', *Journal of Personality and Social Psychology*, vol. 79, pp. 701–721.

Jain, P. and Slater, M. D. (2013). 'Provider portrayals and patient-provider communication in drama and reality medical entertainment television shows', *Journal of Health Communication*, vol. 18, pp. 703–722.

Jensen, K. (2012). *Oregon's doctor to the world: Esther Pohl Lovejoy and a life in activism*, University of Washington Press, Seattle, WA.

Johnson, C. E. (2005). *Meeting the ethical challenges of leadership: Casting light or shadow*, Sage, Thousand Oaks, CA.

Khullar, D. (2017). 'Being a doctor is hard. It's harder for women', *New York Times*, 7 December, www.nytimes.com/2017/12/07/upshot/being-a-doctor-is-hard-its-harder-for-women.html (accessed 1 July 2019).

Leavitt, J. W. (1986). *Brought to bed: Child-bearing in America*: 1750–1950, Oxford University Press, Oxford.

Leavitt, J. W. (ed.) (1999). *Women and health in America*, 2nd edn, University of Wisconsin Press, Madison, WI.

Luchetti, C. (1998). *Medicine women: The story of early-American women doctors*, Crown Publishers, New York, NY.

Marshall, R. K. (1982). *Virgins and viragos*, Academy Chicago Ltd, Chicago, IL.

Moldow, G. (1987). *Women doctors in gilded-age Washington*, University of Illinois Press, Urbana, IL.

More, E. (1999). *Restoring the balance: Women physicians and the profession of medicine, 1850–1995*, Harvard University Press, Cambridge, MA.

Moyer-Guse, É. (2008). 'Toward a theory of entertainment persuasion: Explaining the persuasive effects of entertainment-education messages', *Communication Theory*, vol. 18, pp. 407–425.

Peitzman, S. (2000). *A new and untried course: Woman's medical college and medical college of Pennsylvania*, 1850–1998, Rutgers University Press, New Brunswick, NJ.

Petersen, A. H. (2014). '*Outlander* is the feminist answer to *Game of Thrones* – and men should be watching it', *Buzzfeed*, 4 August, www.buzzfeed.com/annehelenpetersen/watch-outlander (accessed 23 September 2019).

Pringle, R. (1998). *Sex and medicine: Gender, power and authority in the medical professions*, Cambridge University Press, Cambridge, UK.

Roberts, M. J. D. (2009). 'The politics of professionalization: MPs, medical men, and the 1858 Medical Act', *Medical History*, vol. 53, no. 1, pp. 37–56.

Stegall, S. (2016). 'The Beaton: Healing as empowerment for Claire Beauchamp', in V. E. Frankel (ed.), *Outlander's Sassenachs: Essays on gender, race, orientation and the Other in the novels and television series*, McFarland, Jefferson, NC, pp. 97–104.

Théré, C. (1999). 'Women and birth control in eighteenth-century France', *Eighteenth-Century Studies*, vol. 32, no. 4, pp. 552–564.

Tuchman, A. (2000). *Science has no sex: The life of Marie Sakrzewska, MD*, University of North Carolina Press, Chapel Hill, NC.

Ty, E. (2016). 'Melodrama, gender and nostalgia: The appeal of *Outlander*', in V. E. Frankel (ed.), *Adoring Outlander: Essays on fandom, genre and the female audience*, McFarland, Jefferson, NC, pp. 58–68.

Tzu-Chun Wu. J. (2005). *Doctor mom Chung of the fair-haired bastards: The life of a wartime celebrity*, University of California Press, Berkeley, CA.

Ulrich, L. T. (1990). *A midwife's tale: The life of Martha Ballard, based on her diary, 1785–1812*, Vintage Books, New York.

Walsh, M. R. (1977). *'Doctor's wanted – no women need apply': Sexual barriers in the medical profession, 1835–1975*, Yale University Press, New Haven, CT.

Wertz, R. W. and Wertz, D. C. (1977). *Lying-in: A history of childbirth in America*, The Free Press, New York.

White, M. (2000). 'Indy & Dr. Mike: Is boy to global world history as woman is to domestic national myth?', *Film & History*, vol. 30, no. 1, pp. 24–37.

3

Avoiding 'the faddlings of Dr Choake': the professionalisation of medicine in *Poldark*

Barbara Sadler

The BBC television series *Poldark* (2015–2019) is an adaptation of Winston Graham's novels about a Cornish family which begins as the main character, Ross Poldark (Aidan Turner), returns from the American Revolutionary War. The Mammoth Screen production of *Poldark* was adapted for television by Debbie Horsfield and covers the period 1783 to 1802. Significantly, this particular time frame marks the period when the medical profession is beginning to establish itself and progress in medical science has begun to move beyond the 'classical framework' of the body. Up until the mid-nineteenth century, Galenic humoral doctrine prevailed, wherein disease and illness were thought to be caused by 'imbalances of the fluids, or humours, which the Ancients believed to be the constituents of the body: black bile, yellow bile, phlegm, and blood' (Shorter, 2006: 107). Medical historians agree that during this material time most people would treat themselves or obtain remedies from other family members, neighbours, or close friends. It was rare that patients would seek the assistance of a physician. This situation was not merely the result of the fees incurred, but also that the treatments available from the physician were not always efficacious and, in some cases, folk medicines were known to be more reliable. Sumich (2013: 4) points out that the excessive fees of some physicians led to a reputation of greed and in general that 'physicians as a group were plagued with issues of low social status'. What this brings to the foreground is the deep mistrust of physicians. In addition to such opinions, physicians would also need to compete for business with barber surgeons, herbalists, apothecaries, religious healers, and even blacksmiths, who were known to reset broken bones. It is clear Winston Graham had taken care to research the historical background for his characters and storylines and it is within this milieu of numerous lay healers and 'quacks' that the doctors of *Poldark* operate. Graham's focus on family life, the wars of the era, and the centrality of tin and copper mining in Cornwall all allow for some quite detailed and interesting medical storylines to be developed. Through such stories and across all five series, there is a demonstration of the increasing professionalisation of medicine.

This can be evidenced by analysing and charting the rise of Dr Dwight Enys (Luke Norris), whose skills many of the main characters come to rely upon at various points in the narrative. Importantly, Horsfield's adaptation conflates several medical storylines and physicians into the character of Dwight Enys, making her iteration of Enys carry additional meaning.

The doctors of *Poldark*

> *Ross:* Demelza, my friend Dr Dwight Enys.
> *Dwight:* Ma'am.
> *Demelza:* 'Twas you that mended his face? (S1E5)

As Ross Poldark introduces his friend Dr Enys to his wife (Eleanor Tomlinson), and to the viewing audience, it is the doctor's knowledge and surgical skill which act as the marker of his identity. Throughout the five series, the development of Enys's character and narrative offer the viewer a glimpse of the historical development of medicine from the 'free for all' of 'herbalists, midwife-healers, bonesetters and others' (Saks, 2003: 142) to the reliable, educated, and experienced doctors the general public would recognise in the twenty-first century. However, at the time Dr Enys arrives, there is already a doctor working in the area. The resulting competition between the two doctors marks the real circumstances which would have existed.

In *Poldark*'s Cornwall, Dr Choake (Robert Daws) is the embodiment of the upper-class gentleman as physician with little scientific medical knowledge and little concern for patients who could not pay. Even his name is something of a warning. At their very first meeting the dialogue between Choake and Enys sets up their relationship as one of opposites:

> *Choake:* If in doubt, purge. That's our motto. Bleed, boil, blister, sweat. Healing is a science. Few comprehend its mysteries
> *Dwight:* Or its fees ... I merely meant not everyone can afford expensive treatments. (S1E5)

This initial exchange continues with Ross explaining to Choake that Enys is studying lung diseases which prompts Choake to point out that miners rarely pay and that Enys will be 'living under a hedge and dining on thistles'.

As a character, Choake personifies the greedy physician with a somewhat tarnished reputation. He is laying claim to healing as science and aiming to elevate his position within the assembled company. Throughout the seasons, Choake uses a haughty manner and some medical language to maintain and encourage belief in his authority. At first, it appears he is defending his position or his right to make a living from his work, but closer scrutiny illustrates how physicians use such language in their practice and in doing so usher in the birth of medical discourse. In the Foucauldian sense, Choake's declaration of his knowledge (even if it is limited), and his authority because of such knowledge, has the result of bringing his subject position as a physician into being. At the same time, the discourse also produces a subject position for the patient or listener as subordinate to his knowledge/power. Foucault claims that discourses are 'practices that systematically form the objects of which they speak' (2011: 54). In this example, Choake's discourse produces the identity of both the doctor and the patient. Within the *Poldark* narrative, Choake is represented as an incompetent doctor, and yet he is still a professional in that he receives payment for his work. For Choake, he must convince people to trust him and pay for his services and in the programme, he achieves this by presenting himself in a superior way and utilising some medical terms. However, with the arrival of Dr Enys, Choake faces additional competition for work and the underlying narrative towards professionalisation takes some significant steps forward because Enys shows some of the traits contemporary patients would recognise and expect.

During the seasons, the two doctors are represented as physical opposites; Choake is rotund, florid, and wears a rather dandy-like wig, whereas Enys is slender, fresh-faced, and with a full head of thick, natural hair. Enys's extremely good looks only serve to heighten the difference between the two men. Indeed, in the British press he is referred to as Dr Dishy or Dr Dreamy (Shelley, 2018) in a clear reference to the *Grey's Anatomy* (ABC, 2005–) character Derek 'McDreamy' Shepherd. Nevertheless, it is in their chosen profession where the distinctions are most damning for Choake. This is made manifest in their differing approach to patients and the resulting interactions. Fissell explains that 'early modern medicine was dominated by the client' (2005: 92) insofar as the diagnosis was conducted largely from the patient's narrative of events and symptoms. In his interactions with patients, Choake follows this pattern and he is rarely depicted conducting a physical examination of his patients. However, as medical knowledge progressed, Foucault points to a shift in practice where the doctor ceases to ask what is wrong with the patient but rather 'where does it hurt?' (2003: xxi) and then proceeds with a physical examination. This change makes the patient's story almost redundant and shifts power to the hands of the physician. In *Poldark*, this is made manifest in the outbreak of 'putrid throat' (S1E8). Choake is called to Trenwith to attend Francis (Kyle Soller) and Elizabeth Poldark (Heida Reed) and their household. As Choake is leaving, Ross Poldark asks if the family have the dreaded 'putrid throat'. Choake responds incredulously, 'Morbus strangulatorius? What fool gave you that idea?' and states his remedies are applied and 'they are all on the mend'. They are not, but the family survive due to Demelza's attendance and sustained care with the use of herbal treatments. This example serves to illustrate again how Choake uses medical language to display his superiority and even though his confidence is misplaced, his use of medical terminology has the effect of establishing a relationship of power where it is the doctor who can define whether or not an individual is well or ill. In this circumstance, it is the beginnings of professionalisation. In the same episode, Demelza and Julia become ill and Ross fetches Dr Enys to tend them. Dr Enys immediately conducts a physical examination to confirm the diagnosis, and whereas he cannot save Julia, he remains present at Nampara so that the viewer is left with no doubt that he is the embodiment of the 'good' doctor.

Throughout the seasons, Dr Enys has an interesting character arc. When he first appears, he presents as kind and self-effacing; even in his first meeting with Choake (detailed above) he seems almost at pains to ensure his remarks do not cause offence. However, his attraction to and relationship with Keren Daniel (Sabrina Bartlett) in season one have the effect of casting some doubt upon his character. In this way, he reflects the concern patients held that physicians were 'intrinsically immoral, perhaps even atheistic' (Sumich, 2013: 20). He can be interpreted as immoral in his sexual relationship with another person's spouse and even as atheistic in his search for medical knowledge to cure illnesses, when during that historical period some believed illness was a form of punishment from a god for wrongdoing or weakness of character. By interfering with the will of God, physicians were often believed to be anti-religious. Their powers to potentially cure gave physicians a god-like quality which was akin to blasphemy for some. Notably, when Reverend Whitworth is attempting to have his wife committed to an asylum for being mad (S4E4), he points out that the Church's view is that madness is a judgement upon the wicked. Enys refutes this common belief of the time and mentions King George's afflictions and reminds Whitworth it would be treasonous to say the King's madness was a result of evil ways. Throughout the seasons of *Poldark*, Enys is constantly seeking medical knowledge and means to cure, but what can be interpreted as against God within the historical setting is simultaneously evidence of the professionalisation of medicine. After Keren's murder by her cuckold husband, Ross implores Enys to leave the area. When Enys refuses, he admits he has wronged Mark Daniel (Matthew Wilson) but he explains how he cannot leave because the people in the area have been very kind to him and he feels wretched that he has acted inappropriately. His willingness to face the consequences, and his subsequent absolute devotion to his medical work and local people, allow for his character to be restored to the former position of eminence.

In contrast, the position of Dr Choake diminishes as Enys's medical competence is established. Choake is the physician for the wealthier inhabitants of Cornwall and yet this situation appears to exist on the basis that Choake is a gentleman rather than that he has any medical skill. Indeed, Uncle Charles Poldark (Warren Clarke) claims 'Choake is a fool' (S1E4) when Choake suggests to Francis that Charles will recover from his stroke. However, Enys and Choake observe an agreement to not encroach upon each other's clients. This is evidenced when Enys refuses to visit Trenwith as Choake will dislike the interference with his patients. Within the lower social groups, Enys's good reputation for healing surges on as he cures an outbreak of scurvy and fixes Rosina Hoblyn's (Amelia Clarkson) lameness. Even Ross's wife, Demelza, foregoes all help from Choake at the birth of Clowance Poldark. At this point in the plot, Enys is in prison in Quimper and rather than send for Choake, Demelza chooses to give birth without medical assistance at all. This is particularly significant because Ross and Demelza have sufficient funds to employ Choake and this would be the appropriate route for Demelza with her social position being that of a lady. She exclaims, ''Tis more than wise to avoid the faddlings of Dr Choake' (S3E4) as she goes into labour with only her servant Prudie to assist at the birth. Demelza's lack of faith in Choake's skills indicates more trust in shared female wisdom than to agree to the 'faddlings' of an inept doctor. The move to employ male doctors as man-midwife was rooted in distinctions of social class, according to Wilson (1995). Before the mid-eighteenth century, upper-class women would be attended by lower-class women who had experience of birthing. Effectively the lower-class women acted as midwives to aristocratic women, but in doing so blurred the social divide. Wilson points out the birth experience had a 'levelling quality ... a tangible reminder that ladies were mere women. But the man-midwife offered proof of their superior social status' (1995: 191). Indeed, as Demelza goes into labour she states 'Ross wouldn't hear of me birthing alone but what he don't know can't hurt him' (S3E4). In this circumstance, it is the ability to pay for treatment that restores the social status distinction. Moreover, it is the patriarchal order of the time that put Demelza, her body, and her labour into her husband's keeping. She considers Ross's perspective temporarily, but then dismisses it as it would lead to her having to be tended by Choake for the sake of male pride and social status. Thus, this seemingly small scene highlights some important points in the struggle for the professionalisation of medicine and the role of social class and gender in its development.

The triumphs and limits of medicine

From the instant that Dr Enys is introduced to the audience, he is identified as a doctor seeking further knowledge. He is making a 'study of mine diseases' and receives wages from Ross of £40 for attending to workers at his mines. Enys is established as a scholar and professional using shots where he is seen dissecting and inspecting diseased lungs (S1E6), but these shots are fleeting and easily missed. In series two there is no such escape from Enys's thirst for greater knowledge of anatomy. Enys is called by Rosina and Charlie Kempthorne (Ross Green) as there is a dead body washed up on one of the Poldark beaches (S2E6). Enys advises Charlie to take Rosina home and he will bury the body. Instead, he waits for the couple to leave then produces a saw to remove the dead man's leg from above his knee. The good doctor then dissects parts of the leg – in particular, the knee. In series four, after the duel with Monk Adderley (Max Bennett) (S4E7), Ross has been shot and Enys is seen to expertly remove a piece of Poldark's bone in a bloody and graphic scene. Such depictions are at odds with the common misconception of period drama as soothing depictions of the past or 'warm bath tv' (Hunt, 2007). Byrne claims period drama has undergone an evolution of sorts and it is more accepted that programmes such as *Peaky Blinders* (2013–) and *Banished* (2015) offer more realistic scenes which are 'grittier and more corporeal than we are accustomed to seeing on our screens' (2018: 154). *Poldark* is part of this trend, especially when it focuses upon the medical expertise of Dr Enys. In both examples, the bloody scenes are not gratuitous, but serve to highlight Enys's growing surgical skill and knowledge of the body. The removal of the dead sailor's leg on the beach has more than a touch of Burke and Hare, but as a direct result of this questionable theft, the 'good' doctor Enys is able to cure Rosina's lameness. This intervention alone does much to develop Dr Enys's reputation for medical expertise in Cornwall and in a later scene between Ross and Caroline, the stories of Dwight's miracle cure are mentioned as being much talked of in the village.

Enys's medical triumphs earn him good favour with the lower classes swiftly. They are his main patients in the earlier seasons of the show. However, by series three there is a marked increase in higher classes employing Dr Enys's service. It is arguable whether this change is a direct effect of his success in his medical practice or whether it is due to his attachment and subsequent marriage to heiress Caroline Penvenen (Gabriella Wilde). Initially, Caroline mocks his skills by having Enys attend her pet dog, Horace. Enys acquits himself sufficiently to be called upon to assist Caroline herself when a fishbone is lodged in her throat. Thereafter, their courtship develops as does his employ by the wealthier patients in *Poldark*, including the Warleggans. Valentine Warleggan is diagnosed with rickets by Dr Choake (S3E5), but his treatment is to keep Valentine in darkened rooms, with his legs in splints, and take prescribed tinctures which make him vomit. Elizabeth expresses concern about the treatments and motivated by ensuring his son's full recovery, George Warleggan (Jack Farthing) sends for Dr Enys. On his arrival, old Aunt Agatha Poldark (Caroline Blakiston) points out that her advice would be to 'get rid of the splints and get him out in the fresh air'. George dislikes Agatha and comments that Dr Enys 'does not subscribe to old wives' tales'. What is important here is that George is acknowledging Enys's role as a specialist physician and his reputation as recognisably more skilful than Choake's. In the event, Enys agrees with Agatha and prescribes sunlight and fresh fruit and vegetables, which has the effect of attesting to the continued significance of lay healers, especially women. When Elizabeth expresses surprise at the lack of medicine, Enys points out 'Dr Choake's prescriptions often serve his purse not his patients'. In this example, Enys's medical knowledge, good manners, and professional conduct mark him as a type of physician not dissimilar to the twenty-first-century version of a professional medical doctor.

Notably, Dr Enys's encounters with high-status patients increase hereafter. Reverend Osbourne 'Ossie' Whitworth (Christian Brassington) employs him to attend his wife at the birth of their child. After a difficult labour Morwenna (Ellise Chappell) gives birth to John Conan Whitworth. Dr Enys delivers the child and saves the mother (S3E8). However, Enys must intervene later in the episode to prevent Ossie from continuing his marital relations with Morwenna immediately after the birth of their son. At this point in the story, Enys has not long been free from prison in Quimper where he was held as a prisoner of war. Enys's experience in the prison and subsequent release leave an indelible mark on his mental health but also provide the young physician with empirical knowledge of mental health symptoms and treatment. Consequently, Enys describes Morwenna as 'delicate' and continues to insist that Ossie refrain from sexual activity. However, Reverend Whitworth is determined and approaches Dr Enys to assist him in his endeavours to incarcerate Morwenna in an asylum (S4E4) because she still refuses his advances. Enys acknowledges the position, but aims to reason with Ossie: 'As Mrs Whitworth's husband you are of course entitled to put her away, but why would you wish to? She performs her household duties admirably' (S4E4). Ossie insists he requires a physician to sanction Morwenna's incarceration in order that he does not have his religious status damaged. Enys leaves the encounter stating clearly that he hopes Ossie will not be able to find a physician to assist with such an act. In responding in this way, Enys accepts the position that husbands 'have a right' to put their wives in a mental institution. What is expressed here is the common law of coverture, which subsumed a woman's rights to her husband upon marriage. In effect, 'married women had no legal independence from their husbands' (Hodgson-Wright, 2001: 3), nor was marital rape written into UK Statute Law until the 1994 Criminal Justice and Public Order Act. Ossie goes so far as to use the law and religion in his efforts to have Morwenna submit to him: 'We are about God's holy work' (S4E5). Whilst Enys acknowledges the legal position, he refuses to assist and aims to reason with Ossie that in other aspects Morwenna is a good wife.

Later in the same episode, it appears that Ossie may have indeed found a less ethical doctor to assist his aims when Enys is called to Ossie's house and he is confronted by the presence of Dr Choake. Until this point, Choake and Enys have always operated as opposites. However, something unexpected occurs and Choake, breathing anxiously, entreats Dr Enys to provide a second opinion. When Enys requests to examine Morwenna, Ossie objects, but Choake defies the audience's expectations and encourages Enys with a sigh, 'pray do'. Enys duly returns to Choake and Ossie confirming he can find no indication of Morwenna 'losing her reason'. There ensues a discussion between Choake and Enys about the lack of sexual relations in the Whitworth's marriage:

> *Enys:* Choake, I don't deny it's a problem, but is it one we can take any professional steps to resolve? We were asked to confirm a diagnosis that Mrs Whitworth is insane and must be put away, well my answer is no as yours must also be. (S4E4)

This encounter between the doctors marks a change in the dynamic of their relationship, with Enys occupying a clear position of power and authority and Choake accepting Enys's diagnosis and advanced knowledge. Enys's rise is predicated upon his ever-increasing scientific medical knowledge, his commitment to his patient's wellbeing, and his plain-speaking, reasoned explanations for his diagnosis. It is Enys's 'clinical gaze' (Foucault, 2003: 148), the fact that he insists upon examination, which marks him as recognisably professional in the encounter. He refuses to accept Ossie's or Choake's account of what is wrong with Morwenna. He even articulates his professional status by asking if there are any 'professional steps' they could take to resolve the matter. The grudging respect Choake gives Enys is a significant triumph. Enys's success in this scene, and throughout the series, is achieved by consistent demonstration of skills and qualities that a twenty-first-century audience would expect of a twenty-first-century doctor.

Having examined many of the professional triumphs of Dr Enys, it is also necessary to point out the limitations of medical science in the eighteenth century which led to some notable disappointing medical outcomes. In season one, for all his skills and best efforts, Enys cannot save Julia Poldark from the 'putrid throat' or Jim Carter from 'jail fever'. One of the most affecting storylines is his failure to save the life of his own daughter, Sarah. Enys's keen 'medical gaze' exposes a congenital heart defect in his baby (S4E4) but he is aware there is no effective treatment and must accept that she will succumb to the first infection she contracts. The drama in the same episode is heightened, when after a flood at the mine, Enys refuses to stop his vigorous efforts at resuscitation of a miner who appears dead. Enys is aware there is medical hope for the miner and continues with mouth to mouth breathing. The medical detail here is significant because the miner was almost drowned, and this enables the writers to use historically accurate resuscitation techniques which were established in the 1740s (National CPR Foundation, 2017). His professional actions at this point are fuelled and motivated by his despair at not being able to cure or save his own child. A similar conclusion occurs for Lieutenant Hugh Armitage. Armitage was Enys's protégé in Quimper prison. Enys refused to leave his post in the prison hospital which prompted Armitage to offer 'to learn some of your skills if only to give you one hour's rest in twenty' (S3E4). Dwight proceeds to show Armitage certain medical treatments. This has the effect of further developing Enys's claim to professional status in that he is teaching a 'student' his medical knowledge. After the pair are rescued from France by Ross, Armitage becomes ill with a 'brain fever'. Unable to cure him and suspecting Armitage is weakened because he is lovesick for Demelza, Enys can only help alleviate his patient's symptoms by encouraging Demelza to visit him. At this point, it is worthy of note that some twenty-first-century medical doctors have stated their admiration for the series. Roger Jones, editor of the *British Journal of General Practice* comments that 'Dr Dwight Enys and the dreadful Dr Choake represent the opposite poles of diagnosis and treatment' (2018: 451), whilst David Garner, a consultant microbiologist, appears to have great fun working out exactly what infections caused the deaths of the characters in *Poldark*. He states, 'Lt Armitage died from granulomatous amoebic meningoencephalitis' (2018). This appears to indicate the medical storylines are a point of identification for professional medical practitioners which lends further support to the point that *Poldark* has an underlying story to tell of the professionalisation of medicine. It is doubtful that any twenty-first-century doctor would agree that Armitage died as a result of 'lovesickness', although the connection between mental health issues and physical illness has long been noted (Naylor et al., 2012: 5). Enys identifies Hugh's mental health issue as an impediment to his physical wellbeing, but does not have the knowledge or medical language at that point to treat the physical condition.

In the case of Armitage, Dwight does not have sufficient scientific knowledge to provide a cure, but in the case of Elizabeth Warleggan, her death may have been avoidable medically. Despite Elizabeth maintaining that Valentine's birth was premature, George suspects Valentine is not his biological child but that of Ross Poldark. To secure Valentine's inheritance and happiness, Elizabeth seeks to induce an early birth of George's actual child to prove to him that she usually delivers prematurely. This plan is first intimated by Ross when he and Elizabeth meet at Sawle church (S3E8). Years later Elizabeth enacts the plan and seeks help from Dr Anselm (Richard Durden) who operates a practice for society ladies which clearly includes abortions. Anselm is represented as having some knowledge and he conducts his encounter with Elizabeth very professionally, taking notes and providing detailed guidelines for safe use of the medicine and with strict instructions that if there are complications, she should explain the full circumstances to her physician without delay. However, his secretive practice and subject specialism implies that he is a 'bad' doctor, in contrast to Enys.

After a quarrel with George, Elizabeth takes medicine that produces the desired effect and goes into premature labour. Dr Enys attends the birth and a healthy girl is delivered. George and Elizabeth reconcile, but Elizabeth begins to experience violent post-delivery spasms. Dr Choake attends but cannot help, so George summons Enys. Arriving back at Trenwith, Enys speaks to Elizabeth: 'This is a sad change, Mrs Warleggan. I wonder what could be the cause?' (S4E8). Elizabeth does not respond and when she fails to follow Anselm's advice and does not take Enys into her confidence her fate is sealed, and she dies. What is significant is that Anselm suggests that even if complications occur, a recovery is possible. It is not the limit of medical knowledge which leads to death, but Elizabeth's silence. Enys clearly suspects her actions and when he finds the incriminating medicine bottle immediately before her death, he understands what has occurred. Being the benevolent doctor, he removes the evidence, thus preserving her secret and her reputation.

Quimper and mental health specialism

Throughout the five series of *Poldark*, the doctors are referred to as physicians. During the time the story is set, there were only three recognised types of medical professionals within the law: physicians, surgeons, and apothecaries. The physician occupied the highest esteem and rank, as it was the physician who administered the medicine produced by the apothecary and who oversaw the operations of the surgeon (Waddington, 1977: 165). At the beginning of the nineteenth century, there was a change in the professional structure of the medical professions to distinguish solely between general practitioners and consultants. To be considered a consultant there had to be a defined area of medical expertise. The character development of Dr Enys begins to highlight this forthcoming alteration to medical hierarchy as he begins to achieve eminence for his knowledge and treatment of mental health disorders. This interest, knowledge, and skill develops from

Enys's own experience whilst being held as a prisoner of war in Quimper. The prison has an infirmary section where queues of prisoners line up for whatever basic treatments Enys and the other three physicians can provide. These queues of patients and the addition of Hugh Armitage as Enys's 'pupil' in medical matters mark the prison infirmary as a figurative 'clinic'. The 'clinic' in Foucauldian discourse is the teaching hospital. Within this learning space, Enys performs surgery using the most primitive tools made from any material he can find. In one scene he is shown removing a bullet from a patient with tweezers that appear to be constructed from sticks (S3E4). Throughout the horror of his imprisonment, Enys never leaves his post and rarely sleeps. When Williams is shot by the French guards, Enys stares in disbelief and rolls over on the floor in tears of desperation. This point illustrates the degeneration of Enys's own mental health and at the point that Ross appears in the infirmary to rescue him, Enys laughs and believes he is imagining things in his delirium (S3E5). The escape continues at the cost of Captain Henshawe. Enys tends to him on the roadside as they are fleeing the French soldiers. Enys confirms he is dead, and the company continue to their boat and away to the safety of Trecrom's smuggling ship, *The One and All*. Aboard the ship, Enys saves Drake Carne and confesses to Ross that Henshawe was not dead when they left him. Enys justifies his actions, stating, 'unless I lied you would willingly die alongside him and that I could not permit' (S3E5). Enys articulates that he knows he must keep himself busy to prevent the necessity of facing impossible questions of why he was saved and others were not. At this point, Enys knows he is suffering from mental illness.

Enys's return to Caroline and Killiwarren brings the doctor's mental state into sharp focus. Dwight is plagued by flashbacks of his prison experience and when Caroline inadvertently sneaks up behind him, he shrieks and runs and collapses on the floor hunched and clutching his knees.

> *Caroline:* Don't be so girlish … shall I be forced to prescribe hartshorn?
> *Enys:* Opium is more effective.
> *Caroline:* For what?
> *Enys:* Inducing oblivion. (S3E6)

It is evident that Enys is suffering from the trauma of his prison stay and in the grip of what contemporary doctors refer to as post-traumatic stress disorder. Ross recognises the symptoms of distress many men suffer after experiencing the horrors of war and he sends for Armitage to visit Enys. The two spend time discussing their recollections and as Armitage leaves Killiwarren, Enys acknowledges that Armitage has found a cure for his torment. Hugh dismisses this accolade, but notes it is 'not a cure, but the direction by which we may find a cure' (S3E6). At Ross's behest Enys then begins to discuss his trauma with his wife and in doing so begins to cure himself through talk. Jones suggests this 'talk therapy' is '19th-century CBT' (2019: 448). Cognitive behavioural therapy, a contemporary form of talk therapy, addresses problematic behaviour patterns and bears some similar features to the therapeutic conversations adopted by Pinel as 'moral treatment' in mental asylums in Paris in the later eighteenth century (Bynum, 1981). Pinel maintained that talking to the patient enabled the doctor to get to know the person and thus enabled an accurate diagnosis and effective treatment. Enys adopts this talking approach several times with mentally distressed patients.

This personal struggle with mental health matters begins Enys's focus upon this area of medicine as his subject specialism. This has a significant impact when Enys is called to attend the Whitworths' home when Ossie is attempting to have Morwenna committed. Enys's specialist experience provides him with confidence and Choake ultimately defers to him. In this case and in the case of Henshawe's death, Enys holds power over life and death and the ability to declare who is ill and who is not. It is his superior knowledge and skill and his command of medical discourse which separates him from the more 'general practitioners' in the later episodes. Dr Enys acts as a metonymic sign for the rise of the consultant and the reorganisation of the medical professions which occurred in the mid-nineteenth century.

Enys's subject specialism is certainly put to effective use in season five. After Elizabeth's death, her husband George Warleggan descends into a grief that results in him having hallucinations of his dead wife. In an interview for the *British Journal of Medical Practice*, actor Jack Farthing who plays George Warleggan discussed the research he conducted for these episodes, confirming that hallucinations present for up to 80 per cent of older people after the death of their spouse (2019). In the programme, George exhibits symptoms of similar complicated bereavement and he begins to see images of Elizabeth and subsequently begins to engage in conversation with the apparitions. Rather than allow George's grief to damage business relations and opportunities, uncle Cary Warleggan (Pip Torrens) employs Dr Penrose (Simon Thorp). As Jones states, 'The dreadful Dr Penrose, engaged by uncle Cary, considered George to be possessed by animal spirits and subjected him to bleeding, blistering, cupping, sedation, restraint and iced baths' (2019: 448). With the absence of Choake in this series, Penrose occupies the role of 'dreadful doctor' to Enys's 'good doctor'. The brutal treatments inflicted upon George follow the pattern of being identifiable as accurate of the period. In many examples, this is due to the research endeavour of the *Poldark* novelist, Winston Graham. However, season five was written by Debbie Horsfield to bridge the gap left by Graham between the setting of *The Angry Tide* (1977) which is set in 1798–1799 and *The Stranger from the Sea* (1981) which is set in 1810–1811. Horsfield uses hints provided by Graham from the later novels to produce new storylines which account for developments that are apparent in the later books. In addition, the production company, Mammoth, employed a historical consultant, Dr Hannah Grieg, to manage the historical depictions of the setting. The knowledge of such accuracy makes some of the scenes extremely uncomfortable viewing, particularly those of George being provided with vomit-inducing medicine, of bloody cuts from leeches burrowing into his skin, and of him being waterboarded. Many of these treatments were used upon King George III and depicted in Nicholas Hytner's film *The Madness of King George* (1994).

In the Mammoth *Poldark* story, George Warleggan is depicted strapped to his bed in his nightgown after further injurious 'treatments'. However, George manages to escape his restraints and flees across the Cornish fields to Nampara where he peers through the window to see Valentine happily included with Ross's legitimate children in a vision of domestic contentment. This image is clearly too much for George to bear and he wanders to the cliff edge in readiness to end his torment and join Elizabeth. Enys spots George through the window and follows him to the cliff, managing to grab hold of George before he leaps to his death (S5E3). Enys calmly holds George and asks to accompany him back to Trenwith (see Figure 3.1). Once back in Trenwith, Enys questions Penrose and uncle Cary about George's bodily injuries. In the exchanges between the men, Penrose sneers to Enys, 'Call yourself an expert on mental conditions? Sir George is clearly in the grip of animal spirits' (S5E3). In spite of the disparaging tone, the effect

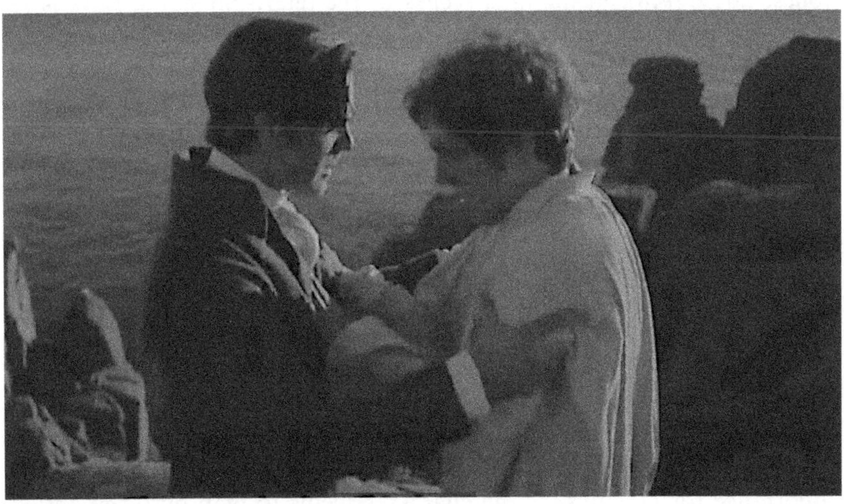

Figure 3.1 'May I accompany you back to Trenwith?' (*Poldark*)

of Penrose's question is to bring Enys's reputation as an expert on mental health matters into being. Enys responds by branding Penrose as 'the only lunatic' and suggests that George requires kindness and patience.

In the scene with George, Enys has full authority as a direct result of his knowledge, and this is recognised by both Penrose, albeit grudgingly, and Cary. His elevation to subject specialist is complete and at this point he embodies all of the characteristics expected of a professional, twenty-first-century doctor: well educated, extensive clinical experience, constantly seeking new knowledge, sound character, good bedside manner, clear subject specialism, and regarded highly enough to teach others. However, Enys is very much at the vanguard of professionalisation. Physicians such as Penrose, Choake, and Dr Behenna were still in circulation with their lack of knowledge, strange beliefs, and willingness to seek profit over patient's welfare. In season five, Enys is duly employed to treat George, who recovers swiftly and reverts to his former habits of business and profit at all costs. The treatment given to George reflects the turning point already heralded by Pinel in France of 'moral therapy' that instead of treating patients with mental health disorders as mad beasts, there was 'a recognition that kindness, reason, and tactful manipulation were more effective ... than were fear, brutal coercion and restraint and medical therapy' (Bynum, 1981: 37).

In later episodes, Enys delivers a paper on mental health to the Royal College of Surgeons. This, in turn, leads to him being called as an expert witness at court. All of these factors would be recognisable as part of the work of a contemporary, professional doctor. However, the impact of the success for Enys 'gave this quiet country doctor a national reputation' (Jones, 2019: 448). In the final scenes of the television series, Enys is set to accompany Ross Poldark to France, where Ross will become a spy and Enys explains he will complete further study 'with the famed Dr Pinel at his mental asylum in Salpetriere in Paris' (S5E8). In subsequent *Poldark* novels not covered by the series, Enys is employed to treat the mental health issues of King George III – a role which must be perceived as sanction of his outstanding medical status.

Conclusion

It is evident that Winston Graham's detailed research provides a foundation for the stories and characters of *Poldark*. The series' historical advisor, Dr Hannah Grieg, confirms that 'the historical context behind the drama is carefully construed in the original novels' (2016). This research has importance for Dr Enys, as the character seems to map onto the known historical developments of the medical profession at the time of the setting.

By following Dr Enys's narrative over the five series, he is represented as a symbol of the move towards professionalisation. Building on Graham's novels, scriptwriter Debbie Horsfield has developed the character in the Mammoth adaptation to depict Enys's own mental trauma as a result of his experience in Quimper prison and this is understood as motivation and empirical knowledge for his subsequent treatment of George Warleggan. Neither aspect is represented in the earlier 1975–1977 BBC TV adaptation of *Poldark* which suggests that the foregrounding of Enys's mental health and trauma is expressing something relevant for contemporary culture in 2015–2019. This cuts to the heart of the necessity of adaptations to refresh the narrative for a new audience and articulate concerns of the era. Mental health trauma and the need for quality health care are currently in public debate.

Viewed in the context of the struggling NHS in Britain, maybe the attraction of the idealised, professional doctor is assuaging some anxieties. The recent damaging scandals of doctors who are serial killers (Harold Shipman) or 'wound with intent' (Ian Paterson) or overprescribe opiates causing death (Jane Barton) are described by Mannion et al. as 'an enduring problem' (2019). Larger-scale misconduct or poor professional practice within an institution, such as the Staffordshire Hospital scandal, Alder Hey organs scandal, and the Liverpool Care Pathway scandal (Stanford, 2012), all have impact upon public trust in the medical profession. The effect is to align contemporary doctors with the misogynistic monstrous doctors which are so often the subject of television period dramas (see Taddeo and Wright in this volume). Dr Enys and Dr Turner from *Call the Midwife* (see Byrne in this volume) stand apart as positive representations which counter the bleak fictional and life-world narratives. Both are kindly and pioneering, both have suffered personally with mental health issues and both take time to listen to their patients.

Luke Norris's performance of Dr Enys is distinctive from other television doctors, and other versions of Enys in the source novels and the earlier BBC adaptation of *Poldark*. The reigning Enys has prevailed in dire circumstances and subsequently flourished to defend and support the disadvantaged and vulnerable. He is a 'good' doctor and a good guy who succeeds. In a brief article in *The Big Issue* (2019) Luke Norris writes about why he considers that *Poldark* became so successful and suggests it is the show's 'gospel of tolerance'. This is an apt description of the actions of Enys championing the poor and vulnerable, challenging the misguided, and continually seeking knowledge and new perspectives himself. Thus, Enys stands apart not just because he is a metonymic sign for the professionalisation of medicine, but because he is the personification of the ideals of the National Health Service. Viewed now within the most recent context of the global pandemic and the sacrifices made by real medical professionals, Enys's character may set a precedent for future depictions of period drama doctors.

References

Bynum, W. F. (1981). 'Rationales for therapy in British psychiatry, 1780–1835' in Scull, A. (ed.) (1981), *Madhouses, Mad-doctors and Madman: The Social History of Psychiatry in the Victorian Era*. Pennsylvania: University of Pennsylvania Press.

Byrne, K. (2018). 'Pathological masculinities: Syphilis and the medical profession in *The Frankenstein Chronicles*' in Byrne, K., Leggott, J., and Taddeo, J. (eds) (2018), *Conflicting Masculinities: Men in Television Period Drama*. London: IB Taurus.

Fissell, M. (2005). 'The disappearance of the patient's narrative and the invention of hospital medicine' in French, R. and Wear, A. (eds) (2005), *British Medicine in an Age of Reform*. London: Routledge.

Foucault, M. (2003). *The Birth of the Clinic*. London: Routledge.

Foucault, M. (2011[1972]). *The Archaeology of Knowledge*. London: Routledge.

Garner, D. (2018). 'Poldark's 'brain fever' – Part 2', *Microbiology Nuts and Bolts*. Available at: www.microbiologynutsandbolts.co.uk/the-bug-blog/poldarks-brain-fever-part-2 (accessed 29 September 2019).

Greig, H. (2016). 'Poldark adviser: How I stripped down history for the screen', *The Conversation*, 5 September 2016. Available at: https://theconversation.com/poldark-adviser-how-i-stripped-down-history-for-the-screen-64700 (accessed 2 September 2019).

Hodgson-Wright, S. (2001). 'Early feminism' in Gamble, S. (ed.) (2001), *The Routledge Companion to Feminism and Postfeminism*. London: Routledge.

Horsfield, D. (nd). 'Greedy banker's, women's rights … The politics in Poldark are as relevant as ever', *Radio Times*. Available at: www.radiotimes.com/news/tv/2018-11-06/greedy-bankers-womens-rights-the-politics-in-poldark-are-as-relevant-as-ever/ (accessed 1 September 2019).

Hunt, T. (2007). 'The Time Bandits', *The Guardian*. Available at: www.theguardian.com/media/2007/sep/10/mondaymediasection.television1 (accessed 20 September 2019).

Jones, R. (2018). 'Medication, medication', *British Journal of General Practice*, October 2018, pp. 449–504.

Jones, R. (2019). 'Life and times; Grief, hallucinations, and *Poldark*: An interview with Jack Farthing', *British Journal of General Practice*, September 2019, p. 448.

Mannion, R., Davies, H., Powell, M., Blenkinsopp, J., Miller, R., McHale, J., and Snowden, N. (2019). 'Healthcare scandals and the failings of doctors: Do official inquiries hold the profession to account?' *The Journal of Health Organisation and Management*, Vol. 33, No. 2, pp. 221–240.

National CPR Foundation (2017). 'What is CPR?' Available at: www.nationalcprfoundation.com/what-is-cpr-cardiopulmonary-resuscitation/ (accessed 11 March 2020).

Naylor, C., Parsonage, M., McDaid, D., Knapp, M, Fossey, M. and Galea, A. (2012). 'Long-term conditions and mental health: The cost of co-morbidities', The Kings Fund. Available at: www.kingsfund.org.uk/sites/default/files/field/field_publication_file/long-term-conditions-mental-health-cost-comorbidities-naylor-feb12.pdf (accessed 10 March 2020).

Norris, L. (2019). 'Poldark actor Luke Norris on the show's "gospel of tolerance"', *The Big Issue*, 26 August 2019. Available at: www.bigissue.com/latest/poldark-actor-luke-norris-on-the-shows-gospel-of-tolerance/ (accessed 17 May 2020).

Saks, M. (2003). 'Bringing together the orthodox and alternative in health care', *Complementary Therapies in Medicine*, vol. 11, pp. 142–145.

Shelley, J. (2018). 'Caroline Enys dumps the dishy, decent doctor and to the second location with Ross. Love Island had nothing on Poldark', *Daily Mail*, 1 July 2018. Available at: www.dailymail.co.uk/tvshowbiz/article-5907095/Caroline-Enys-dumps-dishy-decent-Doctor-n-Poldark-Jim-Shelley.html (accessed 8 August 2019).

Shorter, E. (2006). 'Primary care' in Porter, R. (ed.) (2006), *The Cambridge History of Medicine*. Cambridge: Cambridge University Press.

Stanford, P. (2012). 'Families left grieving and angry by the Liverpool Care Pathway', *The Telegraph*, 29 October 2012. Available at: www.telegraph.co.uk/news/health/9635842/Families-left-grieving-and-angry-by-the-Liverpool-Care-Pathway.html (accessed 10 March 2020).

Sumich, C. (2013). *Divine Doctors and Dreadful Distempers: How Practicing Medicine Became a Respectable Profession*. New York: Rodopi.

Taddeo, J. (2018). '"The war is done. Shut the door on it!": The Great War, masculinity and trauma in British period television' in Byrne, K., Leggott, J. and Taddeo, J. (2018), *Conflicting Masculinities: Men in Television Period Drama*. London: IB Taurus.

Waddington, I. (1977). 'General practitioners and consultants in early nineteenth century England: The sociology of an intra-professional conflict' in Woodward, J. and Richards, D. (eds) (1977), *Health Care and Popular Medicine in Nineteenth Century England*. London: Croom Helm.

Wilson, A. (1995). *The Making of Man-Midwifery: Childbirth in England, 1660–1770*. London: University College London Press.

4

'Infection was Mary's reward': *Harlots* and televising the realities of eighteenth-century English prostitution

Kristin Brig and Emily J. Clark

Introduction

As a period drama, the Hulu show *Harlots* (2017–), about the culture and society of eighteenth-century English prostitution, never set out to portray the history of medicine in Georgian London.[1] It has no physicians, apothecaries, or surgeons. There are no prescriptions, medical texts, or hospitals. Nonetheless, medicine and the body are embedded and constantly analysed within the framework of prostitution, which is, as an act, obsessed with the body. Medicine naturally fits into the plot, exposing how prostitutes and their clients thought about bodily health for professional and personal reasons.

The second episode of the first season functions as a way to think through how period drama intertwines medicine and the body with everyday historical life for twenty-first-century viewers. Through a close reading of this episode, in which characters exploit a woman's illness in a power struggle, we argue that *Harlots* decentres early modern medicine by portraying how syphilis and its potential outcome in death formed a regular part of life for Londoners. Fusing disease and medicine into a period drama without breaking the show's rhythm, this perspective educates the audience about eighteenth-century prostitution and sexually transmitted infections, in a moment when syphilis rates are the highest they have been since World War II.[2] Studies of venereal disease in early modern Europe tend to emphasise the perspective of professional healers or moralist commentators, rather than the sufferers themselves (Arrizabalaga, Henderson, and French, 1997; Bynum, 1987). In contrast, *Harlots* reminds us of the everyday realities of women acting as lay healers and medical experts for themselves and those close to them.

Through its premise, *Harlots* becomes an effective vehicle to transmit the history of eighteenth-century prostitution to popular audiences. It is part of a recent trend in televised period pieces to expose the power dynamics of historical narratives. Scholarship on period pieces, including essays in this volume, has pointed out how series such as *Outlander* (2014–), *Land Girls* (2009–2011), and *Call the Midwife* (2012–) use their settings and plots to challenge traditional and nationalistic narratives (Byrne, Taddeo, and Leggott, 2018; White, 2019). Audiences are receptive to new period pieces because of these often unexpected counter-narratives. In her analysis of ITV's *Foyle's War* (2002–2015) – a murder mystery series centred on a civilian policeman in Hastings, England during World War II – historian Siân Nicholas argued that the show was more relatable, and thus garnered a number of twenty-first-century viewers, because it appealed to the struggles of people on the British home front (Nicholas, 2007). Instead of centring the story on the military and battles, it focuses on everyday people, inverting the traditional World War II narrative. Similarly, *Harlots* removes traditional narratives about Georgian England, particularly the government elite, to instead focus on everyday people, giving the audience a realistic rather than spectacular view of the period.

At the same time, such narratives compel viewers to think critically about traditional historical threads: not all medical experiences happen at the hands of doctors in hospitals and clinics, just as not all work during World War II was performed by the military. *Harlots* uses a similar tactic, writing well-structured plots and characters in unconventional spaces to draw viewers in and urge them to reconsider their preconceived notions about history. Prostitutes and other marginalised persons such as Black Londoners – including enslaved and freed people – and queer people are portrayed in a complex and engaging fashion, granting them more agency as central figures than as sidekicks or liminal characters. In turn, elite figures play simultaneously marginal and powerful roles in prostitutes' lives, revealing deep power dynamics not just between but *within* eighteenth-century English classes and genders.

We will consider Mary Cooper and her place in eighteenth-century medicine and society in two parts. The first section explores Mary's physicality, especially in the space her body occupies and how the episode uses that space to draw viewers' attention to the realities of eighteenth-century prostitution and disease. The second section moves from Mary's body to the people and objects around Mary, reacting to and using her body in particular ways for both Mary's benefit and their own. Through these sections, we particularly highlight the spaces in which early modern English prostitution and illness took place, the different perspectives early modern Londoners had on the 'French Pox' and the kinds of domestic medical practices employed to help Mary in her suffering. Above all, *Harlots* inverts the traditional Western medical narrative with the goal of helping viewers, to whom we refer in the first person in this chapter, reconsider their preconceptions of where, how, and why medicine took place.

The physicality of Mary Cooper

In its second episode, *Harlots* introduces us to venereal disease when one of the main characters, the bawd Margaret Wells (Samantha Morton), mentions that a woman she used to know in the sex trade, Mary Cooper (Amy Dawson), had fallen on hard times, victim to the so-called 'French Pox'. Eighteenth-century prostitutes would have been all too familiar with the disease. As an example, English physician Gideon Harvey wrote a text titled *Little Venus Unmask'd* (1700) on the 'French Pox'. He described this venereal pox as hiding in prostitutes' bodies across Europe, emphasising the widespread nature of the 'French Pox' and the visible 'spots, blotches, and pimples' it caused (Harvey, 1700: 5). Once these symptoms erupted on the victim's body, particularly her face, she became 'unmasked', an outcast pariah in her community that relied so heavily on beauty and health for their livelihood. *Harlots* leans into this narrative by constructing the space which Mary Cooper inhabits to extract a response from viewers. As bystanders, we are both drawn to sympathy for Mary and recoil from her ailment, similar to the response of the show's characters.

We first see Mary at the end of a shadowy alleyway in Covent Garden, sitting against a wall with her face turned away from the camera. The bright sunlight in the open square contrasts with the alley's darkness, demonstrating how far Mary has fallen since she contracted the pox. She no longer belongs to the outside world but rather to this darker atmosphere from which she cannot recover. Although treatments for the French Pox existed at this time, they were largely limited to those who could pay for them, and their efficacy was highly debated. Additionally, patients underwent further stigma and pain through them; mercury notably poisoned bodies while it cured their sores, causing conspicuous hair loss and heavy salivation (Arrizabalaga, Henderson, and French, 1997: 139–144; Siena, 2001: 208). Though her face is turned from the camera, the viewer can still tell that Mary's visage looks sickly, corroborating an earlier conversation between Nancy Birch (Kate Fleetwood) and her two employed prostitutes about Mary's rumoured illness. Nancy had called Mary a 'shining star' who had 'fallen on hard times' (*Harlots*, S1E2). Mary's body placed in the dark alley, sickly face turned from outside society, fulfils this comment. She becomes an outcast to viewers in a single camera shot, perhaps even more quickly than through rumour.

Nancy's girls enter the shot from the left, one standing in front of the alley, the second leaning against the wall slightly removed from the scene. As they debate who would touch Mary's body to bring to Margaret Wells's house per Nancy's instructions, they continue to gaze at Mary's forlorn figure. This gaze is not the male Foucauldian medical gaze we often find in medical history; it is instead a scrutinising, almost economic gaze. The girls know that they will not catch the pox by touching Mary's body, but they *will* have to carry it through the streets. Already medicine has become decentred – the first people to assess Mary's body are her peers, not a licensed medical practitioner.

Gaze and space also feature as contrasting devices meant to emphasise where Mary originated and where she ended up. Though we do not follow Nancy's girls carrying Mary's body through Covent Garden, the next scene shows the girls, now helped by two men, carrying the body and approaching the Wells' front door. Margaret Wells with Nancy's aid pulls Mary upstairs into an empty bedroom, passing her horrified partner William North (Danny Sapani) on the stairwell. Throughout the scene, Mary becomes a more active body, shielding her coughs with a kerchief, delivering muffled responses to the conversation around her. Her face appears with more clarity, the pox marks showing.

The scene cuts to Mary's original bawdy house, owned by upper-class madam Lydia Quigley (Lesley Manville), a sharp contrast to Mary's appearance. Beautiful and full of light, the scene depicts pretty girls gathered around wealthy clientele seeking leisure in women's bodies. The scene is everything Mary is not, at least on the surface: hygienic, angelic, flawless. The camera returns to the Wells' house, where Margaret and a male journalist stand over Mary's diseased body on a bed. The contrast jars, reminding the viewer of the precarities of Georgian prostitution. Quickly moving between the scenes highlights the reality of Mary's fall: if the darkened alley captured Mary's sense of despair and provoked our curiosity and sympathy, the move from beauty to disease spikes our horror, intentionally heightening our shock at Mary's descent.

Throughout these scenes, Mary gains more agency, moving from huddled in a dark alley to mumbling as she moves upstairs to finally screaming while walking and running around the Wells' house. Eighteenth-century bawdy houses were loud and busy places where conversation, pleasure, and physical actions came together over furniture and bodies (Henderson, 1999). Even so, *Harlots* depicts the Wells' house as ordered – everyone has their place, including the clients. As the episode approaches its mid-point, Mary inserts herself into the ordered life of the house, leaving in her wake a parallel increasing anxiety over her place in the house. The morning after her arrival, she interrupts Margaret, William, and one of Margaret's working girls having breakfast in the kitchen. Mary startles the group with her harsh words as she stumbles through the doorway: 'So, you're using me in a fight with Mrs. Quigley. No one uses me unless they pay.' Margaret drily responds, 'Beg your pardon? You'd have died yesterday if it weren't for me.' The other girl leaves as Mary approaches the table, just missing Mary's grip

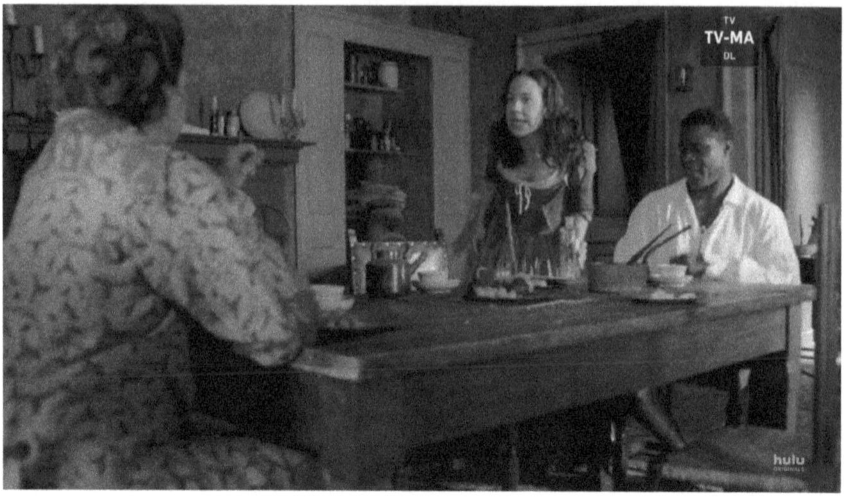

Figure 4.1 Mary demands laudanum, five pounds, and a roast chicken from Margaret at the breakfast table as Margaret's partner, William, watches (*Harlots*)

on the back of her chair. Mary leans towards Margaret, saying, 'I want laudanum. I want five pounds, and a roast chicken. Or I shall walk out into the street and I shall tell how I love good Lydia Quigley.' As she speaks, her face comes close to the camera. The viewers finally see the facial pockmarks, the sweaty hair and brow, and her dishevelled clothing, indicative of her earlier position on the bed (see Figure 4.1).

Through her manipulation of space and ill presentation in this scene, Mary invades this ordered setting and uses that invasion advantageously to negotiate her needs with her caretakers. She knows she is just as useful to Margaret in her illness as she was to Quigley in her prostitution. Her diseased body may no longer be of value for its sexuality, but it can be used as a weapon against the rival madam's reputation. She also recognises that she must disrupt the house's order, and more specifically Margaret's life, to assert agency over the use of her body, replacing beauty and slyness with illness and chaos. Mary creates more disorder later that morning in the house's living room, where all the girls are gathered to wait for an important client's appearance. She enters the room swearing loudly and demanding laudanum. Charlotte Wells (Jessica Brown Findlay), Margaret's daughter and Mary's friend, pulls Mary back to her bedroom, where she presumably gives Mary the laudanum to calm her. Like the pox itself, Mary's presence throws the bawdy house into pandemonium, a secret not easily hidden.

Mary's room courts disorder in a quieter but no less disruptive way. As Charlotte helps Mary back into her bed, the camera takes in the scene: strewn bedclothes where Mary tossed and turned as she lay; a side table with glass bottles and a washbasin recently employed; used candles in disarray. Mary continues coughing while Charlotte tries to make conversation: 'Had some adventures since I last saw you.' Mary responds with a cough and a brief statement: 'You mean I look like a bunna [burner]?' She knows how she appears to Charlotte and prefers to be open about it, anticipating Charlotte's concern. Her body mirrors the disordered room around her, a mess that is difficult to conceal.

The second half of the episode begins when Mary has a brief psychotic break the same afternoon while the Wells' important clients are enjoying themselves, briefly leaving her room screaming before returning to bed quietly. As the night progresses after the psychosis, Mary becomes less and less coherent, gradually losing the agency she once had over her movements. Whereas the disturbed bedclothes had implied Mary's tossing and turning, we now see her tossing in action, groaning with new splotches of blood on her pillow. The camera shifts away to Charlotte's unwanted companion, Mr Haxby (Edward Hogg), praying over Mary's body. The camera swivels back to Charlotte leaning over Mary's now calm body. 'You can stop now', Charlotte says to Haxby. 'She's dead.' The room is still disordered, the body still sickly, but Mary's suffering is over.

Death moves our focus from Mary as a living person to an examination of the materiality of her corpse. As when we first saw Mary hunched in the darkened alley, the scene compels us to gaze on Mary's body through the eyes of Margaret, Nancy, and other prostitutes. Early modern English funeral rites, particularly in lower-class households, consumed the activities of those closest to the deceased. Despite the growing secularisation and professionalisation of morticians throughout the eighteenth century, only the upper and middling classes could afford such funerary services (Gordon and Marshall, 2000; Jupp and Gittings, 2000). As *Harlots* depicts, lower classes continued practising funerary rites in the home with the help of family and friends. The space in which these rites took place was particularly important, which *Harlots* demonstrates through the movement of Mary's body. It first lies on the Wells' kitchen table, where Nancy and Margaret prepare the body for its public wake and funeral. The body, now surrounded by flowers and candlelight, then moves on a board carried by Margaret and Nancy's girls through Covent Garden's streets. Margaret takes this moment to make a poignant statement to onlookers: 'Mary Cooper reminds us of how brief our dance in the candle light can be.' The parade thus serves as a performance to both commemorate Mary's life and draw people's attention to the precarities of prostitution. We, too, become solemn bystanders, watching the parade as it travels across the screen.

As Mary's body moves from public street to semi-private tavern, the episode shifts from procession to funeral and wake. The shift reminds us of the spaces that these women inhabit: Mary's body is prepared for the rites at a bawdy house, not a funeral home; the parade of women performs the funeral in the streets, not down a church aisle; the wake occurs at a communal eating and drinking hall, not at a church altar. Yet there is no less reverence for Mary's body despite these differences. Mary, now lying on another table, seems pure in death. She wears a white shift and make-up hides the marks on her face. The tavern-goers, most of whom followed the parade into the hall, gather around the table. When Nancy begins singing a popular ditty about Mary in a heavy tone, which we explore more deeply in the second section of this chapter, the onlookers join in. Remembrance thus becomes a communal act open to the Covent Garden public, widening the number of participants from private home to public street to community tavern. The viewer, too, is invited to sing along after having heard the song earlier in the episode, turning Mary's wake into a truly public event inside a space shielded from the street and unwelcome eyes.

In fact, the funeral wake, as with the Wells' house, compares to Lydia Quigley's house, Mary's original home. Throughout the episode, Quigley's house on Greek Street is depicted as ordered and clean, everyone in their place to cater to elite clients who expect elite service.[3] The Wells' house and the tavern stand in Covent Garden, which caters to a middling and lower-class clientele who do not expect the polite society of elite bawdy houses. Instead, the wake reminds the viewers of middle- and lower-class Irish wakes. People dance, sing, and drink to celebrate Mary's life as her body remains on the table in the middle of the room. Quigley's house, despite its order and cleanliness, contrasts sharply with this vision; it is almost *too* clean, bordering on lifeless. While Nancy and Margaret take a break from dancing, Nancy looks at Margaret and describes Quigley's house as a morgue because 'there's not a soul' there. This statement disconnects happiness from cleanliness, discounting emerging elite medical theory about hygiene and respectability.[4] Mary Cooper's diseased death brought about a gathering full of life and laughter, while Quigley and her girls sat at home, manufacturing joy for their clients but exuding none organically.

Finally, the women carry Mary's body to Quigley's front door. Lydia Quigley and her son open the door to find the corpse surrounded by flowers and candles with lower-class Covent Garden women standing opposite them in the street. Margaret and Nancy here finally use Mary's body itself for their foremost intention – to unnerve Lydia and ultimately threaten her business. The Covent Garden women stand in the vacant street, Lydia and her son in their comfortable doorway, and Mary lies between the two groups.

As this episode on Mary's illness and death ends, her body serves a greater purpose in exposing twenty-first-century viewers to eighteenth-century prostitution and medicine in two ways. First, prostitutes' bodies were constantly in use, not only by themselves but more frequently by the people inhabiting the spaces around them. At the same time, prostitutes inhabited multiple spaces in both life and death, many times the same ones whether they were culling clients or laid out on a table dead in a white shift. The prostitute's body was a capitalistic symbol, a good traded for currency. Few times did the prostitute actually *own* her own body – in life, madams and customers assumed control over that body, while in death, their bodies often became tools for political, economic, or even medical purposes. Through its re-enactment of eighteenth-century prostitution, *Harlots* opens a window into this otherwise hidden world for viewers, pulling them into the plot and, once there, exposing the harsh yet close-knit realities of prostitution in Georgian London.

The gendered life of Mary Cooper

While Mary's body and her agency are the episode's contested objects, the central focus is on the people around Mary and their perceptions and use of her illness. Early modern venereological theory was crafted within a highly gendered and misogynistic worldview. As many historians have noted, physicians and moralists alike located the source of venereal disease in the bodies of women, especially prostitutes, a result of the particular combination of their female physiology and promiscuity (Siena, 1998). It was the prevailing medical theory by the seventeenth and early eighteenth centuries that syphilis was first concocted within women, particularly women who had sex with more than one man. The womb of a 'Publick woman' was seen as a particularly dangerous fount of moral and literal corruption, a furnace in which diverse seeds mixed, heated, and fermented into poisonous vapours to be spread to others (de Blegny, 1676: 3).

To many, prostitutes represented anxieties about modernity, poverty, and immorality, the transgression of social and sexual boundaries. These fears also overlapped with intense nationalist sentiment. The 'French Pox' was not only so-called because of the supposed transmission from that nation's material goods and people, but because foreign influence began to be taken as pestilent, with the potential to corrupt the very fabric of English life, opening it up to the sins of modernity and excess. Syphilis was related to all things seemingly 'French', hedonistic, and effete (Hentschell, in Siena, 2005: 133–158). In Lydia Quigley's brothel featured in *Harlots*, all things French are on display. The pale painted faces, the rich, lavish fabrics – it is the picture of excess, seduction, and frivolity. Combined with medical theories of the time linking venereal disease to women's leaky, porous bodies, in the eyes of an early eighteenth-century venereologist it would seem clear that syphilis would spring up out of the lush setting. It makes sense, then, that Margaret Wells and the gossip writer she employs attempt to spin Mary's disease as the tragic result of the decay hidden beneath all of Quigley's Golden Square luxury.

While *Harlots* subtly represents these historical fears through rumours locating the seat of venereal disease in the luxurious brothel, the show subverts these fears by demonstrating multiple perspectives on the matter. It notably uses prostitutes, not professional medical practitioners, to tell the story. The ailing Mary Cooper confronts Margaret Wells after being taken into her house, immediately sensing that her body is being used in a fight between the two madams. 'I wasn't even ill 'til I left [Quigley's] house … I caught this pox on Cheapside', Mary scoffs. Beyond an analysis of venereological theory, much of the secondary literature on syphilis explores the dynamics of the patient–healer relationship. Too often, period dramas, much like the histories they draw from, presume the presence of a recognisable, typically male, medical practitioner. In contrast, the characters in *Harlots*, including the sufferer herself, neither call for nor even suggest involving a doctor or a medical practitioner. Such a portrayal, we argue, is more representative of everyday experiences of illness, especially among working-class women in early modern London.

This is not to say that such women would have had no interaction whatsoever with medical practitioners. Their presence is off-screen but suggested by the use of laudanum, as well as condoms, which would have likely been purchased from an apothecary or a medical practitioner who advertised their nostrums for the cure of the venereal disease. As Olivia Weisser and Kevin Siena have shown, medical advertisements of the time demonstrate how many practitioners either directly shipped their cures to patients or sold them through retailers such as booksellers (Siena, 2001; Weisser, 2017). Both authors, however, conclude that this method of third-party sale of venereal medications was prompted by the demand of patients who were too embarrassed to visit a doctor in person. While this is surely the case for many, it also seems to overlook the likelihood that some patients may have preferred to purchase a nostrum for themselves either because of convenience, privacy, or the fact that they were perfectly capable of administering the medicine and treatment as they needed.

Despite the high competition for venereal patients, medical practitioners maintained a level of distrust for their patients, and for women in particular. To finagle a confession of sexual transgression out of their patients seems to have been just as important to these medical men as curing them. Indeed, many saw confession as an essential part of the medical encounter, as though purging the body of sin and pestilence were one and the same (Weisser, 2017: 698–705). As one minister put it, calling to mind the sweating brought on by mercurial treatments, 'for the health of the body, men will purge and sweat ... so the vomit of the soul is the griefe of Repentance' (Taylor, 1618: 112). In light of this, the absence of a physician in *Harlots* seems all the more significant. Mary Cooper does not seek confession or spiritual cure, nor express any shame in her disease. Neither do any of the prostitutes around her. Instead of subjecting themselves to the scolding of a physician, or risking their refusal, the women competently deal with Mary's illness on their own in their home. They demonstrate clear experience and knowledge in medical care, treating Mary with laudanum, and cleaning the sores on her body. When her partner expresses concern about the sick woman being in their home, Margaret Wells says, 'It's the French Pox, Will. You'd have to fuck her to get it.' An exasperated explanation of the nature of transmission indicates the lay knowledge and expertise that these women had picked up in their line of work.

Harlots also cleverly illustrates everyday preventative medicine. After a scene in which wealthy men discuss the rumoured presence of syphilis in the Golden Square brothel, the episode abruptly cuts to a shot of one of the Covent Garden prostitutes cleaning out a condom in a washbasin – a clear and silent reminder that these women regularly understood and used medical knowledge. Condoms were just as important in preventing the transmission of venereal infections as in preventing pregnancies (Lane, 2001: 32–38; Trumbach, 1991).[5]

As a number of recent historians have argued, the majority of medical care in the early modern world was performed in the domestic realm, by women who were not licensed or professional practitioners (Fissell, 2008). By refocusing our attention from stereotypical doctor–patient encounters to laywomen, onto the bedside and care of the body, it becomes clear that the hierarchy of care did not always prioritise the learned physician. This decentring is just as important within popular culture depictions of the past as it is within our history books. *Harlots*, we claim, asserts a historically feminist approach to the portrayal of both sufferers and healers, a perspective appearing more frequently in televised period pieces in the #MeToo era.

Take, for example, a typical healing encounter that is reproduced for the screen in *Harlots*, taking the viewer into what would have been an intimate process of healing that so often went unrecorded. After Mary Cooper has been taken into the Covent Garden brothel and given care, Charlotte Wells goes to visit her. 'Mary, remember me?' Charlotte asks when she sees the sick woman. 'Oh Charlotte', Mary responds, groaning, 'what does a whore have to do to get some poppy in this dump?' Charlotte then sits by Mary's bedside and performs the essential women's healing work of comforting the ill and dying. She cleans her skin, keeps her cool with a wet cloth, and provides her with soothing laudanum. By taking the time to portray such a healing encounter on-screen, taking place between women at the bedside rather than the expected consultation by a physician, *Harlots* asserts the power and authority of women's healing labours.

After Mary's death, the three Wells women are then shown cleaning the corpse, preparing Mary for burial. Another essential task of women is on display in this understated scene, as the characters act as layers-out of the dead. Lucy (Eloise Smyth), the youngest, observing Mary's poxed body, comments, 'We should put some powder on her.' 'Let's not hide what life did to her', Margaret responds. This commentary points to a particular significance of syphilis, its physical manifestation on the skin. To many early modern observers, the exterior of the body reflected its interior, both in terms of physical and moral character. For syphilis, its characteristic skin lesions and pustules, and, in advanced stages, the loss of hair and deterioration of facial and nasal tissue, seemed to confirm theories of moral decay. The dermatological effects provided a seemingly self-evident connection with, among other things, leprosy, along with its long-held moral and social stigmas (Siena, 1998; Berco, 2014). To the women of *Harlots*, though, the lesions on Mary's skin speak to the decay of broader society, of the system that placed each of them into a position of selling sex, of being vulnerable to disease and violence while condemning them for their sins, for their very bodies.

Several times throughout the episode, characters sing a song about Mary, an apparently popular ditty recounting the woman's exploits in a heroic, playful tone. The final line, giving her the title of 'London's Venus, Mary Cooper', proves soberingly prescient by the time the viewer hears the full song, after the once-lauded harlot lays on her pyre of flowers. The goddess of love and beauty came to be shorthand in England for the disease that killed her, especially in the hands of misogynistic medical theorists who placed the seat of disease within the womb itself (Siena, 2001, 218). Using the imagery and language of mythology, Venus was portrayed as the poisonous seductress, the wicked woman responsible for the downfall of man.[6] The song reappears at Mary's memorial, in which the women and locals gather in the pub to reminisce. 'Mary Cooper, Mary Cooper / Leaves her lovers in a stupor / Ridin' high, no man can dupe her / London's Venus, Mary Cooper'. In reclaiming the gendered imagery of Venus, and in the subtle depiction of laywomen's everyday healing work, *Harlots* resists clichéd depictions of venereal infection that play into long-held gendered stereotypes.

To underscore what makes *Harlots*' depiction of venereal disease so significant, let us briefly turn to another portrayal of syphilis in a period drama: *The Frankenstein Chronicles* (2015–2017), a two-season British ITV Encore crime drama set in 1820s London.[7] Taking place in the same city, some sixty years after the setting of *Harlots*, *The Frankenstein Chronicles* takes to heart all the moralising and shame-filled rhetoric surrounding venereal disease. The essential difference between these two portrayals of syphilis comes down to gender. In *Harlots*, we see syphilis from the perspective of women, filling the role not just of sufferers but as lay healers, medical experts, and sex workers. From the male perspective that is prioritised in *The Frankenstein Chronicles*, syphilis serves as a mostly unseen symbol, in order to provide the viewer with a glimpse into stoic masculine interiority.

A single sore on protagonist John Marlott's (Sean Bean) hand nags at him. We eventually discover that he contracted syphilis abroad during the Napoleonic wars, confirming the anti-foreign sentiments in the 'French Disease'. Marlott consults two male medical practitioners, one of whom suggests a mercury treatment, noting that it will lead to 'bad dreams, visions'. Marlott confesses to the doctor that his 'carelessness' infected his wife Agnes (Deirdre Mullins) and infant daughter. After the child's death from the disease, the show suggests that his wife committed suicide by drowning. In Marlott's mercury-induced visions, the two are shot through a hazy lens, less fully-formed characters than angelic reminders of the masculine protagonist's sex-based guilt and silent suffering. As such, his wife shows no physical sign of the disease, but remains 'uncorrupted' to match her moral innocence. Marlott's symbolic sore grows as the series goes on, serving to show the emotional and moral suffering that he increasingly feels but does not express. On the other side of this extreme, a naturopath shows Marlott a patient suffering from tertiary stage syphilis which has caused their nose and palate to collapse. The show makes use of this sufferer not as a character, but as a moralistic monstrosity, an omen of Marlott's future that has otherwise manifested only in his hand (and arguably his mind, though the show's final acts seem to contradict this). Later on, Marlott looks in the mirror and hallucinates his own face eaten away from the disease. These two extremes accentuate the metaphoric message, and are not, it seems, intended to provide viewers with a look into everyday sickness and death in the past.

In contrast to *Harlots*' female-centred, sex-positive – or at least sex-neutral – and harshly realistic portrayal of illness, *The Frankenstein Chronicles*' take on syphilis is decidedly masculine, sex-negative, and metaphoric. Where the characters in *Harlots* internalised and espoused a variety of symbolic meanings from Mary's illness, the show itself makes it clear that syphilis, for all its potential metaphor, is and was a real, painful disease. Marlott's suffering is portrayed as mental, emotional pain, the supposedly deserved punishment for his moral lapse and 'carelessness'. Syphilis is a narrative tool to symbolise his sorrow, guilt, and fear – emotions that remain otherwise repressed beneath a stoic exterior. His wife's experience with the disease is similarly seen only in her expressions of motherly grief, she the innocent victim of her husband's sexual transgression. In contrast, Mary Cooper did not suffer from the pox out of guilt or as punishment for her sins; she was not the martyred victim of a cruel bawd or lecherous cull. She suffered because she contracted an illness endemic to early modern Europe, which ran its course through her body, manifesting in internal pains and external pustules, and led to her death. Ultimately it is clear that syphilis is not a symbol at all – as Mary Cooper herself says, she did not even contract the pox from the brothel. In this way, *Harlots* demonstrates that disease is inelegant, quotidian, and refuses to conform to the expected narrative, and that most health care for the eighteenth-century lower class took place in domestic spaces, not doctors' offices.

Conclusion

As a piece of historical fiction, *Harlots* has artistic freedom to portray events and individuals who remain unfortunately elusive in traditional historical scholarship. It prioritises those individuals and everyday events that, due to the constraints of written sources and the problems of the archive, have been relegated to the margins of our historical memory of the early modern period. Rather than relying on the traditional narrative and prioritising the perspectives of those in power, including licensed male medical practitioners, the creators of *Harlots* have made an important intervention into our view of working-class life, health, and sex in eighteenth-century London. Foregrounding the perspectives of working-class women, the show does subtle work in asserting the authority of such individuals in experiences of health and healing.

The decision to feature a plotline surrounding venereal disease, and syphilis in particular, may seem to be an obvious one on a show about prostitution set in a time period in which this particular disease was widespread, the subject of much debate and condemnation. However, the choice that *Harlots* made to eschew a medical practitioner, indeed the male medical gaze itself, is far more subversive than it appears at first glance. The manipulation of space on the screen, and the ways in which healthy and diseased bodies navigate through it, demonstrate the interpersonal relationships and gendered and class-based power dynamics at play in eighteenth-century sex work, as well as the potential danger and illness running through this world. Furthermore, *Harlots*' staunch insistence on a female perspective on sex and healing presents a crucial and underrepresented view of history, appealing to twenty-first-century viewers' desire for more inclusive and representative portrayals of the past in period dramas. As is made clear in this episode, early modern England was a highly gendered and complex society. In the face of intense social, structural, and physical oppression, women filled a range of roles as healers, prostitutes, preachers, sufferers, antagonists, and allies through which they asserted their own authority, agency, and power.

Notes

1 The show is based on Hallie Rubenfeld, *The Covent Garden Ladies: Pimp General Jack & the Extraordinary Story of Harris's List* (Stroud: Tempus, 2005).

2 For some recent coverage, see Liam Stack, 'Sexually Transmitted Disease Cases Rise to Record High, C.D.C. Says', *New York Times* (8 October 2019), www.nytimes.com/2019/10/08/health/cdc-std-study.html, and 'STIs: Why Is Syphilis on the Rise?' *BBC News* (10 June 2018), www.bbc.com/news/health-44384289.

3 Eighteenth-century Greek Street was the site of respectable bawdy houses for better-paying customers to visit.

4 The Enlightenment spurred new thoughts on public hygiene and order. For more information, see William Coleman, 'Health and Hygiene in the "Encyclopédie": A Medical Doctrine for the Bourgeoisie', *Journal of the History of Medicine and Allied Sciences* 29, 4 (October 1974): 399–421.

5 Condoms were also referred to as 'French letters' in a nod to the previously discussed associations of sexuality and venereal disease with France.

6 The simultaneous medicalisation and eroticisation of the female form recalls the use of anatomical wax Venus figures, popular in the eighteenth and nineteenth centuries. For more information, see Joanna Ebenstein, *The Anatomical Venus: Wax, God, and the Ecstatic* (New York: Distributed Art Publishers, 2016).

7 The show is discussed at length by Andrea Wright in another chapter of this book. ITV's *Victoria* creates a more nuanced but similar scenario surrounding Prince Albert's brother Ernest, who contracts syphilis in season two and undergoes secret mercury treatments at a London physician's clinic. For a deeper examination, see Anne Hanley, 'Why Last Night's VD-Laced Episode of *Victoria* Should Worry Modern Audiences', *The Guardian* (2 October 2017), www.theguardian.com/science/blog/2017/oct/02/why-last-nights-vd-laced-episode-of-victoria-should-worry-modern-audiences.

References

Akilli, S. and S. Öz (2016). 'No More Let Life Divide…': Victorian Metropolitan Confluence in *Penny Dreadful*', *Critical Survey* 28 (1/Spring), 15–29.

Arrizabalaga, J., J. Henderson, and R. French (1997). *The Great Pox: The French Disease in Renaissance Europe*. New Haven: Yale University Press.

Berco, C. (2014). 'The Great Pox, Symptoms, and the Social Body in Early Modern Spain', *Social History of Medicine* 28 (2), 225–244.

Byrne, K., J. Taddeo, and L. Leggott (2018). *Conflicting Masculinities: Men in Television Period Drama*. London: I.B. Tauris.

Cavallo, S. (2007). *Artisans of the Body in Early Modern Italy: Identities, Families and Masculinities*. Manchester: Manchester University Press.

Coleman, W. (1974). 'Health and Hygiene in the "Encyclopédie": A Medical Doctrine for the Bourgeoisie', *Journal of the History of Medicine and Allied Sciences* 29 (4/October), 399–421.

De Blegny, N. and W. Harris. (1676). *New and Curious Observations* [...]. London: Tho. Dring and Tho. Burrel.

Fissell, M. (2008). 'Introduction: Women, Health, and Healing in Early Modern Europe', *Bulletin of the History of Medicine* 82 (1), 1–17.

Gordon, B. and P. Marshall (eds) (2000). *The Place of the Dead: Death and Remembrance in Late Medieval and Early Modern Europe*. Cambridge: Cambridge University Press.

Green, M. H. (1989). 'Women's Medical Practice and Health Care in Medieval Europe', *Signs* 14, 434–473.

Harvey, G. (1700). *Little Venus Unmask'd Being a Discourse of the French Pox [...]*. 6th edn. London: W. Turner at the Angel at Lincolns-Inn-Gate.

Henderson, T. (1999). *Disorderly Women in Eighteenth-Century London: Prostitution and Control in the Metropolis, 1730–1830*. London: Longman.

Jupp, P. C. and C. Gittings (eds) (2000). *Death in England: An Illustrated History*. New Brunswick, NJ: Rutgers University Press.

Lane, J. (2001). *A Social History of Medicine: Health, Healing and Disease in England, 1750–1950*. London: Routledge.

Nicholas, S. (2007). 'History, Revisionism, and Television Drama: *Foyle's War* and the "myth of 1940"', *Media History* 13 (2/3), 203–219.

Poole, S. (2018). *Wasteland: The Great War and the Origins of Modern Horror*. Berkeley: Counterpoint.

Rubenfeld, H. (2005). *The Covent Garden Ladies: Pimp General Jack & the Extraordinary Story of Harris's List*. Stroud: Tempus.

Siena, K. P. (1998). 'Pollution, Promiscuity, and the Pox: English Venereology and the Early Modern Medical Discourse on Social and Sexual Danger', *Journal of the History of Sexuality* 8 (4), 553–574.

Siena, K. P. (2001). 'The "Foul Disease" and Privacy: The Effects of Venereal Disease and Patient Demand on the Medical Marketplace in Early Modern London', *Bulletin of the History of Medicine* 75 (2/Summer), 199–224.

Siena, K. P. (ed.) (2005). *Sins of the Flesh: Responding to Sexual Disease in Early Modern Europe*. Toronto: Centre for Reformation and Renaissance Studies.

Taylor, T. (1618). *Davids Learning, or the Way to True Happinesse*. London: Printed by W. Stansby, for Henry Fetherstone, and are to be sold at his shop in Pauls Churchyard, at the signe of the Rose.

Trumbach, R. (1991). 'The Condom in Modern and Postmodern Culture', *Journal of the History of Sexuality* 2 (1), 95–98.

Weisser, O. (2017). 'Treating the Secret Disease: Sex, Sin, and Authority in Eighteenth-Century Venereal Cases', *Bulletin of the History of Medicine* 91 (4), 685–712.

White, B. (2019). 'Britishness and Others: Representing and Constructing Identity in BBC's *Land Girls*', *Critical Studies in Television* 14 (1/March), 90–105.

Part II

Pioneers, heroes, and villains

5

Feminist doctors and medicine women: the lady physician in the American western

Jacqueline D. Antonovich

In 1993, *Dr. Quinn, Medicine Woman* (1993–1998) premiered on television sets across America. A feel-good western starring Jane Seymour, the show centres on Dr Michaela Quinn, a physician who leaves Boston in 1867 to practice medicine in Colorado. The overarching premise of *Dr. Quinn* rested on two interrelated concepts – the unusualness of a woman physician practising in the American West, and how that unique presence brings civility and modernity to the frontier. Over the run of its six seasons, Dr Quinn wins over sceptical westerners by treating the town's bodies and souls; in doing so, the lady doctor finds professional fulfilment while simultaneously taming the Wild West. *Dr. Quinn, Medicine Woman* found its niche within the family entertainment genre that dominated 1990s television, yet its popularity with American audiences also could be attributed to what Seymour's character represents in the cultural imagination: the 'civilised' white woman on the 'uncivilised' frontier. The show, in fact, followed in the footsteps of several novels, films, and plays produced in the early twentieth century that used the figure of the woman physician to teach morality, promote public health, and advocate for progressive politics. In the simplest terms, *Dr. Quinn, Medicine Woman* was a resurrected character from the imaginations of first-wave feminists, reinvented and repackaged for a 1990s audience.

Tracing the fictionalised female physician in American popular culture is a helpful exercise in examining shifting sex and gender norms throughout the twentieth century. Ever since Elizabeth Blackwell became the first woman in the United States to earn a medical degree in 1847, the 'lady physician' became a powerful political and cultural symbol. She appears in Louisa May Alcott's 1886 novel *Jo's Boys*, in the 1916 film *The Woman in Politics*, and in more recent television shows such as *ER* (1994–2009) and *Grey's Anatomy* (2005–). The 'western lady doctor' in particular became a potent figure in popular culture, especially in the early twentieth century as women's roles in the public sphere began to expand. To first-wave feminists, she represented the possibilities of educated, professional, and politically empowered womanhood (Meade,

2004). To the burgeoning silent film industry, she represented something else entirely: a gender-bending comic foil ripe for exploring sexuality on the untamed frontier. By the mid-twentieth century, however, TV westerns depicted the woman physician not as a feminist reformer or sexual threat, but as a dutiful helpmate for male protagonists. As scholars of the American West have argued, westerns as a genre are powerful fantasies that serve ideological functions relevant to the time period and intended audience (Brauer, 1971; Cawelti, 1971; Slotkin, 1992). In other words, because westerns often evoke a mythic past, they are ideal vehicles for exploring present-day issues from a safe historical distance. The figure of the woman physician serves an important function in this process. Throughout the twentieth century, the lady physician on the frontier became an archetypical character for examining shifting ideological debates over gender, sex, race, and politics.

This chapter begins by examining the real women physicians in the turn-of-the-century American West that inspired their fictionalised counterparts. Although *Dr. Quinn, Medicine Woman* attempted to dramatise a 'forgotten history' of women in the West, the show neglected a more complicated, contentious, and historically significant story of the first women physicians in the region. The chapter then examines fictionalised physicians in three distinct periods. The first, the Progressive Era (1900–1920), explores how feminist writers and silent filmmakers created contrasting depictions of women physicians in the West. Although both groups saw women doctors as powerful symbols of new womanhood, feminists characterised them as guiding lights of morality and modernity, while filmmakers depicted them as comically subverting traditional gender and sexual mores. The second period, mid-century (1950s–1970s), examines women physicians during the heyday of the television western. Following World War II and in the midst of the Cold War, TV westerns became a vehicle for exploring masculinity, violence, and shifting political and cultural climates. No longer feminist political actors or subversive sexual characters, western women physicians were largely relegated to the background, playing helpmates, nurses, or damsels-in-distress to their white-hatted heroes. Finally, this chapter traces the re-emergence of the western woman physician as a feminist symbol in the closing decades of the twentieth century (1980s–1990s). Following the rise of women's history, female physicians underwent a reappraisal from both feminist scholars and popular culture, culminating in the 1990s television show, *Dr. Quinn, Medicine Woman*. In emphasising maternalism, morality, and progressive politics, the show embodied the goals of first-wave feminism, while also embracing a distinct 1990s multiculturalism that elided the racial politics of actual women physicians that populated the region at the turn of the century.

The real women physicians of the American West

After Elizabeth Blackwell graduated from Geneva Medical College of New York in 1849, a select group of women followed her lead, comprising the first generation of female physicians in America. The majority practised medicine in the northeast; however, by the closing decades of the nineteenth century, many women who were born, raised, and educated in the east began looking westward for political and professional opportunities. The popularity of medical climatology, the need for physicians in the region, and the rhetoric of 'freedom on the frontier' lured hundreds of women physicians to western states and territories. By 1900, cities in California, Colorado, and Oregon had some of the highest ratios of women physicians in the nation (Antonovich, 2018).

The majority of the region's female physicians during this period were concentrated in cities such as Los Angeles, San Francisco, and Portland. In Colorado, most women chose Denver as their destination, although Colorado Springs, Boulder, and Pueblo were also popular among women doctors looking to practise in an urban area large enough to attract a sustainable patient population. *Dr. Quinn, Medicine Woman*, set in Colorado Springs, misrepresents the city in two distinct ways: first, Colorado Springs did not exist until 1871, four years after Dr Quinn settles there. Second, and more importantly, because of its popularity as a health destination, Colorado Springs was home to numerous physicians, both male and female. Many women chose to practise medicine in these cities because they offered more professional opportunities than rural towns, but urban areas held an additional advantage: the chance to be part of a community of medical women. Cities like Colorado Springs provided the space to foster collegiality through membership in local women's medical societies and women's professional organisations.

A few women did choose to practise in small mountain, mining, or ranching towns, where they were often the only female doctor, and in some cases the only doctor. Mary Winter Fisher, for example, moved to the rural mountain town of Pagosa Springs in 1895. Dr Fisher's job as a rural medical doctor in turn-of-the-century Colorado was often difficult, and many aspects of her life and career sound straight out of a *Dr. Quinn* episode. She had to ride horseback up in the mountains to make house calls or tend to emergencies. She also had a pet bear named Pickles, who she trained to wrestle miners and cowboys in local saloons. Although Dr Fisher lived an adventurous life worthy of any TV western, her life differed from fictitious accounts in one important way: it was not an isolated one. Like many women physicians in the region, she cultivated connections to the larger medical community and women's professional networks. Dr Fisher worked as the Archuleta coroner in 1911, served as the county health officer, and regularly attended state medical society meetings in Denver (Antonovich, 2018).

Wherever they chose to practise, upon arrival, women doctors established private medical offices, sanatoriums, and hospitals throughout the region. The experiences they gained treating patients informed them of the public health needs of their communities, while also building up their professional reputations. Their medical work in the region fundamentally guided their future political work. From municipal housekeeping to suffrage activism to running for elected office, women physicians leveraged their status as medical professionals to propel their political careers and drive maternalist health reforms. Unlike *Dr Quinn, Medicine Woman*, a show that emphasised multicultural politics, most women physicians in the region used their political power to promote eugenics and advocate for public health legislation based on racial science. It was these women, with their pathbreaking, yet problematic political activism, who would inspire first-wave feminist writers in the United States.

Feminists, filmmakers, and the female physician in the Progressive Era

As female physicians spread out across the United States, the 'lady doctor' increasingly became a common character in turn-of-the-century popular culture. With titles such as *Kitty's Choice* (Davis, 1874), *A Country Doctor* (Jewett, 1884), and *Helen Brent, M.D.* (Meyer, 1892), the mostly women-authored books depicted their main characters as altruistic, middle-class ladies who struggled with choosing between their professional calling and their marriage prospects. By the early twentieth century, the personally and professionally conflicted lady doctor gave way to a new type of character: the politically active woman physician. The female physician gave novelists and filmmakers an entry point for joining the debate over a woman's place in political culture (Bardes and Gossett, 1990). The woman doctor became a symbol for the debate of the day – women's rights and her role in the public sphere.

In 1916, for example, Mutual Film Corporation released *The Woman in Politics*, starring Mignon Anderson. The silent film centres on Dr Beatrice Barlow, a young woman doctor who, once appointed as the health inspector of an eastern metropolis, learns that the city is run by a corrupt political ring. Instead of ignoring the malfeasance surrounding her, she decides to risk her career by trying to expose the political criminals. Dr Barlow's 'puny will', as one reviewer phrased it, succeeds only after she is aided by the governor's private secretary, a young man of 'superior strength and mental resource' (Harrison, 1916). In the film's telling, women physicians possessed the right amount of medical knowledge and feminine altruism to righteously serve in municipal politics; yet, because of their lack of political experience, they needed to rely on the aid of their savvier male counterparts.

If the woman physician became a popular figure in the debate over women's rights, then the woman physician in the American West became its avatar. Western women physicians symbolised the possibility of what professional women could do. By the end of the nineteenth century, as they opened their practices across western states, they joined or even spearheaded successful suffrage campaigns. Beginning in 1869, western states and territories began granting women the right to vote, decades before the ratification of the 19th Amendment. Subsequently, women physicians in the region became political agents of reform, especially with laws concerning women and children. By the end of the first decade of the twentieth century, these women held powerful sway in the minds of eastern feminists because most western medical women were living, working, voting, and reforming legislation in the region, some for decades ('What Does the Franchise Mean to Women Physicians?', 1912: 91–92; 'The Woman Physician Finds Herself', 1919: 256).

Because of their political and professional power, they became popular figures in fictional works. Charlotte Perkins Gilman's use of the western woman physician is perhaps the most famous example. In 1911, Gilman published a one-act play titled *Something to Vote For* in the June edition of her magazine, *The Forerunner.* A pro-suffrage piece, the play centred on a woman physician from Colorado named Dr Strong. While visiting an undisclosed eastern city, Dr Strong was invited to speak at a meeting of an anti-suffrage woman's club on the topic of 'pure milk'. Other guests included the boss of a local milk trust, Mr Billings; a city milk inspector; and a poor Irish American woman whose infant son died of a milk-borne disease. After a series of events where Dr Strong exposes Mr Billings as a corrupt businessman who sells tainted milk, she tells the ladies that if mothers ran the milk business they would 'not be willing to poison other women's babies even to make money for their own', and stressed the need for women to avoid becoming 'apathetic citizens'. Gilman's play concludes with the group of clubwomen converting to the suffragist cause, thanks to Dr Strong, the visiting physician from Colorado (Gilman, 1911b).

It is significant that the protagonist of Gilman's play was a woman doctor from the American West. For Gilman, a feminist activist and social reformer, women physicians in the enfranchised West represented the ultimate possibilities of womanhood unshackled from sexual discrimination. Dr Strong was an educated woman with a professional career, a woman who devoted her life to improving the health and welfare of mothers and children, and unlike Dr Barlow, a woman who voted. Even her name, 'Dr

Strong', is evocative of the power of informed and enfranchised womanhood. For Gilman, female physicians in the American West represented the sublimity of women's citizenship. In fact, Dr Strong was not the first western woman doctor she wrote about. A year earlier, Gilman published the novel, *The Crux*, which includes the character Dr Jane Bellair, who acts as the moral conscience for a group of eastern women who migrate to Denver in the early twentieth century (Friedl, 1987; Gilman, 1911a).

If women writers saw feminist power in the figure of the western lady physician, male screenwriters saw something else – a comedic plot point to explore gender and sexuality. The earliest depictions of western women physicians on film occur in 1910, with the release of two films, *The Lady Doctor* and *The Little Doctor of the Foothills*. Produced by the Powers Company, *The Lady Doctor* featured Pearl White as Dr Julia May. The film follows the 'pretty physician' as she opens a medical office in an unnamed western town with too many men and not enough women. The rough-and-tumble cowboys of the region compete for the attention of Dr May by feigning all sorts of illnesses and injuries. Dr May, however, is wise to their games. As the film progresses, the physician makes the men perform increasingly ridiculous tasks in order to 'cure' them (Lyceum Theater, 1910). The second film, *The Little Doctor of the Foothills*, follows a similar premise. Produced by the Essanay Film Company, the film stars Clara Williams as Dr Cecil Burton. When the residents of Sturgis, Arizona, get word that a physician will be arriving in town to set up practice, they all assume Dr Burton is a man. When the stagecoach arrives with the physician, the townsfolk are surprised to find out otherwise. The men soon flock to see the woman physician, complaining of an array of made-up illnesses. Fed up with their exploits, Dr Burton refuses to see any more patients. When a real medical emergency does occur – a handsome young man shot in the leg – Dr Burton refuses to ride out to see him. His friends put him on a horse and send him to her office, where the doctor realises the severity of his wounds and the error of her ways. As one reviewer writes, 'She binds the wound, very badly for a doctor, it must be allowed, but she makes up for this by nicely sewing up a gaping wound in his heart' ('Essamay's Stock Company', 1910; 'The Lyric', 1901: 16). The film ends with the little *married* doctor of the foothills free to practise medicine without fear of flirtatious cowboys.

The similar plotlines of the two films can tell us much about the western woman physician in the cultural imagination of Americans at the turn of the century. Both films introduce the woman physician as an outsider; an invader of an exclusively male space (the frontier) and an interloper in an exclusively male profession (medicine). These transgressions create sexual chaos because her profession requires her to touch the (mostly) male bodies of her frontier town. In these scenarios, the educated, politically active 'new woman' described by feminist writers is nowhere to be found. Written through the male gaze, the woman physician (and by extension, new womanhood) is not a symbol of the possibilities of empowerment, but of gender subversion; an economic and sexual threat that could only be contained through marriage.

The tension between the 'new woman' as an educated professional or subversive threat is even more explicit in the 1915 film, *The Lady Doctor of Grizzly Gulch*. Produced by Joker Films, the film stars Max Asher as Dr Shultz and Gale Henry as Dr Helen Hurtmore. Set in the small town of Grizzly Gulch, Dr Shultz is the only physician in town until Dr Hurtmore arrives to hang up her shingle. Like the previous films, the women-starved men of the town flock to her office, hoping they will get the pleasure of a physical examination. Feeling economically threatened, Dr Shultz disguises himself as a woman doctor and flirts with the men of the town to draw patients away from Dr Hurtmore. His plan is successful until Dr Hurtmore figures out his ruse and unmasks him. Enraged at being fooled by the cross-dressing doctor, the town's men string up Dr Shultz to a tree to kill him. Although the men were sexually aroused at the idea of a female doctor performing routine physical examinations, a male doctor disguised as a woman offering the same services crossed the line into sexual deviancy. Seconds before he is hanged, Dr Hurtmore intervenes by cutting the rope. The film ends with a wedding between Dr Shultz and Dr Hurtmore. The two merge their medical practices and their hearts ('Aurora', 1910: 2).

These comedies centred on the sexual chaos created by women physicians on the frontier; however, one film took a more serious tone. The 1917 film *The Evil Eye* stars Blanche Sweet as Dr Katherine Torrance, a woman doctor in Baja California. When diphtheria erupts at a local vineyard, Dr Torrance is called in to help curb the outbreak. The Mexican labourers, having never encountered modern medicine before – nor a woman physician – believe she is using black magic. When the workers attack her, the owner of the vineyard rescues Dr Torrance from the 'savage' Mexicans. The film ends with the two falling in love (Long, 1917: 129–132). *The Evil Eye*, like the films before it, positions the woman physician as a love interest, but the role is notable for Dr Torrance's quest to bring scientific medicine to the 'superstitious' labourers. Dr Torrance is written more like the physicians that feminist writers had in mind – a moral woman using science as a tool for modernity. The film is inherently racist in its portrayal of Mexican labourers but would not be objectionable to white feminists of the period, many of whom embraced xenophobic medico-political ideologies (Rensing, 2006). Most white women physicians, in fact, participated in the medical surveillance of marginalised populations in the region (Shah, 2001: 107; Antonovich, 2018). The fictional Dr Torrance, then, was more in line with the health politics of the period and the medical mission of white women physicians on the frontier.

Despite her symbolic popularity among Progressive Era Americans, the western woman physician all but disappeared from popular culture by the 1920s. This withdrawal could be attributed to a few different factors: the end of the reform era that defined the first decade of the twentieth century or the steep decline in women enrolling in medical schools during this period (Morantz-Sanchez, 1985: 248). Women physicians in general became sparse characters in novels and films during this period. One study shows that fewer than five films depicted women physicians between the 1920s and 1940s (Dans, 2000: 121). By the 1950s, however, the invention of a new medium and a revived nostalgia for the Old West brought the woman physician back into the picture.

The television western and the woman physician

In the years following World War II, Americans indulged in a new medium for pop culture consumption: television. In homes across America, middle-class families gathered in their living rooms to watch shows like *The Honeymooners* (1955–1956) and *I Love Lucy* (1951–1957). It was during this 'Golden Age of Television' that the genre of the western found a new home and newfound relevancy as Americans grappled with post-war gender realignment and heightened fears over communism. Historian Richard Aquila (2015: 166) argues that although most westerns produced during this period relied on images of the 'mythic West' and 'conventional heroes' to promote conformity, others used this same genre to explore the anxiety inherent in changing times. The tension between conformity and change is evident in the mid-century western's depiction of women. Television writers mostly restricted its female characters to either 'civilising' roles – wife, mother, or schoolteacher – or women in need of rescue or redemption (Coyne, 2008: 4; Schackel, 1987). The character of the woman physician was often written as both. She was a symbol of modernity, yet deeply timid and sometimes disgusted by the incivility of the Wild West. Unlike in the silent film era, she was unthreatening, politically or sexually. Instead, writers portrayed her as either a reluctant helpmate to the male protagonist or an unassuming but skilled physician.

One of the first TV westerns to feature a woman physician was *Tales of Wells Fargo* (1957–1962) starring Dale Robertson as Jim Hardie. In the 1958 episode, 'Dr. Alice', Hardie finds himself sharing a stagecoach with Dr Alice MacCauley (Diane Brewster). Recently widowed, Dr Alice is on her way to the train station to return to Boston. She tells Hardie: 'I'll be glad to see the end of this country. Indians, outlaws, drunks, gamblers, and dance hall girls.' Hardie asks her to reconsider: 'We need doctors – more so than back east.' She replies that she's no doctor, just 'an expert at tending to gunshot wounds, stitching up knife wounds, and saving the life of worthless murderers'. She informs Hardie she is returning to Boston and does not want to hear about the frontier ever again. In the course of their stagecoach ride, a robbery occurs, a bandit is shot, and Dr Alice refuses to provide medical care to the wounded. Hardie, who acts as narrator of the show, confides to the audience: 'I've never felt so sorry for someone. She was neglecting her oath – when she spoke, she didn't sound like a doctor – she sounded like a frightened woman.' The episode concludes with Hardie convincing the young doctor that she has a moral obligation to treat the people who need her. In a short time, she ends up delivering a baby and saving a man's life. She tells Hardie, 'I've changed my mind – there *is* a need for me in the West.'

'A Taste of Poison', the 1965 episode of the TV western *Branded* (1956–1966), follows a similar arc. Jason McCord (Chuck Connors) is escorting Dr Evelyn Cole (Carol Eve Rossen) to a medical outpost in the desert when they come upon an overturned wagon. After searching the area, they find dehydrated and sun-scorched survivors near an abandoned well. They tell McCord that they cannot drink the water because they fear the Apache men who attacked them may have poisoned the well. McCord directs Dr Cole in how to triage the injured and eventually solves the mystery of the 'poisoned' well. In this episode, Dr Cole is a non-entity, a figure who only provides medical care at the direction of the male protagonist. In both 'Dr. Alice' and 'A Taste of Poison', the writers depict women physicians as frightened practitioners on a hostile frontier – bystanders in a male hero's narrative. Both episodes highlight the need for doctors in the region – a justification for why women physicians are tacitly accepted in the Wild West – but the characters are passive agents of modernity and need the hero's help to acclimate to the violence of the region.

Another common trope in mid-century westerns is that of the woman doctor who proves her worth. In a 1961 episode of *Frontier Circus* (1961–1962) called 'Dr. Sam', the travelling circus hires a doctor named Sam Applewhite (Irene Dunne). When Dr Sam shows up for duty, they discover that she is, in fact, Dr Samantha Applewhite, and the manager threatens to fire her. When one of the performers cracks her skull in a trapeze accident, however, Dr Sam demonstrates her skill by performing emergency surgery on the woman. The 1970 episode of *Gunsmoke* (1955–1975), 'Sam McTavish, M.D.' follows a similar plotline, even using the 'Sam/Samantha' name swap. When Doc Adams (Milburn Stone) has to travel out of town, he sends for a temporary replacement. Of course, Dr Sam McTavish (Vera Miles) turns out to be a woman. The townspeople are sceptical of her abilities but over time, they realise that Dr McTavish can handle even the most difficult patients with ease.

Although mid-century TV westerns share similarities with their silent film predecessors, their differences demonstrate a changing cultural perception of gender. Both position the woman physician as an anomaly and an outsider. In silent films, she is often a sexualised curiosity, while in mid-century westerns, she is largely de-sexed and met with scepticism and hostility. In both genres, the woman physician eventually finds acceptance in her new town. In early films, this acceptance is accomplished through courtship. In TV westerns, it is through proving her medical mettle. There are, however, significant differences. In silent films, the woman physician is always the central character. She is sexualised for comedy's sake but is also emblematic of the Progressive Era's new woman; she is empowered by new political and professional avenues once closed to her. In contrast, the mid-century version of the western woman physician is never the lead character. She merely plays a guest role in a male-centred envisioning of the western frontier. The shift in focus mirrors much of the cultural representations of gender relationships in the aftermath of World War II. Following the war, middle-class (white) women who worked outside the home as part of the war effort forfeited their jobs to returning soldiers (Coontz, 1993). Because emphasis on the male worker dominated cultural discourse, working women became de-emphasised characters in the media.

Silent film and television depictions of western women physicians ultimately failed to capture their political potential the way that feminist fiction writers of the Progressive Era imagined them. In both cases, western women physicians were largely stripped of their political and moral voices and reimagined through the male gaze. The first-wave feminist vision of the woman physician – the one that Charlotte Perkins Gilman wrote about – would not rematerialise until the 1990s, when CBS greenlit a new show about a lady doctor in the small frontier town of Colorado Springs.

Dr Quinn, feminist physician?

The woman physician in the American West is perhaps best epitomised by Dr Michaela Quinn from the 1990s television show, *Dr. Quinn, Medicine Woman*. How did the female frontier physician regain her cultural capital and political significance by the end of the twentieth century? The answer partly lies in the rise of women's history in the 1970s and 1980s, when historians began excavating the history of women physicians in the United States. *Sympathy and Science: Women Physicians in American Medicine* (1985) by historian Regina Morantz-Sanchez was one of the first monographs to emerge from this new avenue of inquiry. In this ground-breaking study, Morantz-Sanchez examines women's roles as healers in early America, then traces their efforts to gain access to medical schools during the nineteenth century. Following Morantz-Sanchez's lead, more historians began exploring the role of women physicians at the turn of the century and beyond. More than just an 'add women and stir' approach to history, these studies demonstrated that women physicians played a critical role in the evolution of modern medicine (Luchetti, 1998; Bonner, 1995; Bittel, 2009; Wells, 2001).

Just as women's historians created scholarly studies of female physicians, trade press biographies of western women physicians began appearing in bookstores across America. In the 1991 biography *Doc Susie*, author Virginia Cornwell recounts the arduous adventures of Susan Anderson, an 1897 graduate of the University of Michigan Medical School who immigrated to Colorado to practice medicine. In the edited volume, *Women Who Made the West* (1980), two chapters are devoted to 'pioneering' women physicians; Judy Skalla examines the life of Dr Ellis Reynolds Shipp in Utah, while Judy Alter explores the Oregon career of Dr Georgia Arbuckle. These popular press accounts follow roughly the same plotline, weaving tales of lone women migrating west, overcoming sexism, and civilising the frontier through medical care. These biographies are significant because they became influential in the eventual creation of *Dr. Quinn, Medicine Woman*. The creator and executive producer of the show, Beth Sullivan, used several of these books to create a composite character in Dr Michaela Quinn (Schwartzbaum, 1994; Jennings, n.d.)

Debuting in 1993, the pilot episode begins in Boston, Massachusetts. When Michaela Quinn's physician father passes away, he leaves his practice to his daughter, a recent graduate of Woman's Medical College of Pennsylvania. When her father's clients refuse to patronise a woman doctor, she decides to relocate her practice to the small town of Colorado Springs, Colorado. Upon arrival, Dr Quinn meets Byron Sully (Joe Lando), a local mountain man, and makes friends with the town midwife, Charlotte (Diane Ladd). After Charlotte is bitten by a rattlesnake and dies, Dr Quinn takes in her three children. The premise of the show established, subsequent episodes focus on the physician adapting to her new life in a frontier town and convincing the townspeople that a woman doctor can successfully practise medicine (see Figure 5.1).

Although created for a 1990s audience, *Dr. Quinn* borrows from the same romance tropes that silent filmmakers embraced at the turn of the century. The series follows several character romances, but at the heart of the show is the budding relationship between Sully and Michaela Quinn. Sully embodies the 'classic' romance hero; he is the strong, silent type with long, golden tresses and a knack for appearing out of nowhere when our female

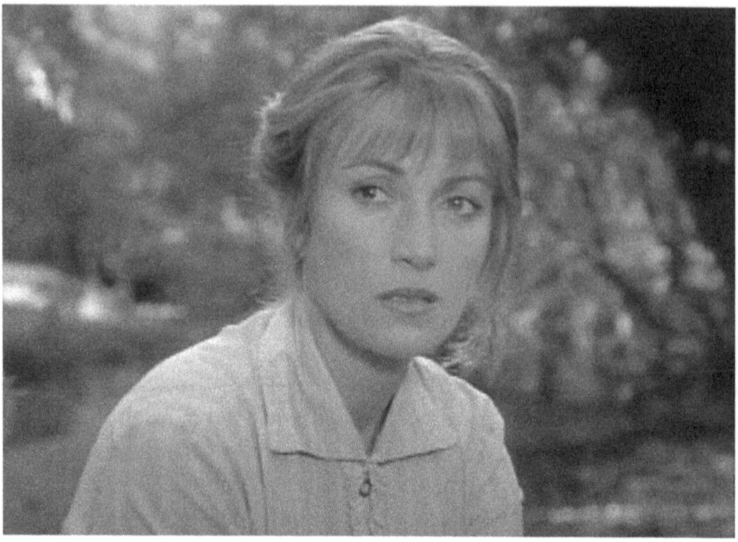

Figure 5.1 Jane Seymour as Dr Michaela Quinn (*Dr. Quinn, Medicine Woman*)

protagonist needs rescuing (White, 2001: 46–47; see Figure 5.2). Their romance is also a Turnerian exploration of the frontier tension between 'civilisation' and wilderness. Sully is a rough-and-tumble mountain man who lives part-time with the Cheyenne, while Dr Quinn is a thirty-five-year-old virgin who must learn to eschew conventional femininity and adapt to the flexible gender roles demanded of women in the 'Wild West'. The match is straight out of a romance novel, yet the show subverts this trope in one important way: Dr Quinn is also a progressive physician who often guides her community through medical, social, and political difficulties (White, 2001: 52).

Despite her leadership role, the series makes clear that Michaela Quinn prioritises family over all else. In the opening credits, the physician narrates: 'I was told a woman doctor couldn't survive alone on the frontier. But I won't give up – and I'm not alone anymore. I've inherited a family, and that may be the biggest challenge of all.' Over the course of its run, the series increasingly focuses on Dr Quinn's attempts to balance career and motherhood. A seemingly modern dilemma (although many women doctors at the turn of the century were married with children), the focus on career/family tensions is another example of how the western genre often reflects contemporary gender anxieties. Just as early-twentieth-century westerns portrayed the sexual tensions over women entering the workforce and mid-century westerns embraced a post-war return to traditional masculinity, *Dr. Quinn, Medicine Woman* grappled with the late-twentieth-century quandary: 'Can women have it all?'

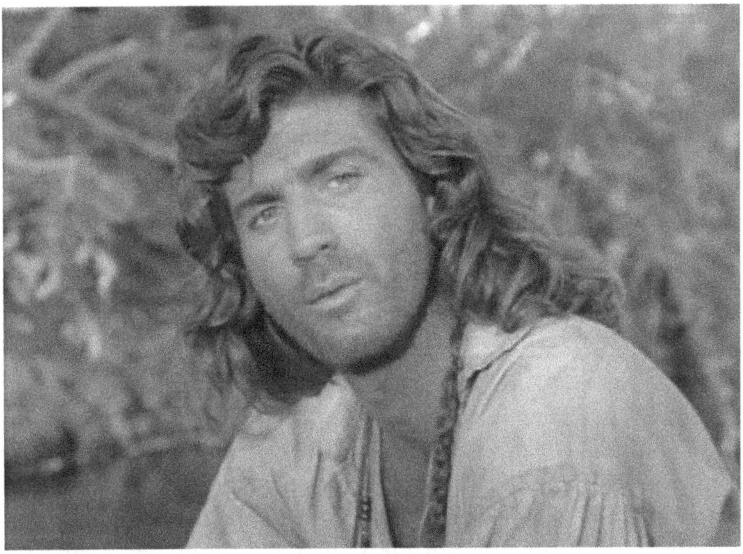

Figure 5.2 Joe Lando as Byron Sully (*Dr. Quinn, Medicine Woman*)

Dr Quinn's struggle to balance career and family is a decidedly 1990s commentary on gender roles, yet its emphasis on women in the public sphere is rooted in a first-wave feminist ethos. As with its feminist predecessors, the show uses the character of the woman physician as a vehicle of progressivism – teaching morals, character, and modernity. Using historical touchstones such as the Civil War, westward expansion, and immigration restriction, *Dr. Quinn* regularly engaged with contemporary concerns such as environmentalism, mental health, racism, and women's rights. The creators of the show populated the town with plenty of recurring characters with whom the show could explore these issues: Loren Bray (Orson Bean), the racist merchant; Hank (William Shockley), the misogynist brothel owner; Jake (Jim Knobeloch), the alcoholic; and Reverend Johnson (Geoffrey Lower), a minister reluctant to embrace progressive ideas. The do-gooder ethos of Dr Quinn did not escape criticism when the show debuted (White, 2001: 47). One TV critic called Dr Quinn a 'politically correct frontier feminist' (Duffy, 1993), while another called the show 'frontier hooey' (Shales, 1993), and *Entertainment Weekly* deemed it a 'feminist western' that 'brought a feminist agenda to the classic Hollywood interplay between cowboys and Indians' (Dow, 1993: 164–165). Despite the disdain of critics, millions of Americans tuned in every Saturday night. At its height in popularity, the show averaged 13.46 million viewers per episode, and it was the forty-ninth most-watched show in America (Brooks and Marsh, 2007).

The appeal of *Dr. Quinn* was due, in part, to what its critics hated the most about it – its embrace of maternal feminism. The show's premise hinged on the idea that women are inherently nurturers and therefore make for compassionate physicians. Michaela Quinn succeeds at both doctoring and taming the frontier because of her special abilities as a woman. This plot device may have irked critics as ahistorical but is in fact reminiscent of first-wave maternal feminism, which argued that women should be allowed into the public sphere precisely because their moral nature could improve society. This argument was also made by women physicians in their fight to enter the profession. Elizabeth Blackwell, for example, argued that women were better suited than men to be family physicians and obstetricians because they possessed the virtues of female sentiment (Morantz-Sanchez, 1995: 196). When Gilman wrote about enfranchised western women doctors and their public health advocacy, she was articulating a vision of medical housekeeping shared by her physician contemporaries. *Dr. Quinn*'s popularity could be partly attributed to a nostalgia for maternal feminism, mixed with more contemporary ideas of womanhood. As media scholar Bonnie Dow argues, by mixing modern and historical concepts of maternalism and feminism, the show creates a sort of utopian feminist western. Indeed, *Dr. Quinn* has none of the violence that characterises past westerns and instead 'threats to the town are internal, and they are transformed, by Dr Quinn's maternal logic' (Dow, 179). Furthermore, because there is no sheriff in town, Dr Quinn's authority is rarely challenged.

Dr. Quinn also appealed to 1990s America for its emphasis on a multicultural West. Jane Seymour, the British actress who played Dr Quinn, emphasised this perspective when reflecting on the show in 2018: 'It's a great way of teaching ... different cultures ... [*Dr. Quinn*] was all about people, the immigration into America. ... We dealt with the Chinese, we dealt with the Jews that were coming in there ... we dealt with slavery and everything' (Smidt, 2018). In addition to the show's white characters, the series featured several characters of colour, including Robert E. (Henry G. Sanders), a blacksmith and former slave; his wife, Grace (Jonelle Allen); and members of the Cheyenne, who live on a nearby reservation. *Dr. Quinn* differed from past westerns that used characters of colour as 'problem[s] to be solved' (Dow, 1996: 175–176). Instead, the show's use of recurring characters of colour provided the physician with a 'ready-made constituency to champion' (Dow, 1996: 175–176). Yet, like much of white feminism of the 1990s, *Dr. Quinn* places its protagonist at the centre of racial conflict, creating a white saviour feel-good narrative for its mostly white audience.

In season two, for example, the writers position Dr Quinn in direct opposition to a white supremacist organisation. In the episode entitled 'The First Circle', Denver banker Jedediah Bancroft (George Further) returns to

Colorado Springs to sell newly constructed homes. When Robert E. accepts the winning bid on one of the homes, Bancroft recruits men of the town into the Ku Klux Klan to terrorise Robert into abandoning his new property. Dr Quinn, incensed by the turn of events, takes a stand against the organisation. In retaliation, the KKK engages in a cross burning in front of Robert's new home. The show culminates in an emotional lecture from Dr Quinn, as she implores the townspeople to reject the KKK, to reject racism, and to welcome Robert and his family into the community. The episode ends with the Klan disbanding and Bancroft leaving town in disgrace.

Aside from the obvious anachronism (the Klan did not surface in the West until the 1920s), Dr Quinn's one-woman fight against white supremacy elides an unsettling truth – most real women physicians during this period endorsed ideas of scientific racism, and used their medical authority to discriminate against minority communities in the region. This is especially true in Colorado, the setting of *Dr. Quinn*, where many women physicians were supporters or members of the KKK. One such physician, Dr Minnie Love, became a leader in the Denver KKK and was elected to Colorado's General Assembly on a Klan-endorsed ticket in 1925. During her time in office, she worked to pass eugenic sterilisation laws, wrote anti-Catholic legislation, and attempted to install Klan members into the state's public health organisations (Antonovich, 2018). The real-life women physicians who populated the towns and cities of Colorado at the turn of the century would not have fought against Jedediah Bancroft's campaign of racial terror. In all likelihood, they would have endorsed it. It is also important to note that the feminist writers who first fictionalised the western woman physician would have also endorsed the medical politics of women like Dr Love. Although Charlotte Perkins Gilman believed western women physicians were the ideal candidates to spread the gospel of progressivism, this ideology also included scientific racism and anti-immigrant sentiment (Rensing, 2006). This relationship between progressivism and racism reveals the Janus-faced ideology of maternalism that underlines *Dr. Quinn*: white women's right to participate in the public sphere and their desire to police marginalised communities. The ultimate anachronism of *Dr. Quinn, Medicine Woman* is its refusal to engage with the racism that dominated the medical world during this period – a philosophy that was embraced by many, if not most women physicians in the region.

Conclusion

Dr Quinn, Medicine Woman aired its last episode on 16 May 1998. Since then, the woman physician on the frontier has all but disappeared from our cultural imaginations. Although westerns have made a comeback in film and television recently, the character of the woman physician is nowhere to be found. It's possible that *Dr. Quinn* has become so ingrained into American culture that any reference to a woman doctor on the western frontier risks parody. One medium where western women physicians are still present is in the genre of historical romance novels. Books such as *Sawbones* by Melissa Lenhardt (2017) or *Hearts Aglow* by Tracie Peterson (2011) depict women physicians in the Wild West and their adventures in finding love with rugged frontiersmen. These romance novels, not unlike their silent film predecessors, focus on love and sex, but are reimagined through the female gaze.

The enduring legacy of the fictionalised woman physician on the frontier, however, is significant for a few reasons. Scholars have rightly pointed out that since men have predominately written for the western genre, women's roles tend to reflect the male gaze. Women characters were (and are) often written as feminine, passive, and dependent on men to protect them from the violence of the frontier. As scholar Michael Coyne argues, 'the genre predominantly marginalized women from the outset' (Conye, 1998). And yet, as this chapter has demonstrated, the character of the western woman physician complicates this narrative, especially when envisioned by women. Western women doctors occupied a unique station in turn-of-the-century America because of profession and geography, and therefore became vehicles for exploring contested sex and gender roles throughout the twentieth century. To early feminist writers, they were active agents of reform, especially where laws concerning women and children were concerned. If feminists saw women physicians as the vanguard for new womanhood, male silent film producers saw a sexual threat in that status. Early westerns depicting lone women doctors on a male-centric frontier used them as comic plot points to explore gender and sex subversion.

By mid-century, the woman physician on the frontier had been relegated to a guest character. Following World War II, TV westerns became platforms for exploring masculinity, violence, and changing political and cultural climates. With constructions of new womanhood no longer a concern, women physicians appeared only as minor characters in several westerns of the time period, appearing only once to aid the main character or to teach the town a moral lesson. It would not be until the 1990s, with *Dr. Quinn, Medicine Woman*, that the political physician returned. The show, created by a woman producer, was inspired by the numerous women-authored biographies of real-life women physicians. Although these biographies served to recover a 'lost' history of women in the American West, their simplistic framework often neglected a more complicated story. Most importantly, these pioneer histories, and *Dr. Quinn* by extension, omit the ways in which mostly white, middle-class women used their medical authority and political power to shape the public health landscape of the region based on prevailing scientific ideologies of race.

That westerns on television and in film also failed to capture these nuances is not surprising. The genre largely succeeds because it simultaneously allows viewers an escape from the complexity of modern life by returning to a 'simpler time', while also constructing contemporary conflicts in a historical context, allowing for exploration from a safe historical distance. This is what made *Dr. Quinn, Medicine Woman* so appealing to the American public. The show was successful precisely because it became a canvas on which to explore contemporary issues of multiculturalism and maternal feminism, without acknowledging the real-life roles women physicians played in perpetuating racism and settler-colonialism through scientific medicine.

References

Alter, J. (1980). 'Pioneer doctor' in Western Writers of America, *The women who made the West*. Garden City, NY: Doubleday.

Antonovich, J.D. (2018). *Medical frontiers: women physicians and the politics and practice of medicine in the American West, 1870–1930*, PhD thesis, University of Michigan.

Aquila, R. (2015). *The Sagebrush Trail: western movies and twentieth-century America*. Tucson, AZ: University of Arizona Press.

'Aurora' (1910). *The Junction City Daily*, 28 June, p. 2.

Bardes, B. and Gossett, S. (1990). *Declarations of independence: women and political power in nineteenth-century American fiction*. New Brunswick, NJ: Rutgers University Press.

Bittel, C.J. (2009). *Mary Putnam Jacobi and the politics of medicine in nineteenth-century America, Studies in Social Medicine*. Chapel Hill, NC: University of North Carolina Press.

Bonner, N. (1995). *To the ends of the earth: women's search for education in medicine*. Cambridge, MA: Harvard University Press.

Brauer, R. (1975). *The horse, the gun and the piece of property: changing the images of the TV western*. Bowling Green, OH: Popular Press.

Brooks, T. and Marsh, E. (2007). *The complete directory to prime time network and cable tv shows, 1946–present*. New York: Ballantine Books.

Cawelti, J.G. (1971). *The six-gun mystique*. Bowling Green, OH: Popular Press.

Coontz, S. (1993). *The way we never were American families and the nostalgia trap*. New York: Basic Books.

Cornell, V. (1991). *Doc Susie: the true story of a country physician in the Colorado Rockies*. Carpinteria, CA: Manifest Publications.

Coyne, M. (2008). *The crowded prairie: American national identity in the Hollywood western*. London: Tauris.

Dans, P.E. (2000). *Doctors in the movies: boil the water and just say 'aah'*. Bloomington, IN: Medi-Ed Press.

Davis, R.H. (1874). *Kitty's choice: a story of Berrytown*. Philadelphia, PA: J.B. Lippincott & Co.

Dow, B.J. (1996). *Prime-time feminism: television, media culture, and the women's movement since 1970*. Philadelphia, PA: University of Pennsylvania Press.

Duffy, M. (1993). 'Dr. Quinn: A terminal case of Goofy', *Baltimore Sun*, 1 January.

'Essamay notes' (1910). *Views and Film Index*.

'Essamay's stock company' (1910). *The Nickelodeon*, July-December.

Friedl, B. (1987). *On to victory: propaganda plays of the woman suffrage movement*. Boston, MA: Northeastern University Press.

Frontier Circus (1961–1962). CBS.

Gilman, C.P. (1911a). *The Crux*. New York: Charlton Company.

Gilman, C.P. (1911b). 'Something to vote for: a one-act play', *The Forerunner* 2 (6), pp. 143–153.

Harrison, L.R. (1916). 'The woman in politics', *The Moving Picture World* 27, 1916.

Jennings, D. (nd). 'Letters to the Editor', *Official Dr. Quinn Medicine Woman Website*. Available at www.drquinnmd.com/faq.html (accessed 9 October 2019).

Jewett, S. (1884). *A country doctor*. Boston, MA: Houghton Mifflin Co.

Lenhardt, M. (2017). *Sawbones*. New York: Hachette Book Group.

Leonard, S. and Noel, T. (1990). *Denver: mining camp to metropolis*. Niwot, CO: University Press of Colorado.

Long, R. (1917). 'The evil eye', *Photoplay*, February–September, pp. 129–132.

Luchetti, C. (1998). *Medicine women: the story of early-American women doctors*. New York: Crown Publishers.

'Lyceum Theater' (1910). *The Dayton Herald*, 25 July, p. 12.

Mead, R.J. (2004). *How the vote was won: woman suffrage in the western United States, 1868–1914*. New York: New York University Press.

Meyer, A.N. (1892). *Helen Brent, M.D.: a social study*. New York: Cassell Publishing Co.

Morantz-Sanchez, R. (1985). *Sympathy and science: women physicians in American medicine*. Chapel Hill, NC: University of North Carolina Press.

More, E.S. (1999). *Restoring the balance: women physicians and the profession of medicine, 1850–1995*. Boston, MA: Harvard University Press.

Peterson, T. (2011). *Heats aglow (striking a match)*. Bloomington, MN: Bethany House Publishing.

Pierce, D. (2013). *The survival of American silent films: 1912–1929*. Washington D.C.: Council on Library and Information Resources and the Library of Congress.

Rensing, S. (2006). *Feminist eugenics in America: from free love to birth control, 1880–1930*, PhD thesis, University of Minnesota.

Schackel, K. (1987). 'Women in western films: the civilizer, the saloon singer, and their modern sister' in McDonald, A. (ed), *Shooting stars: heroes and heroines of western film*. Bloomington, IN: Indiana University Press.

Schwarzbaum, L. (1994). 'TV critics get "Dr. Quinn" wrong', *Entertainment Weekly*, 8 April.

Shah, N. (2001). *Contagious divides: epidemics and race in San Francisco's Chinatown*. Berkeley, CA: University of California Press.

Shales, T. (1993). 'TV preview', *Washington Post*, 1 January

Skalla, J. (1980). 'Beloved healer' in Western Writers of America, *The women who made the West*. Garden City, NY: Doubleday.

Slotkin, R. (1992). *Gunfighter nation: the myth of the frontier in twentieth-century America*. Norman, OK: University of Oklahoma Press.

Smidt, R. (2018). 'Jane Seymour says "Dr. Quinn, Medicine Woman" should be rebooted', *Buzzfeed News*, 5 August. Available at www.buzzfeednews.com/article/remysmidt/jane-seymour-dr-quinn-reboot-profile (accessed 5 October 2019).

'The lyric' (1910). *Fort Wayne Daily News*, 15 July, p. 16.

'The woman physician finds herself' (1919). *Suffragist* 6 (50), 4 January, p. 256.

Tompkins, J. (1992). *West of everything: the inner life of westerns*. New York: Oxford University Press.

Wells, S. (2001). *Out of the dead house: nineteenth-century women physicians and the writing of medicine*. Madison, WI: University of Wisconsin Press, 2001.

'What does the franchise mean to women physicians?' (1912). *The Woman's Medical Journal* 22, pp. 91–92.

White, M. (2001). 'Masculinity and femininity in television's historical fictions: *Young Indiana Jones Chronicles* and Dr. Quinn, Medicine Woman' in Edgerton, G. and Rollins, P. (eds), *Television histories: shaping collective memory in the media age*. Lexington, KY: University Press of Kentucky.

6

The Black doctor on the historical small screen: African American physicians in television period dramas

Kevin McQueeney

Introduction

Starting with NBC's smash hit *E.R.* (1994–2009), American medical dramas have become a staple of television, attracting millions of viewers with their medical emergency tales mixed with the personal lives of the ensemble characters. Many of these shows have featured African American doctors as significant characters. The inclusion of African American doctors in medical dramas mirrors larger trends in the presence of Black Americans on television. Scholars have found that in general, ethnic minorities are severely underrepresented in US television shows, and ethnic minority characters are often portrayed in stereotypical ways. In television's early decades, this held true for African Americans. However, beginning in the 1980s, African American characters began appearing in increasing numbers, and in more complex roles (Atkins, 1992; Baptista-Fernandez and Greenberg, 1990; Warren, 1988). Previously predominantly playing blue-collar workers, African American professionals began appearing on television in the 1980s, including Black doctors like Denzel Washington's breakthrough role as Dr Phillip Chandler on NBC's *St. Elsewhere* (1982–1988) and Bill Cosby as Dr Cliff Huxtable in the ground-breaking NBC-produced sitcom *The Cosby Show* (1984–1992). In twenty-first-century shows, African American characters appear in numbers that mirror the overall percentage of the total population, although they are primarily found on all-Black sitcoms, or in supporting roles on crime and medical dramas (Tukachinsky, Mastro, and Yarchi, 2015).

Similarly, African American characters less frequently portray negative racial stereotypes than in past decades, although anti-Black messages persist (Greenberg et al., 2002). Studies have found that depictions of ethnic and racial stereotypes on television shows help to shape viewers' racial and ethnic attitudes and beliefs, particularly among those with less exposure to racial or ethnic minority groups (Entman, 1994; Fujioka, 1999; Martin,

2008; Mastro, 2009). Negative portrayals of African Americans on television can lead to negative perceptions of African Americans in real life, among white and Black viewers (Ford, 1997).

Some African American characters represent less sinister, but still stereotypical images. For example, many of the Black doctors on medical dramas have often personified a particular trope of the Black professional, as identified by sociologist Herman Gray: the ethos of individual achievement (Gray, 1996). The characters – almost all men – are often depicted as brilliant, singularly focused, and ambitious, with others potentially viewing them as arrogant, and achieving success through their hard work and struggle as an individual.

Beyond partially shaping viewers' conceptions of race and ethnicity in contemporary America, television shows also help to shape their views of the past (Spigel, 1996). While many critics are wary of the historical accuracy of television or movies, historical dramas have proliferated in recent years and are significant sources for learning about American history (Rosenzweig and Thelen, 1998: 98). In the past decade, growing numbers of period dramas have focused on African Americans, with many focused on slavery, as seen in shows like *Underground* (2016) and the remake of *Roots* (2016), and in movies including *12 Years a Slave* (2013), *The Birth of a Nation* (2016), and *Harriet* (2019). As noted by historian Manisha Sinha, the rise in the number of these works, and television and cinema's increasing willingness to present more nuanced and less stereotyped depictions of slavery, potentially will help to counter 'entrenched myths and misconceptions' (Sinha, 2017: 20).

This chapter looks at American period dramas' portrayal of Black physicians on five shows: CBS's *M*A*S*H** (1972–1983), focused on a mobile army medical unit during the Korean War; BBC America's *Copper* (2012–2013), which follows a police officer and his group of friends in the Five Points neighbourhood of Civil War-era New York City; Showtime's *Masters of Sex* (2013–2016), which explores the work on human sexuality by Dr William Masters and Virginia Johnson in the 1950s and 1960s; Cinemax's *The Knick* (2014–2015), which examines the Knickerbocker Hospital in turn-of-the-twentieth-century New York City; and PBS's *Mercy Street* (2016–2017), which details the lives of individuals connected to a Union hospital in Civil War Alexandria, Virginia. This chapter examines how these shows have depicted African American doctors: whether these characters are historically accurate; whether they are nuanced or stereotypical; and how they have contributed to or helped to challenged entrenched historical myths and misconceptions of Black doctors. In other words, what would a viewer learn about the historical role of Black doctors by watching these shows?

Historical accuracy

*M*A*S*H** provides a key starting point to an analysis of the depiction of Black doctors in historical dramas. *M*A*S*H** focused primarily on the members of one of the doctors' residential tents known as 'the Swamp', Benjamin Franklin 'Hawkeye' Pierce (Alan Alda) and 'Trapper' John McIntyre (Wayne Rogers). In the first six episodes, the show also featured African American surgeon Oliver Harmon 'Spearchucker' Jones (Timothy Brown), the only Black doctor in the show's eleven-year run. In his appearances, Jones was largely a supporting character to the hijinks of Hawkeye and Trapper. His most significant role occurs in episode five, in which Trapper and Hawkeye rescue a South Korean girl, Young Hi (Virginia Lee), purchased by an American soldier for use as his personal servant; Hawkeye also challenges the soldier for using a racial slur when referring to South Koreans. Along with Trapper and Hawkeye, Jones helps to teach Young Hi lessons on self-worth and freedom. In one scene, Jones tells Young Hi to look people in the eye when she meets them and that all people are the same. This episode marks the show's first attempt to address more serious issues like racism, which increasingly happens in later seasons. However, Jones would not play a role in these events, as the producers dropped the character after the sixth episode.

For years, rumours abounded over the removal of Jones. Some suggested the producers dropped Jones from the already crowded cast to devote even greater attention to Hawkeye and Trapper. Others believed that producers removed Jones due to controversy over his nickname 'Spearchucker', an ethnic slur for people of African descent; the character in the novel and the movie the show was based on told Hawkeye and Trapper it came from his prowess in throwing the javelin. Finally, in the late 1990s in two posts on an online *M*A*S*H** fan forum, creator and producer Larry Gelbart informed fans that the showrunners removed Jones to reflect historical reality, in this case, the mistaken belief that African Americans did not work as MASH (mobile army surgical hospital) doctors in the conflict: 'Extensive research indicated there were no black surgeons in MASH units in Korea', Gelbart stated. 'We were not interested in empty tokenism' (Gelbart, 1998). The producers of *M*A*S*H** attempted throughout the series run to maintain historical accuracy, with show personnel conducting historical research and interviewing MASH veterans. When they discovered that no Black doctors had served in MASH units during the war, they dropped Jones. However, scholars later disproved this notion. In a 2012 article published in the *Journal of the National Medical Association*, physicians detailed the experiences of Alvin Vincent Blount, Jr, who in 1951 became the first African American to serve in an integrated MASH unit. It is probable that others served as well (Wilson et al., 2012).

While *M*A*S*H** premiered four decades before the other shows analysed in this work, the decision to remove Jones and other attributes of the character reveal many of the patterns seen in the depiction of Black doctors in later historical dramas. First, with some exceptions, the shows are mostly historically accurate and reflect scholarship on the history of Black medical professionals. Historians have disproved the prevalent belief of the time period of the absence of Black doctors that led to the removal of the Jones character in *M*A*S*H**. African Americans have served as physicians and surgeons since at least the late eighteenth century, and the shows in this chapter feature Black doctors. In fact, the writers and actors based the characters either directly on historical figures, or as representative of a composite of Black physicians in the period.

For example, the character Samuel Diggs (McKinley Belcher III), is a volunteer at the Mansion House Hospital in *Mercy Street*. A free person of colour who learned medical skills from a physician for whom his parents laboured as servants in Philadelphia, Diggs hopes to go to medical school and become a doctor. Diggs tells a class of Black children that his role model is Dr David Peck. Peck became the first African American to receive a medical degree from an American medical school – Rush Medical College in 1847 – and then established a practice in Philadelphia (Harris, 1996). Diggs also functions as a proxy for Black physicians who served during the Civil War. Historians have documented thirteen such individuals, three of whom were commissioned officers, and ten of whom were contracted as assistant surgeons. Of the thirteen, seven worked at Freedmen's Hospitals, institutions established to provide care for Black soldiers and refugees (NIH, 2013). Thus, while Diggs is not directly modelled after a singular historical figure, his role as an aspiring Black doctor is based on historical precedent.

Similarly, on *Copper*, Matthew Freeman (Atto Essandoh) is a formerly enslaved African American who learned medical skills from an army physician during his service in the Civil War and later apprenticed under a white doctor in New York City. The producers' decisions to have both the Diggs and Freeman characters learn medicine informally matches the experience of most Black doctors in the period; by 1865, only twenty-three African Americans had medical degrees from American medical schools (NIH, 2013). Although Freeman is an amalgamation of several Black physicians who practised in New York City, in multiple interviews actor Atto Essandoh stated that he based his character loosely on one such individual, James McCune Smith, the first African American to earn a medical degree, from Glasgow University in 1837 (Wagner, 2013; Morgan, 2003).

The Knick is set four decades after *Mercy Street* and *Copper*, and unlike the previous two characters, its Dr Algernon Edwards (André Holland) has a medical degree, having graduated from Harvard University, and previously

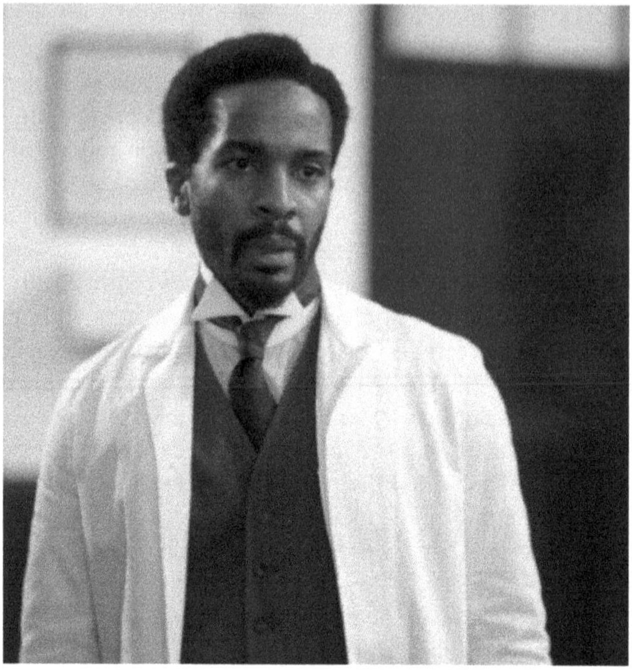

Figure 6.1 Dr Algernon Edwards (portrayed by André Holland) on Cinemax's *The Knick*

worked at hospitals in Europe. This attribute is based on historical precedent: Richard Greener became the first Harvard Medical School graduate in 1870, and many African American physicians, initially unable to gain post-graduate training or employment at a hospital in the US, worked first in Europe. Nevertheless, the show takes some notable historical liberties. In the show, Edwards works at the Knickerbocker Hospital, based on the real Harlem Hospital, although producers moved the hospital's location from Harlem to Manhattan, and changed the clientele from mostly Black to all-white. More importantly, the first African American to gain employment in a New York City hospital, Louis Wright, did not secure his position at Harlem Hospital until 1920; in the show, Edwards starts working at the hospital in 1900 (O'Shea, 2005; see Figure 6.1).

Finally, in *Masters of Sex*, Dr Charles Hendricks (Courtney B. Vance) runs Buell Green Hospital and briefly supervises the pioneering human sexuality researcher and physician Dr William Masters (Michael Sheen). Hendricks informs Masters he has hired him because Hendricks wants Masters to bring white patients to the formerly all-Black hospital. 'The hospital will be integrated', Hendricks tells Masters when the latter states he believes many of his white patients will not use the space. 'We'll move history forward',

Hendricks proclaims; a dubious Masters replies 'I'm afraid history may be outside my purview.'

The real-life Masters never worked at a Black hospital (Maier, 2009). However, Buell Green Hospital is based on St Louis's Homer G. Phillips Hospital, founded in 1937 as the city's only hospital for African American residents. In 1955, Mayor Raymond Tucker ordered the desegregation of St Louis hospitals, although most white people refused to use Homer G. Phillips, a common occurrence for many Black hospitals after federally mandated integration (Wartts, 2008). Hendricks is not based on any single historical figure but is rather a proxy for the African American doctors and activists that pushed for the integration of hospitals nationwide.

Beyond their representation of real-life pioneering Black physicians, the shows discussed accurately detail the struggles of African American doctors in gaining acceptance from white patients and peers. In *Mercy Street*, Diggs believes if he demonstrates his competence he may be able to become a doctor. He initially keeps his medical background secret, and white people take credit for his work. Even after he saves the life of a patient in the first episode, a white nurse, Mary Phinney (Mary Elizabeth Winstead), covers up his involvement from Dr Jedediah Foster (Josh Radnor), a surgeon from an enslaving family who embodies the dismissive and prejudiced views of many white people towards African Americans. When Diggs performs an operation for Foster, who is suffering from drug withdrawal, Foster is at first incredulous that an African American could possess such medical knowledge and skills. The incident helps Foster overcome some of his biased views, and he later offers to write a letter of recommendation for Diggs to attend medical school. In several episodes, Diggs tutors another white doctor who must pass a test to stay at the hospital, and he too grows to respect and support Diggs.

This arc towards acceptance stands in contrast to the real-life Dr David Peck, Diggs's self-proclaimed hero. Peck struggled to attract patients to his practice in Philadelphia and later Pittsburgh, and white physicians shunned him. Due to this professional ostracism, in 1852 Peck moved to Nicaragua, where he died during civil conflict in 1855 (Harris, 1996). Diggs is used to tell a more redemptive and rose-coloured tale of the experience of aspiring Black doctors than was often reflected in the historical record.

Freeman of *Copper* and Edwards of *The Knick* have less positive plot lines. Like Diggs, Freeman must keep his forensic aid in solving crimes secret and instead give credit to his friend, Irish American police officer Kevin Corcoran (Tom Weston-Jones). In the second season, he discovers the cure to a deadly pathogen threatening the city, but he has to let a white professor take credit. Throughout the series, Freeman faces continuous racism, and he even accuses Corcoran and his other white friends of contributing to the suppression of African Americans.

The Knick uses some of the same plot devices as *Mercy Street* and *Copper* on racism. The hospital's white chief surgeon, John Thackery (Clive Owen), initially opposes the hiring of Edwards, and refuses to work with him, as do other white doctors; many white patients also refuse to be treated by Edwards, leading him to consider quitting. Throughout the first season, Edwards faces constant snubs and prejudice, and continuously has to prove himself. Like the Diggs character in *Mercy Street*, Edwards flips the roles on white doctors with his superior medical knowledge, talking several white surgeons partially through a medical procedure on which he wrote an article, then refusing to divulge the rest unless they let him complete the operation.

Similar to the Diggs storyline, Edwards wins over Thackery by showing his medical prowess, explaining to Thackery a new medical procedure he has pioneered with equipment he created. Like Jedediah Foster in *Mercy Street*, this incident not only leads to an acceptance of Edwards – including allowing him to participate in surgeries – but a seeming overcoming of his racism. By the second season of *The Knick*, Thackery and Edwards have become allies, working together on a new experimental treatment for syphilis and drug addiction, and Thackery joining Edwards to provide care for African Americans assaulted by a mob of white people. When Thackery enters rehabilitation for drug addiction, Edwards becomes acting chief surgeon. Despite the refusal of some white doctors to work under him, Edwards expects to be named the permanent chief. However, even when he presents his positive report to the board on the improvements to the hospital under his several months of leadership, the all-white board informs Edwards that they will not consider him for the permanent position and will seek a white chief. Later, he approaches Thackery to seek his support in the hospital allowing the first surgery on a Black patient; Thackery, though, refuses, showing the limitations of his evolving views on race.

That same season, Edwards discovers that another white doctor at the hospital – Everett Gallinger (Eric Johnson) – is performing vasectomies on boys with mental development disabilities as part of the eugenics movement. When Edwards presents this information to the board, the all-white members not only express their support of eugenics, but inform Edwards that new investors – the hospital is planning to move to an uptown location, closer to wealthier patients – do not want a Black doctor on staff. The series finale offers some relief for Edwards. An inheritance from a recently deceased family friend provides Edwards with the funding to start his own drug rehabilitation clinic, but it is far from the more optimistic ending of Diggs in *Mercy Street*.

The struggles the shows depict for Black physicians is historically accurate. Most medical schools refused to admit Black students through the mid-twentieth century; many hospitals refused to hire Black doctors; and many local medical associations denied admittance to African Americans. African

Americans fortunate enough to become doctors – over 900 by the 1890s – faced many of the incidents of explicit and implicit racism from white doctors, patients, and others as those shown afflicting Diggs, Freeman, and Edwards (Ruffin, 2017).

In *Mercy Street*, *Copper*, and *The Knick*, the frustration over racism leads to angry confrontations, with negative consequences for the characters. In season one of *Mercy Street*, Diggs threatens a white man, Silas Bullen (Wade Williams), for sexually assaulting Aurelia Johnson (Shailta Grant), a black laundress and Diggs's romantic partner. Bullen frames Diggs for a crime he committed, leading to Diggs's assault and near lynching at the hand of three Union soldiers. In *Copper*, Matthew Freeman threatens a white storeowner who directed racist insults at his mother-in-law, and throws an axe through the shop window; later, the storeowner and a group of his white friends assault Freeman in retaliation. In *The Knick*, Edwards's frustration over continued racism and denial of his position as chief surgeon boils over into a bar fight, in which a white man damages his eye, ultimately limiting his abilities as a surgeon in the following episodes. In the final episode, Edwards confronts the eugenicist Everett Gallinger, who tells Edwards that the Black doctor fighting him will only prove his eugenics thesis that African Americans are 'like an animal' correct. To add literal injury to insult, Gallinger then assaults Edwards, further damaging his eye.

The symbolism of these incidents is transparent. The characters struggle with limitations imposed by a racist society. When they confront oppressors, they are subject to violence with little recourse, a sad historical reality. The everyday threats of violence African Americans faced in these periods is present in all three shows: the near lynching of Diggs; the assaults on Freeman and Edwards; and the mob violence against African Americans that leads to Thackery and Edwards working together. Of all the shows, *Copper* most explicitly details the damaging effect of this violence, both physically and psychologically. The show reveals that white people lynched the brothers of Freeman's wife Sara during the New York City draft riots of 1863. In a moving incident in season two, Matthew Freeman leads other African Americans in tearing down the lamppost from which white people hanged Sarah's brothers, a fleeting moment of catharsis. Later, the Freemans discover that Sarah is pregnant. However, even this moment of joy is tinged with bitterness: the Freemans worry about bringing a child into the world and subjecting it to the same racial prejudice and violence that caused the deaths of Sarah's brothers. Sadly, it is revealed in the second season that Sarah has miscarried. This is a particularly striking symbol of the physical manifestation of the damage of racism, particularly as Freeman is a doctor, but can do nothing to save his unborn child. Similarly, in *The Knick*, the brilliant surgeon Edwards is unable to prevent the further deterioration of his eye, not only affecting his vision, but his very livelihood and identity as a physician.

While these shows demonstrate how barriers and everyday threats of racism and violence affected Black physicians as they did most African Americans, they also address how African American experiences were far from monolithic. Diggs is a free person of colour who received professional training – albeit informal – and has the opportunity for formal higher education. It is through his work at the hospital and the relationships he develops there that he learns about the lives of enslaved people, who experienced much harsher conditions than his own. In season two, Diggs travels to the Foster family plantation and witnesses first-hand the lives of enslaved people. Diggs learns from these and other enslaved or formerly enslaved individuals, and forms friendships and even romantic relationships with formerly enslaved people.

The Freeman and Edwards characters help reveal African American class division, as well. Although Freeman was once enslaved, his position as a doctor with a private practice leads to tension with some of his patients. In season two, a Black father of a child he is treating accuses Freeman of becoming like the white people through his status as a doctor and doing their bidding. Similarly, Edwards lives in a low-quality tenement building, primarily with low-income and uneducated labourers. Some of these neighbours view Edwards as elitist due to his education and status. In season one, he attends a dinner held by his parents' wealthy employers, with his parents still working there as servants, and he as the only Black guest. In the next episode, a Cuban patient accuses Edwards of purposely using convoluted words to make him feel stupid during a procedure. Through these incidents, the shows unpack a complex issue. Freeman's and Edwards's positions as physicians provide them with a sense of pride and accomplishment. Diggs hopes one day to reach that same status. As will be discussed in further detail in the following section, many African Americans looked at Black doctors as community leaders. Yet, that same status marker, and the position of potential greater privilege and economic stability, also separated them from the experience of most African Americans. While not main plot points, these juxtapositions of using the characters to show how Black doctors were both different from and similar to other African Americans – particularly the ever-present danger of racism and violence, regardless of status – is an important historical lesson.

Historical absences

Despite their efforts to accurately portray historical figures and the difficulties faced by Black physicians, several elements are noticeably absent from the shows. First, none include Black women as doctors, and Black nurses are mostly absent. Several women feature in *Mercy Street* providing medical care, although not as doctors. Belinda Gibson (L. Scott Caldwell) is a formerly enslaved house servant who also works at the hospital and treats African Americans with herbal remedies. Gibson represents enslaved individuals who used folk remedies, herbal medicine, and spiritual healing measures, passed down from generation to generation, and often originating in Africa (Covey, 2007; Fett, 2003). Charlotte Jenkins (Patina Miller), is a formerly enslaved woman who runs the 'contraband' camp, including providing care for those afflicted by smallpox, a significant health issue for African American refugees during the war (Downs, 2012). The Jenkins character was based on Harriet Jacobs, a prominent abolitionist and advocate for the refugees – she and her daughter Louisa worked in 'contraband' camps in Alexandria and Washington and led fundraising drives for the refugees – who rose to fame with her memoir about her enslavement, hiding, and freedom. On *M*A*S*H**, Lt Ginger Bayliss (Odessa Cleveland) is a nurse who appears in twenty-two episodes.

The exclusion of Black women as physicians on these shows partially reflects historically low numbers. *Mercy Street* and *Copper* are set before or just after the first Black woman, Rebecca Lee Crumpler, earned a medical degree in 1864 (Gates and Higginbotham, 2004: 199–200). Although fewer Black women than Black men became physicians in the periods covered in the shows, the decision to focus primarily on Black male doctors reveals a willingness to address one group of outliers – the Black male pioneers – while ignoring their female counterparts. Similarly, the role of women as lay healers is only addressed in *Mercy Street*; as nurses only in *M*A*S*H**; and Black midwives are absent. The lack of African American women as medical providers in the shows reflects larger problems of the underrepresentation of Black women on television shows in general, and more specifically in professional roles (Smith-Shomade, 2002).

Second, the characters have little connection to activism. As previously mentioned, through their professional status, African American doctors became community leaders, including in the Black freedom struggle as seen in the lives of several of the historical figures that served as models for the television characters. David Peck and James McCune Smith were both prominent in the abolition movement. Smith helped found the National Council of the Colored People with Frederick Douglass and wrote the introduction to Douglass's *My Bondage and My Freedom*. Smith used his scholarship – he became the first African American published in a medical journal – to refute ideas of scientific racism. Louis Wright was a leading advocate of civil rights, joining the NAACP as a medical student, writing for *The Crisis*, pushing for the end of segregated hospitals, and serving as the chairman of the NAACP (O'Shea, 2005).

Despite this historical legacy, the shows largely downplay the activism of the characters, only hinting at their involvement in the Black freedom struggle. In *Mercy Street*, Diggs tries to help his romantic partner rescue her family from slavery, and becomes involved with a refugee camp for freed people. In season two of *The Knick*, Edwards starts to forge a connection to the Black freedom movement through a rekindling of his relationship with his estranged wife Opal Edwards (Zeeah Abrahams). Opal brings Edwards to hear a speech by D.W. Garrison Carr (Ntare Guma Mbaho Mwine) – a stand-in for civil rights leader and intellectual W.E.B. DuBois. Carr challenges his audience members to no longer accept prejudiced treatment and fight for Black equality. Edwards's increasing interest in Carr's message leads the doctor to take a more assertive stance on equality at the hospital. Carr suffers from a hernia and wishes to have Edwards operate on him at the hospital, which still bars Black patients. This leads to Edwards's unsuccessful effort to seek permission from the hospital board to allow the surgery, and in doing so integrate the hospital. Unfortunately, the show ended without returning for a third season, and this burgeoning connection to the nascent civil rights movement in the early twentieth century is never fully explored.

Masters of Sex most explicitly explores the civil rights movement through the character of Dr Charles Hendricks. Hendricks has hired William Masters to bring white patients to the Black hospital to help implement integration. Masters, however, is more interested in continuing his studies on human sexuality than in implementing integration. Masters puts up flyers at the Black hospital seeking patients for his studies. An angry Hendricks tears down the flyers and informs Masters that he does not want African Americans participating in the study due to the history of medical experimentation and exploitation, a historical reality (see Washington, 2008). Masters tries to explain – to both Hendricks and a reporter from the *St. Louis Chronicle* – that he hopes to use the study to help challenge racial stereotypes about African Americans. Ultimately, Hendricks asks Masters, unwilling to meet Hendricks's demands, to leave the hospital. While Hendricks is the character most connected to activism, he is also the least developed character. The show does not reveal much about Hendricks, and he appears only briefly in three of the show's forty-six episodes.

Thus, the role of the Black physician as an activist connected to the larger Black freedom movement largely remains on the fringe in these shows. The shows focus on the characters' individual struggles to overcome racism and gain acceptance as doctors. Further seasons of *Mercy Street* and *The Knick* may have explored connections to the collective movements for abolition and civil rights, as seemingly hinted at in the last episodes of their respective second seasons, but were never realised as their networks did not renew the shows.

Relatedly, although *Masters of Sex* briefly included Buell Green Hospital for three episodes, and Thackery and Edwards treated victims of the white mob violence at the all-Black Minetta Hospital, Black hospitals, Black medical schools, and Black patients are conspicuously absent. This latter omission is most striking in *The Knick*, which is based on a real-life hospital that predominantly served African Americans, but producers changed it to an all-white hospital which the Edwards character tries unsuccessfully to integrate. Other Black doctors are largely absent too, partially reflecting the historical dearth of Black physicians, but also based on writers' and producers' decisions about focusing on one character as the stand-in for all Black physicians in the period. The segregation of health care led African Americans to create Black medical schools, starting with Howard University in 1868; Black hospitals, starting with Chicago's Provident Hospital in 1891; and Black medical organisations like the National Medical Association in 1908. While *Mercy Street* and *Copper* are set prior to these events, *The Knick* and *Masters of Sex* – which are set in the key period from the creation of these institutions through the national health care desegregation movement – only obliquely make references without explaining the significance of places like Black hospitals. This critique is perhaps unfair, as the producers of these shows intended them to be historical dramas, not educational programmes. Still, this is a missing and significant piece of the historical experience of African American doctors.

Conclusion

The myth of the missing Black doctor that led to the removal of Oliver Jones from *M*A*S*H** has been repudiated by historical scholarship, and television historical dramas have followed suit. Shows like *Mercy Street*, *Copper*, *The Knick*, and *Masters of Sex* have all featured Black physicians.[1] These characters are largely nuanced, complex, and historically accurate. Through these characters, based on real-life figures, viewers can learn about many obstacles that African Americans faced in becoming doctors, including rejection by white peers and patients, and everyday racism and violence. The shows also detail the persistence and courage that was required to challenge these limitations and hint at their roles as community leaders and activists.

There are problems with some of the portrayals, of course. In some ways, the characters analysed in this chapter follow some of the tropes of the Black professional detailed by Herman Gray and seen in contemporary medical dramas: the exceptional, brilliant, ambitious individual achieving success through personal dedication and hard work. The characters are all men, reflective of the continued underrepresentation of Black women in television shows, particularly in professional roles. Additionally, the characters analysed in this work are primarily significant characters in an ensemble, but not the main characters in the shows, who are all white. *The Knick* is the exception, with Edwards and Thackery as co-leads. Finally, the roles of the Black doctors as leaders in the Black freedom movement is largely absent, and instead, the shows focus primarily on the characters' singular struggles against oppression.

Although most British period dramas feature white doctors, American producers can possibly look to several British shows that include people of colour as physicians and address several critiques discussed in this chapter. BBC One's *The Indian Doctor* (2010–2013) starred Sanjeev Bhaskar in the title role as Dr Prem Sharma, an Indian doctor recruited by the National Health Service to serve as a general practitioner in a small Welsh town in the 1960s. Two other shows featured Black women, albeit in supporting roles. Kananu Kirimi played Dr Joan Makori, a Nigeria-born doctor who serves as a locum (temporary) physician on the staff at St Aidan's Royal Free Hospital in the 1960s, in series five and six of ITV's *The Royal* (2003–2011). The seventh season of BBC's *Call the Midwife* (2012–) premiered the character of Lucille Anderson (played by Leonie Elliott), a Jamaica-born nurse who becomes a midwife in East London in the 1960s; similar to Dr Sharma in *The Indian Doctor*, the Anderson character represents the Caribbean nurses brought by the National Health Service to England in the 1960s. It is the author's hope that new American historical dramas follow the lead of these British shows, as well as many of the positive aspects of the series analysed in this chapter. A show centred on Dr Rebecca Lee Crumpler, the first Black woman to earn a medical degree, would, for example, provide fascinating subject matter for television. Crumpler's life as a pioneer in a field where she encountered racism and sexism, and her advocacy for the Black community for decades, is certainly deserving of greater attention and would make for a compelling show. As a historian and an avid consumer of period dramas, I look forward to seeing the future depictions of Black physicians on the American historical small screen.

Note

1 Black doctors are still missing from numerous historical dramas, particularly westerns like *Deadwood* (2004–2006), *Hell on Wheels* (2011–2016), and *Hatfields & McCoys* (2012).

References

Atkins, D. (1992). 'An Analysis of Television Series with Minority-Lead Characters', *Critical Studies in Mass Communication* 9, pp. 337–349.

Baptista-Fernandez, P. and Greenberg, B. S. (1980). 'The Content, Characteristics, and Communication Behaviors of Blacks on Television', in B. S. Greenberg (Ed.), *Life on Television: Content Analysis of U.S. TV Drama*. Norwood, NJ: Albex, pp. 13–21.

Covey, H. (2007). *African American Slave Medicine: Herbal and Non-Herbal Treatments*. Lanham, MD: Lexington Books.

Downs, J. (2012). *Sick from Freedom: African-American Illness and Suffering during the Civil War and Reconstruction*. Oxford: Oxford University Press.

Entman, R. (1994). 'Representation and Reality in the Portrayal of Blacks on Network Television News', *Journalism Quarterly* 71, pp. 509–520.

Fett, S. (2002). *Working Cures: Healing, Health, and Power on Southern Slave Plantations*. Chapel Hill, NC: University of North Carolina Press.

Ford, T. E. (1997). 'Effects of Stereotypical Television Portrayals of African Americans on Person Perception', *Social Psychology Quarterly* 60, pp. 266–278.

Fujioka, Y. (1999). 'Television Portrayals and African American Stereotypes: Examination of Television Effects When Direct Contact is Lacking', *Journalism & Mass Communication Quarterly* 76, pp. 52–75.

Gamble, V. (1995). *Making a Place for Ourselves: The Black Hospital Movement, 1920–1945*. Oxford: Oxford University Press.

Gates, H. L. and Higginbotham, E. B. (2004). *African American Lives*. Oxford: Oxford University Press.

Gelbart, L. (1998). 'Spearchucker & Klinger', alt.tv.mash, 12 July. Available at https://groups.google.com/forum/#!topic/alt.tv.mash/SWEG0NInUOg (accessed 27 July 2019).

Gray, H. (1996). 'Television, Black Americans, and the American Dream', in V. T. Berry and C. L. Manning-Miller (Eds), *Mediated Messages and African-American Culture: Contemporary Issues*. Thousand Oaks, CA: Sage Publications, pp. 131–145.

Greenberg, B. S., Mastro, D., and Brand, J. (2002). 'Minorities and the Mass Media: Television into the 21st Century', in J. Bryant and D. Zillman (Eds), *Media Effects: Advances in Theory and Research*. Hillsdale, NJ: Lawrence Erlbaum Associates, pp. 333–351.

Harris, M. (1996). 'David Jones Peck, MD: A Dream Denied', *Journal of the National Medical Association* 88 (9), pp. 600–604.

Maier, T. (2009). *Masters of Sex: The Life and Times of William Masters and Virginia Johnson, the Couple Who Taught America How to Love*. New York, Basic Books.

Martin, A. (2008). 'Television Media as a Potential Negative Factor in the Racial Identity Development of African American Youth', *Academic Psychiatry* 32, pp. 338–342.

Mastro, D. (2009). 'Effects of Racial and Ethnic Stereotyping', in J. Bryant and M. B. Oliver (Eds), *Media Effects: Advances in Theory and Research*. Hillsdale, NJ: Lawrence Erlbaum Association, pp. 325–341.

Morgan, T. (2003). 'The Education and Medical Practice of Dr. James McCune Smith (1813–1865), First Black American to Hold a Medical Degree', *Journal of the National Medical Association*, 95 (7), pp. 603–614.

National Institute of Health (2013). 'Binding Wounds Pushing Boundaries: African Americans in Civil War Medicine'. Available at www.nlm.nih.gov/exhibition/bindingwounds/exhibition.html (accessed 23 July 2019).

National Institute of Health (2003). 'Dr. Rebecca Lee Crumpler'. Available at https://cfmedicine.nlm.nih.gov/physicians/biography_73.html (accessed 23 July 2019).

O'Shea, J. S. (2005). 'Louis T. Wright and Henry W. Cave: How They Paved the Way for Fellowships for Black Surgeons', *Bulletin of the American College of Surgeons*, 90 (10), pp. 22–29.

Rosenzweig, R. and Thelen, D. (1998). *The Presence of the Past: Popular Uses of History in American Life*. New York: Columbia University Press.

Ruffin, H. (2017). 'Daniel Hale Williams'. Available at www.Blackpast.org/aah/williams-daniel-hale-1856-1931 (accessed 11 July 2019.).

Sinha, M. (1997). 'Slavery on Screen', *Dissent* 64 (2), pp. 16–20.

Smith-Shomade, B.E. (2002). *Shaded Lives: African-American Women and Television*. Piscataway, NJ: Rutgers University Press.

Spigel, L. (2001). *Welcome to the Dreamhouse: Popular Media and the Postwar Suburbs*. Durham, NC: Duke University Press.

Tukachinsky, R., Mastro, D., and Yarchi, M. (2015). 'Documenting Portrayals of Race/Ethnicity on Primetime Television over a 20-Year Span and Their Association with National-Level Racial/Ethnic Attitudes', *Journal of Social Issues* 17 (1), pp. 17–38.

Wagner, C. (2013) 'Ato Esaandoh Proud of Copper Role', *Chicago Tribune*, 7 July.

Warren, N. (1988). 'From Uncle Tom to Cliff Huxtable, Aunt Jemima to Aunt Nell: Images of Blacks in Film and the Television Industry', in J. C. Smith (Ed.), *Images of Blacks in the American Culture: A Reference Guide to Information Sources*. Westport, CT: Greenwood Press, pp. 135–165.

Wartts, A. (2008). 'Homer G. Phillips Hospital (1937–1979)'. Available at www.blackpast.org/african-american-history/homer-g-phillips-hospital-1937-1979/ (accessed 23 July 2019).

Washington, H. (2008). *Medical Apartheid: The Dark History of Medical Experimentation on Black Americans from Colonial Times to the Present*. Norwell, MA: Anchor.

Wilson, K. L., DeBeatham, W. L., Danner, O. K., Matthew, L. R., Bacon, L. N., and Weaver, W. L. (2012). 'The Forgotten MASH Surgeon: The Story of Alvin Vincent Blount Jr, MD', *Journal of the National Medical Association*, 103 (3–4), pp. 221–223.

7

When women were nurses: gender, nostalgia, and the making of historical heroines

Aeleah Soine

Introduction

In the first episode of the German television drama *Charité* (2017), two young nurses rush a patient through the corridors of the Charité hospital in Berlin alongside staff surgeon, Dr Emil Behring (Matthias Koeberlin). The year is 1888, and Behring has not yet formulated his Nobel Prize-winning diphtheria antitoxin, but even as a humbly trained military surgeon, his ego is formidable against the hospital's nursing superintendent, Matron Martha (Ramona Kunze-Libnow), a Protestant deaconess who explains to the young Sisters and wage-earning nurses that 'the body must heal itself with good nursing and God's help' (see Figure 7.1).

So, viewers are not surprised when she attempts to intervene in the doctor's planned appendectomy, pointing out that the invasive and still experimental procedure is unproven to be more effective than cold wraps, and predicting that surgery may kill the patient faster. Behring criticises the matron's *Halbwissen* (superficial knowledge), and Matron Martha steps aside to allow the doctor, nurses, and patient to pass.

The viewer has seen this story before. Dr Behring removes the patient's appendix, holding it up victoriously before a lecture hall filled with medical students. He plays the heroic young physician representing the march of medical progress against the clutches of disease and religion. Yet, there are also hints of doubt sewn into the narrative. Despite Behring's earlier hubris, he admits to his (all-male) medical students that the experimental appendectomy procedure has not been done successfully more than a few times. Even after the surgery is complete, he warns that the patient still has only a 20 per cent chance of survival. Meanwhile, other distinguished physicians at the hospital struggle to make sense of the Crown Prince's declining health, misdiagnosing him as cancer-free. Nonetheless, the celebration of German medicine continues at the International Medical Congress in 1890, when Dr Robert Koch (Justus von Dohnányi) prematurely declares he has found a 'tuberculin' treatment for tuberculosis. Matron Martha relents and

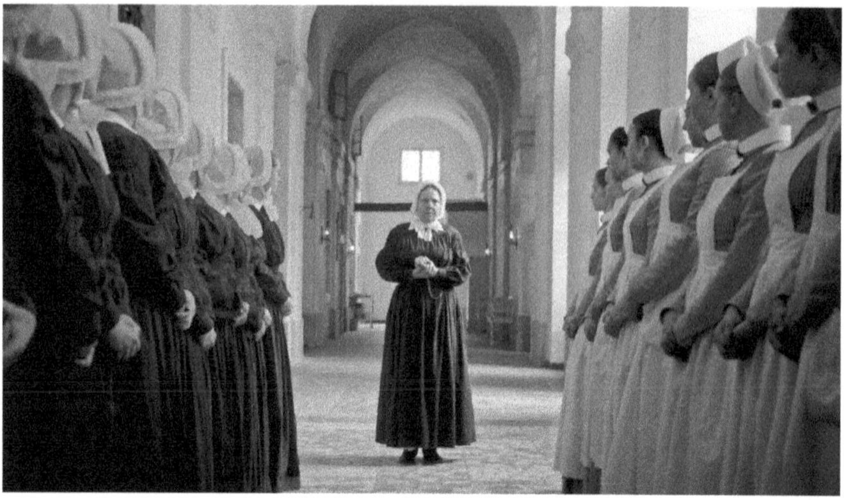

Figure 7.1 Matron Martha addresses deaconesses and nurse aides (*Charité*, 2017, S1E1)

allows him to treat young Sister Therese (Klara Deutschmann). When she does not recover, her relapse is even more intense before she succumbs to death. These real scientific setbacks elicit sympathy for Matron Martha's critical attitude toward the ego-driven masculinity that characterised the late nineteenth-century medical revolution (S1E4). While physicians sought out revolutionary cures, the nurses were cautiously refining their expertise in palliative care: observing patient conditions, carrying out treatments, preventing infection, and easing both physical and psychological pain. Their daily work was integral to the success of medical triumphs. Yet, as the series ends with real and fictional postscripts, it is only the doctors and their wives who are memorialised for their contributions to medical and social progress.

Adapting the complexities of historical health care to an hour of weekly public viewing is no small feat. Hospital-based series contribute to public historical consciousness and literacy by both disseminating a multi-dimensional experience of space, time, and people in the past and also facilitating an emotional connection to the human condition of those who lived, worked, and struggled in familiar ways through unfamiliar circumstances. The fictitious exchange between the deaconess matron and the well-recognised historical titans of medical history serves to uphold a truism in media and popular culture depictions of nurses – historical and contemporary. The tensions between tradition and progress, religion and science, nurses and doctors, women and men serve to drive dramatic television storylines, but often, they also serve the audience's nostalgic desire to imagine the past as it might have been rather than deepening its understanding of how it really was.

In fitting with the themes of this collection, this chapter considers the dramatised role of historical nurses as members of ensemble medical casts and as general representations of women in period dramas. It highlights three characteristics of the recent transnational cohort of nurse-centred historical dramas: (1) the recreation of historical hospital settings and field stations, (2) the heteronormative, racialised, and class-based assumptions that nurses, in particular, represent women in general, and (3) the portrayal of historical hospital life through the lens of twenty-first-century gender norms, contradictions, and nostalgia. Despite the aim of illuminating lesser-known regional or national locations and events, television depictions of historical nurses remain recognisable across time and place. When departures from these established formulas do occur, they reflect intentional choices by the creators, writers, and directors to create common ground between historical and contemporary expectations. By engaging with theoretical and empirical studies of gender, nostalgia, and the historical representation of nurses, this chapter illuminates how creators and audiences have collaboratively reimagined the past as a transnational social commentary for the present.

Where are the nurses?

Between 2008 and 2018, television networks and streaming services delved into the historical stories of real and fictitious nurses in original drama series in the United Kingdom, United States, Germany, Spain, and Australia. In December 2006, the long-running British *Casualty* series (1986–) reset the contemporary emergency department 100 years in the past for a one-episode TV special called *Casualty 1906*. Between 2008 and 2009, two more limited runs continued the premise in *Casualty 1907/1909* (*London Hospital* in the USA). In 2011, the Edwardian period drama *Downton Abbey* (2010–2015) returned for its second series, as the estate was transformed into a convalescent hospital (as was its real-life inspiration of Highclere Castle) during World War I. Receptive British audiences were perhaps not surprising as the country was celebrating the centenary of Florence Nightingale's death in 2010 and planning for major World War I commemorations to launch in 2014. Yet, the sudden proliferation of hospital period dramas in the following six years was also evidence of broader transnational commercial strategy and positive audience reception.

This chapter analyses original drama series centred around historical hospitals, with nurses featured prominently in the ensemble casts. All of the series under examination have female protagonists representing nurses in the eras between the 1860s and the 1920s. *Mercy Street* (USA, 2016–2017), *Casualty 1900s/London Hospital* (UK, 2006–2009), and *ANZAC Girls*

(Australia, 2014) are based upon the memoirs and records of real women. *Charité* (Germany, 2017), *Downton Abbey* (UK, 2010–2015), *The Crimson Field* (UK, 2014), and *Morocco: Love in Time of War* (Spain, 2018) are fictionalised accounts of nurses among semi-fictional characters and spaces.

The historiography on medical period dramas is still developing, often as a form of public history engagement by scholars in popular or public news forums. Nursing historians have begun to recognise the consequences of and patterns among popular representation of their profession in both historical and contemporary perspectives. Sandy Summers and Harry Summers have analysed contemporary media portrayals of nurses, primarily in the US context, including in Hollywood films and on American television. They find that references to nurses are often used as a foil against female physicians to illuminate gender inequity and prejudice against women in medicine, without considering the inaccurate or injurious effects such juxtapositions have on nurses and their own profession (Summers and Summers, 2014: 78–79).

Many of Summers and Summers' critiques hold true for historical depictions too. The validation of competent historical nurses through the suggestion that they harbour aspirations for medical education follows contemporary prejudices rather than historical realities. As German historians of nursing Isabel Atzl, Suzanne Kreuzter, and Karen Nolte wrote in their public review of the German *Charité* series, 'the depiction of nurses is devastating – not only because it contradicts the historical circumstances of the nineteenth century, but because it continues to reinforce perceptions of nursing as an essentialized female activity that at no time does justice to the importance of nursing work and harms nurses to this day' (Atzl et al., 2017). In other cases, scholars have been invited to be actively engaged in the creation of the television series. *Casualty 1900s* drew upon historical individuals and case records from the Royal London Hospital archives. Jane Schultz, who literally wrote the historical monograph on Civil War hospitals, blogs about *Mercy Street* on the PBS website, alongside notable scholars in the history of the American Civil War, women, African Americans, and medicine.

Nevertheless, the faithful recreation of hospital settings has often lost sight of the forest in the painstaking detail of its trees. Historical nursing dramas still generally lack a critical gender perspective that questions the simplistic heroising or villainising of certain kinds of nurses, or women, against each other. Nurses' memoirs have valorised elite women's voluntary experiences at the expense of undermining the professional nurses and working women's labour, who were less likely to leave such robust records of their experiences. Replicated in these series, in which all the main characters stem from aristocratic or upper-middle-class backgrounds, it falls upon the supporting characters to facilitate critical dialogues about the socio-economic, gender, racial/ethnic, and ideological diversity that existed within historical hospital spaces.

The hospital as historical space

In the spring of 1862, as army head nurse Mary Phinney (Mary Elizabeth Winstead) of *Mercy Street* arrives for the first time in Civil War Alexandria (Virginia), the camera spans the street view of unattended stretchers with dirty, still bleeding, injured soldiers lining the promenade around the main entrance. Hucksters peddle prosthetic limbs, as severed human body parts fall out of a loosely wrapped tarp being thrown out of a second-storey window. A makeshift banner hangs crookedly by string to read 'Union Hospital' just below the fading stencilled bricks that have long marked the iconic Mansion House luxury hotel (*Real Stories*, 2017). Based upon Phinney's own account, surviving photographs, and part of the building now recreated for the public as a museum, the Mansion House hotel is recreated with meticulous pride in detail (*Real Stories*, 2017). The effort has the desired effect, as the audience enters the building for the first time with Mary, it sees the chaotic foyer wrapped narrowly around the grand staircase – so bustling with the din of people that we do not know where to look first. There are no signs or uniformed staff; patients are found on makeshift cots, the floor, or on the staircase being attended to by nuns, pastors, or yet unidentifiable personnel – if at all. The operating room employs handsaws and an orderly holding a gold-framed mirror as a spotlight; a hysterical patient wields firearms and demands release from 'this death house' (S1E1). Against the greyness of these bodies is the backdrop of delicately patterned and brightly papered walls, some of the still-hanging art, and coloured stained glass over the staircase.

It is surely not by accident that so many historical hospital dramas open with a visual tour of the space before introducing any of their characters. The recreated hospital setting quietly affirms or challenges the historical assumptions of contemporary viewers. The Mansion House hospital set conveys the *ad hoc*, overburdened, and unprofessional system of military medical and nursing care in the 1860s. It is the earliest among these cases of historical television recreation. In *Charité*, the Charité Hospital of Berlin (another iconic, well-documented, and preserved space) is introduced in 1888 at the height of the revolutions in bacteriology and medical science. However, when the Emperor tours the hospital, he is not drawn to the freshly scrubbed wards of laudanum-subdued patients or to the social reform presentations aimed at serving the poor; rather he demands to be escorted to the hospital stables, where, indeed, Doctors Behring and Koch are carrying out cutting-edge medical research with rabbits and horses (S1E2).

The hospital wards, by contrast, remain feminised domains in depictions throughout the nineteenth and twentieth century. At the Charité, there are Protestant deaconesses and untrained attendants working for wages. By 1906 in the London Hospital of *Casualty 1906*, the equipment gleams more modern and the interior hospital spaces shine brighter in contrast to the greyness surrounding the impoverished suffering patients waiting impatiently at the gate in the East End London street. The matron and ward sisters, now organised as a hierarchy of well-trained nursing staff, still begin the day with prayer and ward checks (S1E1). While physicians make occasional rounds, they are more often found performing their authority and expertise in the operating or lecture theatres – masculine spaces filled with male medical students hanging on their every word. Only occasionally is there a crossover: the 'interfering strumpet' (a.k.a. the head nurse), who dares to venture into the cellar of the steward (*Mercy Street*, S1E2), the morphine-addicted physician who requires a nurse's discreet aid to detox (*Mercy Street*, S1E4; *Casualty 1909*, S1E1–2), the nurse taking lecture notes hidden in the back (*Charité*, S1E3), or a female medical student shooed away from the lecture-hall seat reserved for her own oral exam (*Charité at War*, 2019, S1E1).

By World War I, prominent hospital institutions are largely left behind as the setting for television dramas. *Downton Abbey* and *Morocco* continue to show the triumph of transforming unintended spaces into well-functioning hospital wards. There is a fiction to these spaces that reflects the story perhaps more than the space itself. In *Downton Abbey*, rooms are transformed into dorms and recreation spaces for convalescent officers in 1917. While the family ponders where they will sit, the intrusion into their space is modest and bloodless – an occasional ping-pong ball in the earl's newspaper (S2E3–6). By contrast, the hospital in *Morocco* is forged from an abandoned school building, transformed in a montage of scrubbing and new furnishings sent by ship from the Queen of Spain (*Morocco*, S1E1). When the new hospital is robbed, the Spanish ladies rip up and boil their petticoats for clean bandages (S1E3). These are not unique acts, but reminiscent of similar montages of Australian nurses in *ANZAC Girls* proving their professional dedication by sweeping away mice and bugs in an orphanage turned hospital and stripping off their 'personal things' for bandages (S1E2).

Other war-time medical dramas are set in field hospitals and other makeshift spaces that communicate to the audience the generic interchangeability of the backdrop: a British field hospital of tents somewhere in France (by the sea) in *The Crimson Field* offers as little precision about the location as the many outposts in *ANZAC Girls* separated by land or sea. In both cases, nurses often live and work in tents – some furnished with under-bed chamber pots; others showcasing daily tasks such as showering and doing laundry as a source of dramatic fodder and comic relief. Flora (Alice St Clair), the VAD (voluntary aid detachment) nurse, shakes a severed thumb out of the laundered linens she is about to hang out to dry (*The Crimson Field*, S1E1). Sister Olive (Anna McGraham) chops off her long hair and cracks the layer of ice formed over her morning water bucket (*ANZAC Girls*, S1E3). As days turn into months and years of deployment, these spectacles show, yet remain free from the burden or responsibility of really feeling, the ever-present cold, the smell of disinfectant mingling with decaying flesh, or living with the sound of bombs in the background for more than a minute or two.

Beyond the hospital, the common use of CGI technology that accompanied the new wave of programmes in 2014 had the ability to recreate landscapes representative of historical context. In the introductions to both *ANZAC Girls* and *The Crimson Field*, stylised red poppies spread across the screen – indicative of both blood and romanticised memory. Occasionally sprinkled with depictions of fields filled with white crosses or distant battle scenes lighting up the sky, the series are nevertheless much more reliant on dialogue and emotion than graphic depictions of war injuries such as shell shock or amputations. While the moderation of violent and bloody images of war makes the story accessible to a broader audience, the sanitation of war can tend toward a political rather than humanitarian critique: the British military failing to procure rations and supplies for the ANZAC nurses, the traditional hierarchies obstructing medical and social innovation and progress, or the individuals who overzealously serve country over humanity. Yet, viewers are left with a certain brightness or dream-like quality that seems to reassure them that what they are seeing is not quite the entirety of what was real.

Ladies, sisters, and labourers

In the first episode of *ANZAC Girls*, Matron Grace Wilson (Caroline Craig), a historical Australian nurse leader, is joined by four young women from Australia and New Zealand in 1915. The nurses are instantly recognisable in their light blue dresses, white aprons, and head scarfs. It is the uniform standard, with little variation, of television nurses from the working nurse aides in the Charité hospital in 1888 Germany to the Spanish Red Cross lady nurses of the Rif War in 1921 Morocco. Only the American Civil War nurses, who predate the Red Cross nursing tradition (introduced in 1864), wore their own class-specific clothing, while Catholic sisters and Protestant deaconesses continued to wear distinctive habits or uniforms. Even as late as 1964, British nurse-midwives still wore light blue dresses under scarlet cardigan sweaters, reminiscent of the long blue dresses and scarlet capes from fifty years earlier (*Call the Midwife*, 2012–).

The timeless appearance of television nurses supports a well-worn script. Across the eras, the protagonist is well-intentioned but lacks knowledge and experience; the experienced nurse is cynical, short-tempered, and sometimes devious; nurses are inhibited from forming romantic relationships, but the plotlines are driven by sexual tension and innuendo. Unlike the myriad of other women's roles that might be (but only occasionally have been) featured in drama series, nursing narratives offer a celebration of women's intellect, independence, and adventure without uncomfortably challenging mainstream viewers' assumptions about their embodied femininity, whiteness, heteronormativity, or respectability.

Other hospital labourers are distinctively marked as inferior by their transgression of these norms. The absence of male nurses or attendants is conspicuous. Men in nursing were common in history, especially in German hospitals of the nineteenth century. Martin Schelling (Jacob Matschenz) in *Charité at War* is an important exception, as a Nazi-era nurse, whose presence reflects some of the gendered division of labour within nursing. His duties lead him to interact more with male medical students and patients than the female nurses who assist in surgery, take care of children, or clean the wards. Male orderlies appear more often in these series, but generally as dimensionless representations of marginalised colonial subjects, slaves/freedmen, and non-heteronormative characters among ensemble casts.

By engaging contemporary discourses on gender and nursing, television writers and producers have recentered their narratives on women as heroines and witnesses in history. Yet, the stories of nurses are still often resolved in ways that ambivalently reify rather than diversify the historical representation of nurses and hospital workers, who did not share a uniform experience as women, and were further differentiated among volunteers, professionals, and workers.

Volunteers

Most nurse protagonists featured on television are inexperienced volunteers. In *Downton Abbey*, Lady Sybil's first cooking lesson reveals that not only can she not boil an egg, but she also does not know how to turn on the water tap (S2E3). Likewise, in *Mercy Street*, when Mary Phinney arrives at Mansion House, she admits to Dr Foster (Josh Radnor), 'Blood makes me uneasy.' To which, he dryly responds, 'You'll need to overcome that' (S1E1). Generally, that is exactly what volunteer nurses do. Through instinct or sheer force of will, lady nurses become generally competent – even indispensable – with little if any formal training. While bolstering the character development of the protagonist, these narratives also portray nursing as something any woman can put her mind to do without regard to the theoretical and practical training required of professional nurses.

The tensions between professional and volunteer nurses are well-recognised at the foundation of nursing drama. In *The Crimson Field*, three unacquainted voluntary aid detachment (VAD) nurses are sent to a field hospital in France in the autumn of 1914, after a brief training course. Kitty (Oona Chaplin) seems unfit for military discipline; she even smokes cigarettes, which 'gives an impression', as her new colleague notes. Flora wears rosewater scent and fails bedmaking. Rosalie (Marianne Oldham) is preoccupied with the linen cabinet, which she hopes will save her from encountering a naked male body in the course of the war. These 'very adorable darlings', as one doctor calls them, pose a threat to the hard-won training and military rank of the trained and state-certified Sisters (S1E1).

Indeed, as the volunteers eventually admit to themselves, they have gone to war to escape the daily miseries of aristocratic privilege. Both the British VADs and the Spanish Red Cross ladies of *ANZAC Girls* and *Morocco* reckon with this truth as they experience independence from their families for the first time. Engagements are broken, parent–child bonds are severed, society scandals ensue. Yet, this is no less true for Emma Green (Hannah James), in *Mercy Street*, a southern belle, whose family continues to live adjacent to the hospital they used to own. She starts visiting the hospital under the auspices of lending support to the Confederate soldiers she grew up with, but gradually embraces the sense of purpose she feels as an official army nurse. Mary Phinney, her mentor, is less naïve. Her aristocratic title (as Baroness von Olnhausen) meant little in antebellum New England; she came to the war to fight for abolition, she'd already seen sickness and death. Yet, her presence still valorises the role of elite women's charity over the trained professional nurse and paid hospital labour.

Professionals

In contrast to the elite young women cast in a historicised yet timeless coming-of-age story, the particularities of their professional foils are at first glance more intended for comedic relief than representations of historical villainy. Consider *The Crimson Field*'s Sister Quayle (Kerry Fox), the highly decorated British professional in World War I, who is not only distraught by the imposition of briefly trained voluntary aid detachment nurses, but by her own loss of rank after losing a promotion to her own protégé. At first, it is not only that her adherence to strict military discipline scares the inexperienced volunteers, but she steals a cake from one of them, lying about giving it to the soldiers while eating it alone in her tent at night (S1E1). Similarly, British nurse Anne Hastings (Tara Summers) in *Mercy Street* is first seen in the American Civil War at the Mansion Hotel hospital demonstrating proper casting techniques and regaling her audience with her first-hand accounts of Florence Nightingale's war nursing wisdom. Later, however, driven by jealousy and bitterness she schemes at great lengths to embarrass the new head nurse while hypocritically defying her own Victorian moral codes by openly carrying on a sexual relationship with a surgeon and covertly swigging liquor out of her flask or even the medicinal bottles (S2 E1).

Yet, over time the comedic tone turns dark. In *The Crimson Field*, Sister Quayle's passive-aggressive antics turn tragic as she defies orders and sends a severely suffering shell-shock victim back to the front. It was done in a silent passing moment, a deferred horror over several episodes. When he returns past the point of medical assistance, she expresses not so much remorse as a misplaced sense of disloyalty (S1E6). In *Mercy Street*, Hastings redeems herself perhaps in the end, but only by turning her penchant for tormenting others onto a more deserving target. Her revelation of dismissal by Nightingale introduces an element of empathy for her, as does her late efforts to reconnect Phinney with Dr Foster (S2E3). However, there is more here to examine than wayward petty jealousies and comedic intrigues. Across the historical medical dramas examined here, the professional nurse – marked with scarlet capes, medals, or credentials – is cast as the villain. Trained and certified nurses of the British Empire in World War I wore distinctive scarlet dress capes that distinguished them from volunteer nurses, but as Australian Sister Elsie (Shepherd) Cook (Laura Brent) learned in *ANZAC Girls*, the professional military nurses of the Queen Alexandria Imperial Nurses resented working alongside ANZAC nurses, whether their teacups were not aligned uniformly or because they dared to wear the scarlet cape *only* as reservists and 'colonials' (S1E4).

Across decades, languages, classes, and countries, this comparative transnational analysis suggests that professional ambition for women remains implicitly regarded as treacherous and lonely. British matron Grace Carter (Hermione Norris) of *The Crimson Field* and Australian matron Grace Wilson of *ANZAC Girls* shine as professional leaders precisely because of their acceptance of such social limitations. Both command authority in their insistence upon high standards and hierarchical duty. Yet, Carter must be continually reassured by Lieutenant Colonel Roland Brett (Kevin Doyle) that she has earned the position and vacillates in her decisions behind closed doors. Wilson wins the begrudging respect of the male military hierarchy from the top command to the male orderlies below, as she too is suffering alongside the nurses with the death of her brother and the privations of the desolate Lemnos Island. Like the matrons and young career nurses before them, both have sacrificed personal relationships, Carter leaving behind an Indian sepoy from her younger life in the colonies (*The Crimson Field*, S1E5) and Wilson waiting until age seventy-four to marry (*ANZAC Girls*, S1E8). What makes them good nurses and matrons reifies the essential notions of nineteenth-century femininity: the embodied nature of women's caring capacity, and the self-sacrifice of their own relationships and families.

Workers

Behind the recognisable iconography of crisply uniformed female nurses, there was also a diverse workforce within a hospital or field station. In American Civil War hospitals, the staff 'consisted of a broad spectrum of women; those of higher class and racial standing worked alongside those without privilege, even though the former were usually appointed to jobs of greater status and responsibility' (Schultz, 2007: 4). As a genre, historical medical dramas have challenged the male doctor and female nurse binary by emphasising the intricacy of hospital social hierarchies structured not only by gender, but also by its intersections with race and ethnicity, religion, class, and sexuality.

In *Mercy Street*, three former slave women demonstrate the roles women of colour played in hospital life, which are uncredited as nursing. The Green family housekeeper (and former slave), Belinda (L. Scott Caldwell), understands cooking and homoeopathic treatments, which she does in the hospital kitchen and among the former slaves. Charlotte Jenkins (Patina Miller), a social reformer from the North, sets up a smallpox quarantine tent and school. Finally, Aurelia (Shalita Grant), a 'contraband' African American laundress, is extorted by the crass steward, Silas Bullen (Wade Williams), for what meagre trinkets of worth she has, and then by rape, for empty promises of assistance in finding her separated family.

Despite these nuanced portrayals of African American women, there is still the problem represented by the comedically redeemed steward, who is bludgeoned to near-death twice, and then finds God, and tries to make amends. Such reconciliations were nearly universal for the characters in the Mansion House hospital, who have all turned into abolitionists and allies by the final episode. Yet, the year is only 1863, and the war continues. Most Americans did not so easily accept the inclusion of former slaves into the national community, and the rape of a woman cannot just be erased by a reunion of her family. When the war ended, the white volunteer women were compensated with war pensions for their nursing service; wage-earning cooks, laundresses, and orderlies were not.

Among British period dramas, the racial and cultural diversity of the Empire is both ever-present and politely ignored. *ANZAC Girls* represents the nature of imperialism unevenly. Sister Alice (Georgia Flood) objects to her beau Harry (Dustin Clare) glorifying the war as an opportunity for Australian nationhood, but she too can only see the suffering and futility of the Australians. While making clear that the Australians are the forgotten and derided 'colonials' of the British Empire, the peoples of Egypt and the Ottoman Empire are simultaneously not only forgotten but rendered as though they did not even exist. Instead, they are seen as exotic spaces through the eyes of young, elite, white nurses abroad for the first time, recreated in keeping with theorising of the 'imperial imaginary', which explains how travel narratives could simultaneously embrace the exoticism of colonial spaces without giving agency to the people living in those spaces (Kaplan, 2006). *ANZAC Girls* shows Australian nurses racing camels, touring the Pyramids of Giza on dates, and meandering through bazaars. There are no named Egyptian characters, just 'stall holders' and 'street urchins' (S1E1).

Morocco similarly shows sweeping landscapes, bazaars, even the interior of a modest family home. North Africans are generally cast as enemy combatants; only the hospital orderly, Larbi (Daniel Lundh), is shown as more, though his role too is primarily as part of the Spanish imperial imaginary. We know little about Larbi except that he comes from modest circumstances, cannot read, and has family members actively working against the Spanish. Yet, he becomes wrapped up in a mutual infatuation with Magdalena (Anna Moliner), the Spanish woman who has delayed her society wedding to volunteer as a nurse in Melilla. The limited appearance of male orderlies represents both the subordination of racial and ethnic masculinities as well as the often still dimensionless development of colonial subjects among the characters in ensemble casts.

In these historical medical dramas, the nurses are principally representing women in general, not the nursing profession. Nursing uniforms, titles, and relationships provide a proxy for complex social hierarchies of gender, race, class, and ethnicity, but the nurses cast as heroines in historical medical dramas remain homogeneously drawn from the records of elite white women.

The gender dynamics of hospital life

Like other historical and contemporary dramas, the plot is driven less by history than by personal relationships, though none of these series succumbs to the gender stereotyping of the leading physician as villain and antagonist to the nurses. In the universe of the female-driven historical medical drama, men are constituted instead as the objects of a contemporary female viewer's romantic fantasy. In *Morocco*, Dr Fidel Calderon (Álex Garcia), medical officer of the Spanish Red Cross hospital in Melilla, puts his faith almost instantly in Julia (Amaia Salamanca), an upper-class woman whose preparation for nursing work consisted solely of flipping through the pages of a slim nursing manual handed to her on the train. Despite being engaged to other people, Julia and Fidel fall in love. When Julia's fiancé is saved from prison, he is quite forgiving of what he can see was a romantic tension lingering in his absence, and they reconcile. However, it is when he wants her to return to Spain with him that she turns toward the doctor who sees her as an effective nurse and partner rather than just a wife (S1E12).

In these series, the attraction of the male physician is rooted in his role as a supportive professional mentor. In *Charité*, Ida Lenze (Alicia von Rittberg) slowly overcomes her adolescent betrayal at the hands of Dr Behring, who broke off their engagement when her father died, but who then singularly supports her medical interests and study in Switzerland. In *Mercy Street*, Mary Phinney is at first horrified by Dr Jed Foster's (Josh Radnor) ambivalence to emancipation and callous attitude toward the Black hospital workers, yet his patient support of her inexperienced nursing skills and leadership endear him to her, and vice versa. Although Phinney and Behring are real historical figures, these romances are fiction. London Hospital staffers, Ethel Bennett (Charity Wakefield) and Dr Millais Culpin (William Houston) of *Casualty 1900s*, did marry in real life. However, the story of their courtship following Dr Culpin's support for Bennett's medical education is fictional. The real Bennett did not pursue a medical education but became the matron of a British hospital in Shanghai (Friend, 2008).

The contemporary viewer's aversion to women sacrificing themselves to well-recognised historical limitations on women's professional opportunities is further demonstrated in storylines in which romances fail. In *Casualty 1907*, Sister Ada Russell's (Sarah Smart) beau supports her continued career at the London Hospital by choosing to practise medicine elsewhere, but as she continues to rise through the ranks, she faces an ultimatum between profession and marriage, choosing nursing. In *Charité*, Ida Lenze similarly believes she can reconcile career and marriage with Georg Tischendorf (Maximillian Meyer-Bretschneider), a medical student more in love with photography and art than medicine, but his indulgence of her medical study aspirations turns out to be insincere in the face of his father's disapproval. So, she too chooses her career over marriage. Even in the historical romance *Outlander* (2014–), Claire is a World War II army nurse, who travels to and from eighteenth-century Scotland, only to accept an estranged marriage while she pursues medical school and a career as a surgeon in 1950s Boston (S3E2–3).

Certainly, women in history did make such difficult choices against the grain of convention and gender norms, but medical dramas have normalised these exceptional stories as foregone conclusions. This nostalgia for what might have been not only distorts the lived experiences and narratives of real people but whitewashes the gendered constraints and challenges that defined the historical experiences of nurses. Even in the realm of fantasy, female characters are severely limited in the roles they are allowed to play: nurse, physician, wife. The choices of paths do not reflect historical norms or individual stories, but they have become a common archetype. Wives sit on the sidelines, nurses live like nuns, and smart nurses become doctors, in 1892, 1909, or 1948.

While the major character romances fulfil heteronormative expectations of the historical fiction genre, there are also glimpses of illicit relationships that defy expected historical boundaries of race, ethnicity, class, or heterosexual desire almost universally among the larger ensemble of characters in this new generation of historical medical dramas. There is notably one queer character clearly identified in almost every show. In *Mercy Street*, a young girl joins the Union army in disguise and falls in love with her 'brother-in-arms'. Caught in the act, Dr Foster is horrified by their 'unnatural state' until it is revealed that she was cross-dressing (S2E4). In *Call the Midwife*, Midwife Patsy (Emerald Fennell) falls in love with nurse Delia (Kate Lamb) but the two must conceal their romantic relationship under cover of friendship. In *The Crimson Field*, Flora recognises that Peter (Jack Gordon), an orderly, is a gay man, noting bluntly that she recognised it because her brother is too, but warns him urgently that he needs to be more careful (S1E6). In *Charité at War*, Martin Schelling provides a clearer case for the dangers of homosexuality in the past. He was not only gay but charged as a sex offender and sent to the front where he lost his leg, was discharged, and then forced to become an informant for the Nazi regime. He is also the only example, across all the historical medical dramas examined, of a male nurse.

Finally, the storyline of Sister Therese in *Charité* bears special mention for grappling with the illicit love she has for Ida. Not only is it a violation of her vows of celibacy, but she becomes convinced that God is punishing her for her sinful desires and dies of tuberculosis believing that the disease was a punishment and that her death will usher her into Hell. Left speechless perhaps for the only time in the series, Matron Martha seems to confront the true implications of such religious dogma. These gendered scripts certainly speak more to the contemporary expectations of viewing audiences who want to be simultaneously swept away by historical romance without historical gender prejudices extinguishing the attraction.

Nostalgia

A widely recognised phenomenon of recent years has been the way in which Netflix has used its video-streaming service to target a generation of consumers seeking to reconnect with the youth culture of the 1980s and 1990s

(Pallister, 2019). What is less known, at least in the US, is the global production strategy that has driven Netflix to produce 100 foreign-language original series per year as of 2020. In an interview, Erik Barmack (vice president at Netflix for international originals) confirmed that this vision was not only bold in its scale, but in its intent to create 'feel good' content around strong female characters and non-English speaking niche audiences (Hopewell and Lang, 2018). Streaming programmes were comprised of 47 per cent women among major characters compared to 43 per cent on broadcast programmes (Lauzen, 2017).

The attempt to distribute and market strong female-driven characters as a bridge between local and global audiences is evident in *Morocco*. While the Rif War of 1921 is undeniably regional in its historical resonance, the focus of the series on Red Cross nurses evokes widespread global recognition of an icon that is by intent interchangeably local, national, and international. The same might be said of *Charité* in Germany, as few non-Germans might boast recognition of Berlin in the 'year of three emperors', but its depiction of women and nursing also resonates with contemporary sensibilities.

Apart from the victimisation of Nurse Martin, the nurses in *Charité at War* represent the worst of the Nazi regime. Sister Käthe (Susanne Böwe), the kindly children's nurse, proactively takes steps to report and deport the baby of two doctors she works closely with. Sister Christabel (Frida-Lovisa Hamann) is a true believer who chooses to spy on her colleagues. The same is true of Charlotte (Miriam Stein), in *Generation War* (2013), a newly minted nurse who joins a German Red Cross hospital during World War II only to slide into a loveless affair with an older physician and then the unthinkable betrayal of a Jewish colleague. None of these characters is the main protagonist or a real person, posing a question of what narrative purpose they were created to serve. When Dr Sauerbruch (Ulrich Noethen) of *Charité* asks his colleagues to remember their Hippocratic Oath, Nurse Christabel reminds him of their oath to the Führer, which underlines how fictional nurses have become a sort of moral bellwether. Nurses certainly did become agents of the state in the course of World War II as did military officers and public health officials. However, once it is historically plausible to cast female protagonists as physicians instead of nurses, those characters who remained 'mere' nurses become less likely to be included in redemptive storylines.

These series are a product of recent television industry interest in telling global but universal stories of strong female characters. Historical nurses are appealing in this role because they may be cast as young, independent, yet unthreatening and familiar to cross-cultural viewers in established genres of medical, war, or romantic dramas. Lisa Wolfinger, the creator of *Mercy Street*, affirmed her intent to tell a more uplifting Civil War story led by strong female characters who confront issues that resonate with contemporary audiences, such as sexism and racism (Hautzinger, 2017). The first British medical dramas were proof of the concept that female-centred ensemble casts could draw an audience. Both *Casualty 1900s* and *Downton Abbey* cast a balance between men and women with the leading storylines arguably skewed toward the female characters: not directly representing the average woman of the 1910s, but presenting fictional coming-of-age stories that connected the public commemorations of the Great War with contemporary gender sensibilities in search of independent female characters. The subsequent wave of programmes (and seasons of *Downton Abbey*) were even more intentionally helmed by women writers and directors, and notably more ambitious in reframing historical narratives to illuminate the experiences of non-white, immigrant, queer, and religious characters. Restoring the agency of women in diverse ways relieves these television series of the burden of representing gender as it was rather than how we wish it might have been. Yet, these historical narratives also bear responsibility for their revisionism. Critics point out how *Mercy Street* softened the portrayal of Confederate attitudes on slavery or *Charité at War* redeemed German collaboration with the Nazi regime with all the major surviving characters coming around to resist Nazi eugenics. Even *Call the Midwife*, a nuanced long-running series about post–World War II British nurse midwives, perpetuated a kind of white woman and welfare state saviour narrative in the initial series following a young professional nurse navigating the impoverished London community of Poplar in the early era of the National Health Service.

The simplistic rendering of hospital personnel into heteronormative, heroic Western narratives of scientific and social progress might be unpacked effectively through frames of historical memory and nostalgia. Historical nursing may harken back to a 'simpler time', but it is hard to imagine much to be nostalgic about in the daily hospital work of the past. These recent historical series challenge or redefine popular interpretations of nostalgia within media studies. Scholarship on nostalgia emphasises the relationship of the present to memories of the past, that is, a reconnection of identity and meaning within one's own individual or collective timeline (Routledge, 2015). The genre of historical period dramas is more complicated. Viewers do not have personal emotional connections to the past being depicted, nor do they likely seek a return (even in fantasy) to a world plagued by epidemics or lacking antibiotics and pain-relievers.

Instead, we might describe a form of counterfactual nostalgia. While contemporary viewers do not identify directly with the distant past of the nineteenth and early twentieth centuries, historical recreations can appeal to the way things never were. Counterfactual nostalgia offers an audience comfort in seeing the past through the lens of what might have been. By combining contemporary viewers' social values and anxieties with revisionism of actual historical persons or events, the fictional narratives choose to amplify, consolidate, or minimise aspects of the historical record to tell a 'true' or 'true-ish' story that resonates with contemporary values. Thus, television depictions of nursing history as women's history reflect the intentional historical engagement of writers and creators to draw upon iconic images and well-worn public narratives to revisit the perspective of women or lesser-represented points of view in the past. This new generation of media representation has the potential to create a transnational dialogue among nineteenth- and twentieth-century nursing narratives, or it may remain satisfied to re-sow gender stereotypes and inspirational symbolism that further seek fantasy rather than deeper humanity from the past.

References

Atzl, I., S. Kreutzer, and K. Nolte (2017). 'Nachtrag zur Serie "Charite": Das Klischee der einfältigen Krankenschwester' [Online]. Available at: www.faz.net/-8xnyx-8xou4 (accessed 21 September 2019).

Friend, D. (2008). '*Casualty*'s Culpin Was a Local Hero | East London and West Essex Guardian Series' [Online]. Available at: www.guardian-series.co.uk/news/2183859.casualtys-culpin-local-hero/ (accessed 3 October 2019).

Hopewell, J., and J. Lang (2018). 'Netflix's Erik Barmack on International Growth, Creating Global TV – Variety' [Online]. Available at: https://variety.com/2018/tv/global/netflix-erik-barmack-international-production-global-tv-1202976698/ (accessed 3 October 2019).

Kaplan, C. (2006). 'Imagining Empire: History, Fantasy and Literature'. In Catherine Hall and Sonya O. Rose (Eds), *At Home with the Empire: Metropolitan Culture and the Imperial World.* Cambridge University Press.

Lauzen, M. (2019). 'What We Know for Sure about Women in Television – Women's Media Center' [Online]. Available at: www.womensmediacenter.com/news-features/what-we-know-for-sure-about-women-in-television (accessed 3 October 2019).

Mercy Street (2017). 'Meet the Bloggers' [Online]. Available at: www.pbs.org/mercy-street/blogs/mercy-street-revealed/meet-our-bloggers/ (accessed 28 September 2019).

Mercy Street (2017). 'Real Stories: People and Places' [Online]. Available at: www.pbs.org/mercy-street/uncover-history/real-people-places/mansion-house-carlyle-house/ (accessed 28 September 2019).

Pallister, K. (2019). *Netflix Nostalgia: Streaming the Past on Demand.* Lexington Books.

Routledge, C. (2015). *Nostalgia: A Psychological Resource*. Routledge.
Schultz, J. (2004). *Women at the Front: Hospital Workers in Civil War America*. University of North Carolina Press.
Summers, S., and H.J. Summers (2014). *Saving Lives: Why the Media's Portrayal of Nursing Puts Us All at Risk*. Oxford University Press.

8

Heroic childbirth and *Call the Midwife*

Katherine Byrne

Now in its ninth series, and with viewing figures which frequently exceed ten million, *Call the Midwife* remains one of the BBC's most popular and most long-running series. This show's success can be attributed to its combination of *Downton Abbey*-esque cosiness and nostalgia ('cake and Horlicks', as one reviewer scathingly noted) with the gritty and detailed focus on televised childbirth which recalls BAFTA award-winning docudrama *One Born Every Minute* (Herman, 2014). Based on a bestselling series of books by a former midwife, *Call the Midwife* sets out to construct the NHS as part of British heritage, reminding the modern viewer of the importance of free health care at a time when it has been under attack by austerity politics. In doing so, however, it has courted controversy, inviting debates about the politics of fertility through contraception and abortion plots which have received mixed reviews from feminists and conservatives alike (FitzGerald, 2015). In addition, as this chapter will discuss, with its emphasis on the 'heroic' natural birth and the courageous 'labour' of women it reflects the position of the midwifery profession in regard to their championing of vaginal delivery (Takeshita, 2017). Birth has long been a much-contested area (Mander and Murphy-Lawless, 2013) and the Royal College of Midwives in Britain has been at the centre of controversy in the last few years concerning the relationship between their anti-intervention position and birth complications and mortality (Sandeman, 2017). As this chapter will explore, then, this seemingly 'cosy' television series is in fact right at the centre of the ongoing debates surrounding obstetrics and female choice, reminding us that not only is the womb still a contested and politically charged space, but the Sunday night period drama slot is too.

Birth on television

As a number of critics have discussed 'the noughties have seen the emergence of graphic representations of childbirth within the public sphere.

Childbirth is now visible across a range of popular media; most notably … as mass entertainment in televisual forms' (Tyler and Baraitser, 2013: 7). This increase in the screening of birth on television can be seen in soap operas but is most often apparent through reality shows like *The Midwives* (BBC, 2012–) and, most famously, the aforementioned *One Born Every Minute* (*OBEM*). Much has been written about this show's representation of birth, which is so graphic O'Brien Hill has convincingly compared it to the iconography of pornography (2014: 192) and which has been accused of making women more 'anxious about the process of giving birth' (Tyler and Baraitser, 2013: 7). Other critics have condemned the way it and similar hospital-set dramas 'overwhelmingly represent women as passive subjects, visualized through representations of women on their backs, with limited if any input in decision-making during labor' (De Benedictis et al., 2018). Writing about real-life health care, Tania McIntosh has argued that the process of giving birth has become a 'battleground between mothers, physicians and midwives', and it seems its representation on television is no exception.

Yet, although often discussed alongside *OBEM*, *Call the Midwife* (*CTM*) seems to have avoided many of these criticisms, perhaps because the show's ideology aligns itself with the dominant feminist ideas surrounding maternity. It is not only lovingly nostalgic about midwifery as a profession, but it also mostly represents (and by implication advocates) what would be termed 'natural', unassisted birth. Since the 1970s, feminists have largely embraced 'natural childbirth as a path to empowerment in the face of patriarchal obstetric authority' (Michaels, 2018: 54). As Louise FitzGerald has discussed, *CTM* has constructed itself as a feminist show through a concentration on women's vocations and friendships, a largely female cast, and some significant contraception and abortion plotlines, and we might add to this its embracing of natural childbirth (2015). All of this seems to render it important feminist television (for Caitlin Moran, it is *the* most feminist show on television [2013]) even though some critics have reservations about this. FitzGerald for example, argues that while the show 'might "live" feminism through its thematic focus on issues that affect women, it does not speak about feminism' (2015: 257). For her, the show's focus on pregnancy and birth reinforces age-old value systems about women: it 'reaffirms post-feminist notions of women as only ever the bearers of any form of cultural power if and when associated with birth' (2015: 257–258). This seems to me inarguable, and furthermore, as this chapter will suggest, the *type* of birth the show represents is also problematic for women. Unassisted birth with minimal pain relief, with the mother fully and consciously present, is the birth consistently advocated as normal by the show, as it is by the midwifery profession. However, this downplays the inability of most contemporary women to give birth in this way, and the risks and problems associated with this type of birth, as well as the psychological cost of this ideal. The show's birth representations do change and evolve over the nine seasons, however, and I will examine here how that can be considered a response to changes in UK maternity policy in real life.

Takeshita is one of the critics who consider that this programme, unlike many others on TV, represents birth in a positive, helpful, and women-friendly way. As they describe it, the show 'counteracts the dominant technocratic model of birth by showing that midwifery-assisted homebirths are normal and medically sound' (2015: 8). This is something that the other medical shows on our screens do not do, due to their hospital setting and their focus on more dramatic, and consequently more problematic, births. Indeed, much of *CTM*'s 'cosy' warmth and charm comes from the repeated screenings of positive, non-medicalised births in which mothers and midwives work together to triumphant effect:

> The feel-good emotional responses these scenes solicit from the audience are perhaps the strongest aspect of *Call*'s counter-narrative against the dominant portrayal of childbirth, which denies that women can rely on their own internal and physical strengths to achieve a positive birth outcome. (Takeshita, 2017: 8)

As Takeshita notes here, most episodes – at least in the first few series – follow a very similar format which becomes reassuringly familiar to the regular viewer (9). There are on average two or three births per episode, and the first, usually soon after the opening credits, is a straightforward natural birth that only takes up a few minutes of screen time while Vanessa Redgrave's grandmotherly voice narrates. This serves to remind the viewer of the daily business of a midwife's profession and reinforces the idea that most births take place with minimum intervention. The other plotlines in each episode tend to involve some more problematic pre- or post-partum narratives, exploring social as well as medical issues with the mother or her home or family, which tend to be resolved with the help of the midwives by the end. It is notable, however, that however dark and complex their circumstances might be, the births themselves are mostly straightforward and successful. Takeshita notes that 'the show integrates occasional inevitable maternal and infant death in its stories' (8) but while that may be the case, actually it is extremely rarely, over the whole nine seasons, that there have been issues with the birth itself or the care provided. Even on the very rare occasions when a baby dies, the midwives are absolved from blame. For example, S2E2 features an early cot death which throws suspicion on Cynthia as attending midwife, but this is later proved to have been caused by atelectasis, and hence is an unavoidable tragedy. One of the few other occasions where infant mortality is dealt with, the (infamous) Christmas day episode in 2017, did feature a stillborn baby, but on this occasion, the child comes back to life a short time later. Such a plotline is appropriate fare for a holiday special, but it does avoid the likely reality of such an event and distracts from any sense that birth is filled with risk for mother or child.

Instead, the overall message of the show aligns with the 'social model' of birth: as MacKenzie Bryers and Van Teijlingen describe it, this is

> founded on the idea that childbirth is a natural physiological event: that is, the majority of pregnant women will have a normal and safe childbirth with little or no medical intervention and that those women who are not expected to have a normal childbirth can be predicted and selected. (2010: 490)

This is exactly the message of *CTM*: there are, over the seasons, several mothers whose births require extra care – one woman with a badly deformed pelvis in season two is an example – but if they have attended their ante-natal sessions this is identified and planned for well in advance. Anyone else is able to give birth safely with only midwife assistance and to cope well (with only gas and air, usually) with the pain involved. This social model is in contrast to the prevailing 'medical model' of maternity, which sees pregnancy as a dangerous business that needs to be closely medically monitored (to provide assistance as early as possible should problems arise). This debate between two very different points of view has been at the heart of maternity care for decades: not all midwives might subscribe to the social model, nor every physician to the medical, but generally, the divide is along professional lines. The medical model is personified by shows like the BBC drama *Bodies* (2004–2006), which is set in an obstetrics unit and in which almost all the births involve much drama, intervention, and risk to mothers and babies. *CTM* has a very different message and one which seems all the more concrete and believable because of its regular repetition and because it is framed within careful representation of historical accuracy. The show, after all, prides itself on its realistic portrayal of the working class of the period, and of the medicine of the time (indeed, its writers insist that even the miracle return of the dead baby has had its precedent in real life [*Radio Times*, 2017]). The nostalgic fashion, music, and local community feel of the show are not allowed to distract from its gritty, disturbing plotlines: those which deal with illegal abortion, for example, are not only highly unusual to see on primetime TV but also completely undermine any sense that this is gentle, cosy Sunday night television. Yet what seems a diversion from this grittiness, or perhaps even from accuracy, is its insistence upon these positive, natural, minimum intervention births.

In these natural home-birth scenes 'repeated countless times, normalizing midwifery-assisted birth and weaving it into the fabric of everyday life of the community' (Takeshita, 2017: 9) there seems to be a determined sidelining or underplaying of the increasingly interventionist nature of birth in the second half of the twentieth century. The later seasons, which enter the 1960s, do acknowledge the greater numbers of women who chose to give birth in hospitals by this time, but continue their emphasis on natural birth. (Indeed, season nine features regular complaints about the overcrowded hospitals and the often-rushed treatment they provide, thus showing how much better midwife-led care is.) Throughout the show, gas and air is pretty much the only pain relief shown, for example, and forceps are hardly ever mentioned or used even though they were commonly – if still controversially – wielded by obstetricians from the eighteenth century onwards. Real-life midwives, while not allowed to use forceps – and often disapproving of them, aware of the damage they could inflict – were long accustomed to helping with forceps deliveries throughout the twentieth century (Towler and Bramall, 1986: 224). In contrast, on the show intervention of any kind is something the midwives are almost always able to avoid. Sometimes this is simply because they have no choice in the matter: often births are shown to be taking place in unorthodox circumstances, with no assistance available, and those attending can only rely on their own experience and skill. On other occasions, however, even the most dangerous births can be delivered naturally. Shoulder dystocia occurs several times over the series, for example, but this usually requires only a shift of position and an extra effort on the part of the midwife to deliver the baby, and the same is true of numerous breech presentations (see Figure 8.1).

But not content to show that complex births can be managed by midwives, the series is also keen to remind the viewer about the potential physical and mental cost of intervention. When forceps are finally mentioned, in S7E5, they are part of a plot in which a prospective mother is left suffering from tokophobia because she has been so traumatised by their brutal use in a previous delivery: 'Baby was stuck. The next thing, the doctor came in and my legs were strung up … he stuck these metal things inside me, Nurse, and I was screaming but he just kept on pulling. He ripped it out of me.' So terrified is this mother that she contemplates suicide rather than give birth again, but Lucille (Leonie Elliott) is able to reassure her that needing forceps for her second child is unlikely and that she can deliver at home; by the end of the episode, a successful unassisted birth (with no sign of pain relief, even) has been managed by the midwives. The message of the show is clearly that the best, least traumatic births are natural births, and they are an experience a mother can be thankful for: even this mother is afterwards deeply grateful to Lucille for her help and support. In contrast, intervention is presented here as trauma, even abuse. Hence the show aligns itself with, and advocates for, the widely held view of the midwifery profession and its preferred model

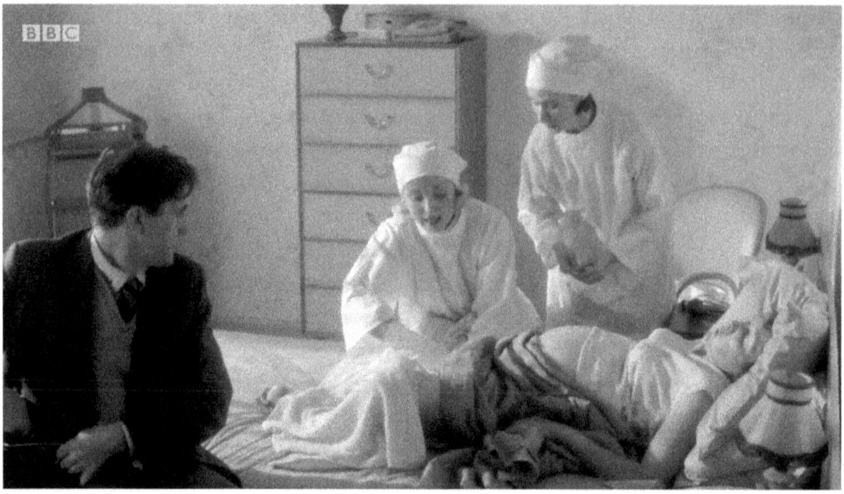

Figure 8.1 The midwives manage a difficult birth without other intervention (*Call the Midwife*)

of birth. This is unsurprising given its source text and the real-life midwives who are consultants on the show and an important part of its production, but such an ideology is not straightforward and not without problematic implications for mothers, as the next section will discuss.

'At the heart of our profession': *Call the Midwife* and the Royal College of Midwives

Call the Midwife has very close links with the profession it represents in a way that seems unusual for a TV show: it has been used to discuss, debate, and even advertise midwifery as a profession. It is rare now to see a discussion on the profession in the media that does not reference the show, and surely no other television programme is used as a recruitment for a non-TV related undergraduate degree, as, for example, at the University of Northampton. The discussion of the show by staff and students at this university is revealing because it does not only draw on the show's popularity, but also acknowledges that it still sets the standard of aspirational care for the profession. This contrasts with the more medicalised, impersonal model of most medical reality shows, of course: 'the close relationships that evolve between mother, family and midwife throughout her pregnancy and childbirth [in *CTM*] is what is at the heart of our profession and is recognised in the drama of 60 years ago by practicing midwives today' (Pendleton, 2018). In other words, this profession has not changed very much in ideological terms over the last sixty years. What we might consider part of the show's nostalgic appeal – surely any new mother watching mourns for a time where her midwife's help encompasses the many forms of care we see on screen – is, according to this perspective, unnecessary, for the profession today still shares the same values.

This is of course a view which does not allow for the increasing economic and social pressures on the NHS today, however, and indeed not all present-day midwives would couch their vocation in such positive terms. Midwife and author Leah Hazard, for example, condemns *Call the Midwife* as a rosy portrayal of an increasingly complex and demanding job: 'It seems almost sacrilegious to criticise a programme that has become something of a national treasure, but when I look at the relentlessly efficient, smartly smocked heroines of *Call the Midwife*, theirs is not a world that I recognise.' Hazard suggests that rather than being valued in the way the show suggests, midwives are vilified in a society that condemns their views on natural birth, or relegates them to a subservient profession:

> Either way, there's a heady whiff of the witch trials of yore, when wise women (including more than a midwife or two) became the focus of their communities' suspicion, ultimately paying for their knowledge with their lives. Midwives have always existed at that dangerous nexus of female power and fragility – and our presence in that space remains as troublesome now as it ever was. (Hazard, 2019)

Hazard's comments remind us of the issues that have dogged midwifery for hundreds of years, and the way it has been undermined by struggles about knowledge, power, and gender. Her use of the witch trials metaphor, in particular, reveals the profession's anxiety about its public perception and status, increasingly under threat from obstetrics, and from the 'medical model of birth' discussed above: 'Midwifery has been in a state of flux or crisis in many developed countries. Since the 1970s midwives have been concerned with the erosion of their role by the medical profession … midwifery has been marginalised by the language of risk' (Van Teijlingen et al., 2004: 150). With this in mind, *Call the Midwife* seems to be aware that it carries a weight of responsibility as an advertisement for a struggling, often undervalued profession. And this advertisement is working: apparently, applications to midwifery courses are up 16 per cent in the UK since the show first aired (*The Lady*, 2015). Hence the idealised, 'relentlessly efficient' midwives Hazard complains about above – dedicated, professional, and knowledgeable at all times, even when beset with personal difficulties – are advocates for this job whose real prospective midwives wish to emulate. Heidi Thomas has stated she is proud to have 'shone a light on midwifery' but in fact *CTM* has done much more than shine a light: it has become the public face of the profession. It is also, however, notable as a litmus test for that profession's problems and policies.

The midwifery profession and its reputation may have long faced challenges as suggested above but they have arguably never caused such controversy in the UK than over the period of *Call the Midwife*'s eight-year running time. In 2005, the Royal College of Midwives launched the 'Campaign for Normal Birth', an initiative to promote 'natural' childbirth without intervention, in the face of growing concerns about its increasing medicalisation. The consensus of the profession in these years was that 'the neutralising of the labour experience through anaesthesia and bypassing of it altogether in elective caesarean section is a grave development in the evolution of human childbirth' (Walsh and Steen, 2008) and the campaign set out to reverse this trend. It was not exactly a new policy, more an attempt to influence decisions surrounding birth to make an increasing emphasis on, and push for, birth with minimum intervention. The RCM's guidance pamphlet for midwives, 'ten top tips for a normal birth', revealed a strong bias against the use of any technology because it 'gets in the way':

> What we begun to understand [*sic*] about the remarkable new technologies of labour and birth is that one technological intervention is likely to lead to the need for further technological intervention and so on, creating a 'cascade' of intervention ending in an abnormal birth. We need to ask ourselves 'is it really necessary?' (Jokinen, 2008)

In this rhetoric, an assisted birth is an 'abnormal' birth, problematic terminology with psychological implications for those many mothers who end up birthing with technological aid. This policy only really became the focus of media attention when evidence emerged that it may have brought about 'a culture of midwives promoting normal childbirth "at any cost"' (*National Maternity Review*, 2016: 32). The investigation (beginning in 2013 but with its findings published in 2015), into failings at the university hospitals at the Morcambe Bay Trust explored the events which led to the preventable death of sixteen babies and one mother over a nine-year period from 2004. The resulting scandal brought about a backlash against the natural birth movement, as it appeared that in this particular case a specific group of midwives (calling themselves the Musketeers) were acting with too much autonomy and prioritising their profession's desire for minimum intervention over the safety of their patients. It does not necessarily follow that RCM policy in general was to blame, and indeed the focus on minimum intervention, and the associated rhetoric, continued after the Morcambe Bay report was published in March 2015. For example, the RCM magazine in autumn 2015 mentions 'natural' birth some 113 times. As a result of the Morcambe Bay findings, however, change was sought in the maternity care sector. In 2016 Baroness Julia Cumberlege led the National Maternity Review, for example, and the previous year the Each Baby Counts initiative had been launched by obstetricians in the UK to investigate causes of infant mortality and severe brain injury in newborns. This is an ongoing survey, but has identified that there are continuing shortcomings in perinatal care in the UK and that 'in 71% [of cases of problematic births eligible for the study] at least one of the independent reviewers considered that different care might have made a difference to the outcome' (2018). In response to this, the British government have committed to a campaign to improve the maternity provision which does seem to be failing some families. Perhaps as a consequence of all this media attention, or perhaps it was itself aware change was necessary, in August 2017 the RCM announced that it was changing its language and no longer using the term 'natural births' (and removing the now-controversial 'ten tips' quoted above, from its website), while still maintaining its stance that as little intervention as possible was the best way to have a baby. RCM guidance now places a real emphasis on patient choice and support irrespective of birth decisions and includes advice to women who have had a caesarean section.

If *Call the Midwife* is a successful marketing campaign for the profession, then, it has never been needed more than over the last couple of years. The show does, however, reveal complicated and constantly evolving responses to all these events and the debates which surrounded them. It is apparent that it, too, has changed some of its representations of birth following the real-life controversies, and over the last two seasons, it now regularly features assisted births. It still, however, reveals deep ambivalences regarding any birth that is not natural – but those are implicit rather than overt.

Increasing interventionist births in seasons eight and nine

Season eight places intervention immediately on the agenda in episode one, in which Dr Turner (Stephen McGann), rather than the midwives, is seen delivering a baby: in itself an unusual occurrence, and particularly so here because he does so with forceps. The circumstances which surround this are clearly represented as highly exceptional, however, for, unknown to her medical attendants, the mother is carrying triplets, and hence her identity as a more high-risk case has been missed. This is significant as it undermines previous RCM beliefs that potentially difficult births can be identified in advance. The first two babies are delivered normally, however, reinforcing the show's usual message. After delivering the head, the mother gasps that 'she had forgotten what that bit felt like' but making clear that 'nature knows what to do', Nurse Crane (Linda Bassett) responds that 'the body remembers'. Intervention is unnecessary because 'Mother doesn't need our help. She's doing magnificent work here all on her own' (*CTM*, S8E1). It is only the third baby who proves much more difficult to get out and requires the doctor – previously standing by unneeded, as he is with so many births on the show – to take over. In contrast to the forceps plotline of the season before, this procedure is reassuringly straightforward: a local painkiller is given, no episiotomy is required (it would likely have been automatically performed in real life) and the baby is quickly and safely delivered. This normalisation of intervention feels like a watershed moment for the show's birth policy, but it comes with some caveats and reservations. For example, the camera lingers on the tray of instruments as though contrasting their traumatically pathological appearance with the usual towels and aprons that are typically the only props apparent at a *CTM* birth. In addition, the dialogue which accompanies this delivery renders forceps 'acceptable' because the mother's body has already laboured, and experienced birth, not once but twice. Hence it is legitimate that she can now hand over to the doctor, without feeling that she has fallen short in any way: 'you are going to get all the help that we can give you … you've done so much hard work. You leave this to us now.' The unspoken implication here is that intervention is necessary only in extreme circumstances – like undiagnosed triplets – and is non-traumatic only when the mother has already worked for, and experienced, the joys of a heroic birth.

By the next season, a year later, intervention seems to be becoming more quotidian: S9E7 opens with a complete change of the expected format, when, instead of the natural midwife-led birth we have seen so many times, the first scene is a forceps delivery carried out by the young doctor. Once again this feels like a totally new departure for the show, which here implies that assisted birth is routine and helpful. The mother, declaring happily that she could kiss the doctor, is just as pleased as though she had delivered the child herself, and there seem to be no repercussions, emotional or physical, for her or her baby. Later in the episode, however, this is undermined by a related plotline concerning the same doctor, who we learn is a prescription drug addict. At his next birth, he panics and performs an unnecessary episiotomy: he is reaching for the forceps when his attending midwife, horrified, has to intervene and herself delivers the baby successfully. This poor decision making is partly a result of his being under the influence of narcotics, but the previous birth implies that this is also partly habit: because he previously needed to use intervention, and did so successfully, he now thinks all births require them. Ultimately, then, intervention as a first rather than a last choice is born of arrogance and fear. As the angry mother declares, 'you [men] are all scared little boys'. The contrast between male obstetricians

– Dr Turner aside – whose shortcomings can have such damaging consequences for the mothers in their care, and the dedicated and experienced midwives, is made clear by this episode. The line between helpful intervention and unnecessary trauma are blurred here, and by the episode's end, the memory of the previous, non-traumatic procedure is more or less erased by its successor. *CTM* may now acknowledge intervention as a normal procedure, but it will not wholeheartedly condone it.

Call the Midwife and caesarean section

Up to this point I have been discussing mainly forceps-related intervention in *CTM*, but of course more politically loaded still is its representation of the intervention most controversial today: caesarean section. Generally, as with other interventions, the show seems to be determinedly shying away from the procedure, with a tiny number of these kinds of births screened. This is even though it became more common in the late 1950s and through the 1960s, with rates of C-sections in the UK almost doubling over the decade (from 2.7 per cent in 1958 to 4.5 per cent in 1970 (Savage, 2007). Of course, these figures are still not high by today's standards, where one in four babies are delivered this way: indeed, as though to reassure contemporary anxiety about C-section becoming too common, the show seems to be at pains to remind us of a time when it was not. As with forceps – but probably with more historical accuracy – C-section is reserved for a few unusual cases only. Notably, those cases are represented as a necessary, and usually predictable (in line with the 'social model of maternity') response to a particular maternal condition. Those who have C-sections on the show are usually identifiable from the outset of their pregnancy as having a particular pathology that makes a natural birth not only difficult but impossible: in one instance a twisted pelvis which has led to multiple miscarriages in the past, another a mother with dwarfism (S6E2). In the former, the voiceover at the end of the episode reminds us of the miracle of modern science which has saved so many lives, yet again, as with the forceps delivery I suggested above, the sub-verbal content of the episode views the procedure rather differently. This is largely because the mother is 'removed' from the birth: always shown either unconscious on the operating table, or not shown at all, with the birth taking place off-screen. Given that C-section was performed under general anaesthetic at this time, this can be considered an accurate reflection of real-life practice, but the show makes a specific choice not to show the baby delivered alive (the camera always leaves its well-being ambiguous until later), or hear it cry, which need not be affected by the consciousness of the mother. In this sense, it is an operation, not a birth, and this makes a dramatic contrast with the vital, present, heroic births which usually fill the show. In S3E7, for example, a C-section saves the life of a baby with a cord prolapse, but not only is the mother unconscious for the birth, but afterwards the rules of the hospital, and her need to recover from major surgery, mean that she is not allowed see her child for some time, nor is she or the viewer told it is alive. It is only until the compassionate Jenny (Jessica Raine) visits her, against hospital policy, that she learns that she has delivered a healthy baby: 'you have a son ... I can't believe they didn't tell you' (S3E7). All these C-section hospital births feature a dramatic contrast between the personal care of the midwives – who are always the ones to let the mother know the outcome of her operation – and the hospital staff, who see her as a 'specimen' (S6E2) and/or are cold and unfeeling (as in S5E4, where a stillborn, thalidomide baby is cruelly abandoned by doctors after a C-section birth).

Such reservations seem understandable given that for midwives caesarean sections were the worst type of birth, 'bypassing' the labour experience completely and totally medicalising an event that could be a natural, organic experience (Walsh and Steen, 2008). They are also, of course, to be avoided in financial terms: in Britain, they currently cost about £700 more than a vaginal birth, a very real concern given the struggling nature of the NHS (this figure does not, however, take into account compensation paid for medical negligence during birth, which is nine times higher for vaginal birth). These anxieties seem to be echoed in *CTM*, to the extent that it deliberately shies away from the procedure even when the plot seems to demand one. The 2019 Christmas special, for example, deals with Dr Turner's failing confidence in his ability to perform under pressure, and reveals a need to confront his traumatic past in World War II, and prove to himself that he is still young and with a steady nerve. This nerve is tested to the utmost by a problematic birth in the outer Hebrides, in a storm that prevents the removal of the mother to hospital. The plot seems to be building towards a medical crisis and surgical procedure to be dealt with by Dr Turner. Instead of the C-section the viewer half expects, however, it turns out to be acute appendicitis which the mother is suffering from, and the birth itself is 'normal' and successfully attended to by the midwives. Typically (for the show) heroic, the mother seems able to put her own suffering aside for the birth, telling the midwife that her final contractions are 'no longer pain ... they are power': even in a pathological crisis, the female body 'knows what to do'. Only after a successful delivery is complete is she operated on by the doctor and he removes her appendix, also in her own home. This rather unlikely scenario seems to make plain the show's continuing commitment to natural childbirth even when the demands of the plot require a surgery scene. A famous article from *The Times* in 1970 argued that 'to suggest we go back to the days of home confinement is like asking a modern surgeon to remove an appendix on the kitchen table': this episode, in a rather tongue in cheek way, does both.

This said, however, it is possible to see a gradual change in the representation of C-section in the show as it progresses, especially after the Morcambe Bay report and the gradual changes in RCM policy it generated. Series six, for example, may be still unwilling to positively represent the procedure in hospital at home in the UK, but abroad it is a different story. This series opens with a two-part Christmas special in which the midwives travel to South Africa in order to help with a rural mission hospital there. As its somewhat belligerent lead physician (Sinead Cusack) informs them to their surprise, C-section is a common and necessary procedure here:

> Too many of our mothers were malnourished as children so we see a lot of very narrow pelvises ... the witch doctor can't save them, but we can, with forceps or a Caesarean. Babies are precious here ... These women are poor, and they are black, and they live in a society that is gradually stripping them of any freedoms that they ever had. So motherhood is everything. It is status, purpose, life itself. And we have to help it to happen. But medicine is never about doing what's easy. It's about doing what's essential. (S6E0)

The normalisation – even redemption – of intervention here contrasts significantly with what takes place at home in the East End, but it is notable that it is 'essential' procedure for these women: without it, many of them, including one we see later in the episode, would die. This is factually accurate: pelvic size due to malnutrition still makes birth dangerous for many women in sub-Saharan Africa today (Munabi et al., 2016) and *CTM* uses its temporary relocation there as an opportunity to make C-section plots take centre stage, while still keeping them, geographically and ideologically, far from home. There is still a heroic – particularly so because it takes place in the middle of the desert – natural birth screened in this episode, but the holiday special's culmination and drama come in a dangerous and unconventional C-section performed not by a doctor but by a midwife. It is Trixie (Helen George) who here wields the scalpel, having witnessed a number of the operations since her arrival in South Africa, and willing to take huge risks since the doctors are away. Significantly, the debate between her and Sister Julienne (Jenny Agutter) over whether intervention is permissible feels like a debate about the role of midwives within modern maternity care as a whole:

> 'You are right ... if we don't intervene, the uterus will rupture. Constance needs a caesarean section. Without one, neither she nor the child will survive. And there's no one here who can do that for her.'

> 'We have no choice. We have to operate ourselves.'
> 'We are midwives, Nurse Franklin. I don't normally wish we were doctors too, but I do today.' (S6E2)

Trixie's response, that she has seen many caesareans and is 'skilled enough and desperate enough', asserts that she is capable to do all that a doctor can, and the successful operation proves her right. This feels like a particularly feminist moment in the series because it is one of the very few occasions where the characters overstep their (usually very clearly defined) professional roles. At no other point in the drama do the midwives, usually so fulfilled in their vocation, express any 'wish [to be] doctors too', even with the increased authority and status that would accompany that, in the real world at least. Of course, in a way reminiscent of the happily docile staff at *Downton Abbey* (2010–2015), they are so valued and respected in their current positions they have no need to wish for more! But in this episode Trixie, arguably one of the most complex and rebellious characters in the show, has already articulated frustration with the status quo. She has rallied against the kind of patriarchal society which values women only for their reproductive power, following her discovery of a phantom pregnancy in a woman who desperately wanted to bear a child: 'Don't you see why this has happened? Because she's been forced into a wretched, narrow, filthy life, where her only worth comes from what she can grow in her womb. She wanted that baby so badly her body started lying to her' (S6E2). It is the rural, traditional society of South Africa that Trixie is condemning, but what she says is equally applicable to many of her own patients at home. Indeed it recalls FitzGerald's concern, quoted at the start of this chapter, that women have always only had any real power when they are associated with birth, and that is as true for contemporary society as it was in the 1960s. Negra argues that post-feminist culture mobilises discourses of nostalgia to negotiate tensions between its impetus to 'cast women as subjects of their own self-determination' (2009: 107), and competing imperatives to restore traditional gender roles, especially at times of crisis. *Call the Midwife*'s key characters exactly dramatise these tensions: Trixie becomes a self-taught surgeon in this episode, which also features an influential female physician (Cusack), but on her return home to London is restored to her traditional gender-prescribed role as midwife. Significantly, it seems to be through plots associated with caesarean section that the show interrogates the status quo most overtly; the midwives clash and argue with male physicians in all the hospital plots I mentioned above, too, but when they return to the usual core business of natural birth, the tensions and resistance of surgical birth seem to be happily forgotten.

Conclusion

When Helen George, the actor who plays Trixie in the show, gave birth recently she revealed in a *Radio Times* interview that she did so via an elective caesarean because of what she'd 'learnt on *Call the Midwife* ... working on the show means that lots of people tell you their horror stories' (Lang, 2018). The interviewer 'nearly choked on their tea', so surprising was this admission from someone who we expect to have internalised the experiences she acts. Significantly, George clearly felt she had to defend her choice and she did receive a lot of online vitriol for sharing it: a reminder that maternal choice in childbirth remains as controversial as ever. This chapter set out to explore some of these controversies and the ideologies which surround this highly popular show, and the changes that have occurred within it over its many series. It is unsurprising, given its provenance, that *CTM* represents unassisted vaginal birth as both the norm and the ideal, but I have tried to argue here that this is not without its issues. As O'Brien Hill argues, most mothers 'are shown to be heavily invested in both the good mother myth and the ideals of the natural childbirth movement', irrespective of their background and social class, with a resulting 'pressure to achieve a "natural birth"' (2014: 200). *Call the Midwife* adds to this pressure through its valorisation of natural birth, and its recurrent anxiety about all kinds of assisted birth. Forceps or C-section delivery may be often avoided or evaded by the show, both in terms of plot and camera attention, but in real life these are often an unavoidable reality or (especially in the latter case) a constructive choice for many women, George among them. *CTM* is a nostalgic period drama, of course, and it could be argued its primary goal is to entertain, or at most to teach about the past, not to inform or shape maternity policy in the present. This show does have a deep influence upon a wide range of viewers, however: not only parents but future and current midwives are affected by its representation of the profession, as the discussion here has shown. Hence its politics do matter, especially given the turbulent and hotly contested state of midwifery in the UK over the last few years. The show does appear to have done much to redeem a profession that has historically been vilified or sidelined, partly because it is female-dominated, and it reminds the audience of the value and importance of its contribution to society. The problem remains, however, that it is largely unwilling to challenge midwifery's continuing assertion that natural is best, even if that means long-term physical or emotional implications for mothers who do not manage to – or even wish to – achieve a 'heroic' birth.

References

Anon. (2015). 'The *Call The Midwife* factor', *The Lady*, https://lady.co.uk/call-midwife-factor (accessed 2 August 2020).

De Benedictis, S., C. Johnson, J. Roberts and H. Spiby (2019). 'Quantitative insights into televised birth: a content analysis of *One Born Every Minute*', *Critical Studies in Media Communication*, 36:1, pp. 1–17.

FitzGerald, L. (2015). 'Taking a pregnant pause: Interrogating the feminist potential of *Call the Midwife*', in Leggott and Taddeo (eds), *Upstairs and Downstairs: British Costume Drama Television from The Forsyte Saga to Downton Abbey*. Rowman and Littlefield, pp. 249–263.

Griffiths, E. B. (2017). 'How realistic is that *Call the Midwife* Christmas stillborn storyline?' *Radio Times*, www.radiotimes.com/news/tv/2018-12-21/how-realistic-is-that-call-the-midwife-christmas-stillborn-storyline/ (accessed 2 August 2020).

Hazard, L. (2019). 'My life as a midwife is nothing like it's portrayed on TV', *The Guardian*, www.theguardian.com/society/2019/apr/27/midwife-midwives-nothing-like-tv-smiling-angels-hi-tech-cheerleaders (accessed 2 August 2020)

Herman, D. (2013). 'Horlicks for Chummy: Britain's romance with cosy TV nostalgia', *New Statesman*.

Jokinen, M. (ed.) (2008). *Campaign for Normal Birth: Top Ten Tips*. Royal College of Midwives.

Lang, K. (2018). '*Call the Midwife*'s Helen George on pregnancy, childbirth and women being shamed for choosing to have C-sections', *Radio Times*, www.radiotimes.com/news/tv/2018-06-20/call-the-midwifes-helen-george-on-pregnancy-childbirth-and-women-being-shamed-for-choosing-to-have-c-sections/ (accessed 2 August 20).

Mander, R. and J. Murphy-Lawless (2013). *The Politics of Maternity*, Routledge.

MacKenzie Bryers H. and E. Van Teijlingen (2010). 'Risk, theory, social and medical models: A critical analysis of the concept of risk in maternity care', *Midwifery*, 26:5, pp. 488–496.

Michaels, P. A. (2018). 'Childbirth and trauma, 1940s–1980s', *Journal of the History of Medicine and Allied Sciences*, 73:1, pp. 52–72.

'Midwifery care in labour guidance for all women in all settings' (2018). *Royal College of Midwives*, 1 (Nov 2018), www.rcm.org.uk/media/2539/professionals-blue-top-guidance.pdf (accessed 16 March 2020).

Midwives Magazine. Royal College of Midwives, Autumn 2015, www.rcm.org.uk/media/2673/midwives-autumn-2015.pdf (accessed 4 August 2020).

Moran, C. (2013). 'Call the radical feminist', TV review in *The Times*, www.thetimes.co.uk/article/caitlin-moran-on-tv-call-the-radical-feminist-f765chg72wq (accessed 16 August 2020).

Munabi, I. G. et al. (2016). 'Association between maternal pelvis height and intrapartum foetal head moulding in Ugandan mothers with spontaneous vertex deliveries', *Obstetrics and Gynecology International*, vol. 2016.

National Maternity Review: Better Births (2016). www.england.nhs.uk/wp-content/uploads/2016/02/national-maternity-review-report.pdf (accessed 16 March 2020).

O'Brien Hill, G. (2014). 'The older Mother *in One Born Every Minute*', in I. Whelehan and J. Gwynne (eds), *Ageing, Popular Culture and Contemporary Feminism: Harleys and Hormones*, Palgrave Macmillan, pp. 187–202.

Pendleton, J. (2018). 'What message does the BBC's 'Call the Midwife' deliver about the profession?' *University of Northampton News*, www.northampton.ac.uk/news/what-message-does-the-bbcs-call-the-midwife-deliver-about-the-profession/ (accessed 16 March 2020).

The Royal College of Obstetricians and Gynaecologists (2018). *Each Baby Counts*, www.rcog.org.uk/globalassets/documents/guidelines/research--audit/each-baby-counts/each-baby-counts-report-2018-11-12.pdf (accessed 16 March 2020).

Sandeman, G. (2017). 'Midwives to end campaign to promote 'normal' births', *The Guardian*, www.theguardian.com/society/2017/aug/12/midwives-to-stop-using-term-normal-birth#:~:text=Midwives%20are%20to%20end%20their,medical%20interventions%20feel%20like%20failures (accessed 16 August 2020).

Savage, W. (2007). 'The rising caesarean section rate: A loss of obstetric skill?' *Journal of Obstetrics and Gynaecology*, 27:4, pp. 339–346.

Takeshita, C. (2017). 'Countering Technocracy: "Natural" Birth in *The Business of Being Born* and *Call the Midwife*', *Feminist Media Studies*, 17 (3), pp. 332–346.

Towler, J. and J. Bramall (1986). *Midwives in History and Society*. Croom Helm.

Tyler, I. and L. Baraitser (2013). 'Private View, Public Birth: Making Feminist Sense of the New Visual Culture of Childbirth', *Studies in the Maternal*, 5 (2), pp. 1–7.

Van Teijlingen G. L. et al. (2004). *Midwifery and the Medicalization of Childbirth: Comparative Perspectives*. Nova Publishers.

Walsh D. and M. Steen (2020). 'The role of the midwife: Time for a review', *Midwives Magazine*, reproduced on RCM website, www.rcm.org.uk/news-views/rcm-opinion/the-role-of-the-midwife-time-for-a-review/#:~:text=Holism%20requires%20a%20midwife%20to,experience%20of%20labour%20and%20birth.&text=The%20relationship%20between%20the%20midwife,experiences%20of%20pregnancy%20and%20birth (accessed 4 August 2020).

9

'Physician, heal thyself': the good doctor of *When the Boat Comes In*

James Leggott

Created and mostly written by the South Shields-born writer James Mitchell, the BBC's historical drama *When the Boat Comes In* (1976–1981) was an immediate ratings and critical success when first broadcast in early 1976. It has historical interest as the first long-running series on British television to be set (for the most part) in north-east England, and its representation of an economically disadvantaged industrial town had an important role in shaping the image of the region's history, culture, and dialect in the popular imagination, even if it was stereotyped in some quarters as 'flat caps on every corner' (Hutchings, 1996: 274). This chapter will consider how the series weaves medical plots and themes into its tapestry of interwar political and social history, and pay particular attention to one of its central characters, a young doctor whose radical ideas about practice put him at odds with his family and community (see Figure 9.1).

To be fair, *When the Boat Comes In* is probably not remembered as much for this doctor figure as for its intriguing central character, Jack Ford, who was charismatically played by James Bolam, already a household name in the United Kingdom for his work in TV comedies and dramas. Over the course of four series shown between 1976 and 1981, comprising a total of fifty-one episodes of around fifty minutes' length each, the show demanded investment in the character's fluctuating financial and romantic fortunes. He is introduced in the opening episode, upon his return from World War I (via Russia) back to his depressed hometown of Gallowshields (a fictional name, but clearly reminiscent of South Shields), which offers few opportunities other than tough work in the local shipyards and coalmines. By the end of the first series, he has risen to the position of district secretary of the (shipyard) fitters' union, but his boundless ambition and steeliness propel him through cycles of entrepreneurial fortune and failure in the following decade. By the time of the fourth and last series, he has returned to Britain from America after losing his bootlegging fortune in the Wall Street Crash, but soon is rich again and mingling with London high society, before he is killed in Civil War-era Spain following a bungled gun-running mission.

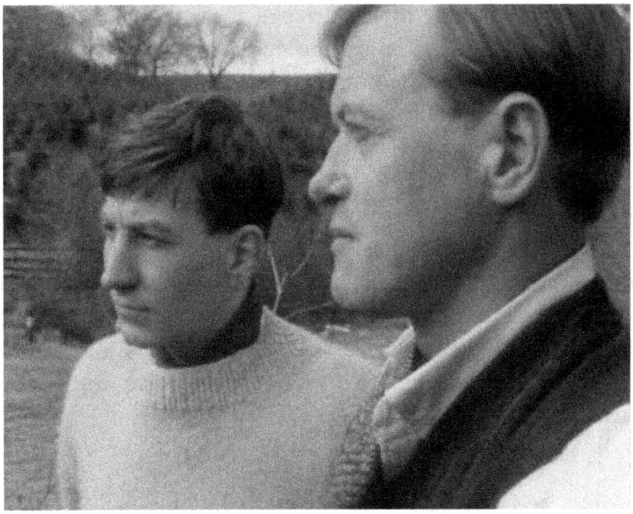

Figure 9.1 Billy Seaton and Jack Ford (*When the Boat Comes In*)

Given that the characterisation of Jack Ford is one of the main pleasures of *When the Boat Comes In*, it is unsurprising that the show has tended to be conceptualised by way of his appeal and peculiarity. Bolam's image features prominently, for example, across the artwork for the VHS and DVD releases, and the manner in which he provides a 'highly distinct male image for the British screen in the 1970s' (McNally, 2007: 119) is the main focus of the only substantial academic writing on the series to date. In her article, 'The Geordie and the American Hero: Revisiting Classic Hollywood Masculinity in *When the Boat Comes In*', McNally argues that the portrayal of Ford as aspirational charmer had 'little in common with standard cinematic or televisual depictions of the British working man' (McNally, 2007: 107), and was more akin to the 'American hero' of classic Hollywood cinema. Indeed, even the character's proper name, John Ford, carries clear associations of the archetypes of strong masculinity associated with the western genre.

However, this chapter is less concerned with the singularity of Jack Ford than the way this character is repeatedly contrasted in the show with the 'good doctor', Billy Seaton, and the emphasis throughout (with the exception of the final series) upon medical debates and concerns. The way in which numerous plotlines turn on health crises and conditions can of course be understood as dramatic necessity; having introduced a core group of sympathetic characters, the writers of continuing drama are duty-bound to generate scenarios of jeopardy and peril – and here we have work accidents, problematic pregnancies, mental breakdowns, and so forth. There is even an occasional mordant streak to the matter-of-fact incorporation of hospitals, clinics, injuries, and death into the ongoing drama; for example, one episode has a character's uncle giving an (accurate) racing tip as his dying words in hospital, although fate intervenes to prevent the bet from being placed. The incorporation of medical and health concerns into long-running period dramas is hardly unique, and *When the Boat Comes In* sits comfortably within a tradition encompassing the likes of *Poldark* (1975–1977; 2015–2019) and *Downton Abbey* (2010–2015), as discussed by others in this collection. But I would argue that the health-related aspects of *When the Boat Comes In* are not just historical colour, or simply used for generating melodramatic plot developments, but rather are crucial to the show's (occasionally didactic) conceptualisation of conflicts between collectivism and individualism, and between socialism and capitalism.

Jack Ford, the Seaton family, and the Gallowshields poor

Typical of the 'studio' production style of the era, the show's themes and plots take shape through lengthy scenes of dialogue, many of which involve Ford on the make, negotiating a better deal for himself or others, or turning happenstance into an advantage. The show's creator has observed that:

> In the days about which I am writing there were two ways out of the appalling economic mess: one was to change the world, the other to change yourself. And to change yourself you needed charm and wit and, I suppose, a fair helping of bluff. (Mitchell, 1976: 26)

The viewer is often led to wonder, as a particular scene or storyline gets underway, whether Ford's actions are for self-interest, self-preservation, or negotiations on behalf of his brotherhood of fellow soldiers or workers; the code of the 'marra' – a Northumbrian dialect term for close friends and work pals (Jackson, 2019: 2) – is much invoked in conversation. In his cultural history of north-east English identity, *The Northumbrians*, Dan Jackson notes how the history of the region's people is 'one where mutuality has always been more cherished than individualism' (Jackson, 2019: 3), and this notion of collectivism have been attributed to the area's particularly strong martial traditions as much as to its inherently strenuous forms of manual labour and concomitant ideals of masculinity.

Much of the dramatic interest of *When the Boat Comes In* comes not only from the way Ford's actions and behaviour pivot between philosophies of mutuality and individualism, but also how his strategies of social and economic betterment contrast with those of the show's other recurring characters: the Seaton family. As introduced to us, and Jack, in the first episode, the Seatons are comprised of mining father Bill (James Garbutt), housewife mother Bella (Jean Heywood), and three grown-up children: miner Tom (John Nightingale), school-teacher Jessie (Susan Jameson), and – particularly relevant to this collection – a medical student named Billy (Edward Wilson), whose character and storylines will be shortly discussed in detail. By the close of the series, almost all of these characters will have attained a degree of material success. However, along the way, they are all affected in some way by health-related problems or incidents, whether directly or indirectly.

Following a brief courtship with Ford, the school-teacher Jessie, initially a socialist firebrand, marries her patrician, Tory-voting head-teacher, Arthur Ashton (Geoffrey Rose). As the series progresses, she becomes increasingly enervated, and is bed-ridden for a stretch with a condition explained as anaemia, which complicates her pregnancy. Although this may have been a pragmatic necessity given the real-life pregnancy of the actress, it is hard not to give a feminist reading to the way her husband – and the programme itself – confines and sidelines her, eventually shifting her off-screen altogether when her husband insists upon a move to a teaching post far away from Tyneside. In early episodes, her brother Tom makes the difficult and damaging decision to be a 'scab' during a miners' strike, so as to provide for his wife Mary (Michelle Newell), who is dying of tuberculosis, for which, as his medical student brother Billy says, there is no treatment, apart from the right food and climate: only a 'boss's wife' would have any chance of recovery. Significantly, it is only when Bill Seaton, the family patriarch and former miner, becomes a 'boss' himself that he is able to afford the pioneering orthopaedic surgery that allows him to walk again following the pit accident that broke his back in the first place – for Bill used the compensation money from the pit owners (brokered by Jack Ford no less) to set up the first of a successful chain of shops. This concern with the inequalities of medical treatment is given significant emphasis, as I will discuss shortly, through the storylines concerning Billy and his commitment to free clinics. But it is often conveyed with subtlety, such as when Jack's first wife Dolly (Madelaine Newton) suffers a miscarriage and is offered private hospital treatment paid for by the businessman with whom Jack is entering a relationship.

The storyline concerning Bill's injury, treatment, and recovery also illustrates how a long-running show with such well-established character relationships as *When the Boat Comes In* can take pause to capture the material, lived experiences of medical procedures. The mechanics of getting patients into hospital is often dwelled upon, such as the commandeering of Rolls Royce cars as makeshift ambulances, or the necessity for a doctor to accompany a patient for referral purposes. There is a detailed sequence showing

Bella carefully packing her husband's bag for the operation, with the objects in question – 'proper soap' and 'two separate flannels' – shown in the foreground of the screen, whilst the irritable Bill in the background chides her fussing; as other scenes have shown, he has been more concerned about the practicalities of life insurance policies. Bella insists on him taking his own pillow, as the ones in the hospital are 'like doorsteps: they won't wash 'em'. There follows a lengthy scene showing the arrival of the ambulance, the placing of Bill on a stretcher, and Bella's caring act of subterfuge as she smuggles the aforementioned pillow into the ambulance, contravening the edict against it (for reasons of possible contamination). Bella is established early in the series as the voice of superstition and fear with regard to medical procedures, at one point shrugging off her own crippling pain as mere 'colic', until it is eventually diagnosed as appendicitis: 'there's nobody sticking their knives in me', she despairs.

These plotlines involving Bill and Bella, and other characters, falling ill have an important structural purpose too, in balancing other stories of a more drily 'corporate' nature. The episode depicting Bill's admission into hospital also features the culmination of a complex boardroom plot involving Jack Ford and the wealthy entrepreneur Sir Horatio Manners (Basil Henson) in a hostile take-over of an engineering firm. In the traditional manner of the continuing drama format, episodes of *When the Boat Comes In* tend to feature two or three plot threads, and here the rather cerebral take-over plot is leavened somewhat by the scenes encouraging the viewer to share in the Seaton family's sentimental and financial worries over the hospitalisation of a loved one. This particular storyline also exposes the delicate politics of family consent where illness and treatment are concerned, and of power within the typical working-class Tyneside household. Once Billy hears of a potential treatment for his father, there are debates about whether this should be pursued, or conveyed to him; his wife, as we might expect, has no desire for anyone to 'stick knives' in her husband, and argues that as she has managed him adequately so far, so he should not be told. Similarly, after his operation, Bill insists that certain details about the procedure should not be conveyed to his wife.

Beyond the Seaton family, *When the Boat Comes In* depicts a community beset by health risks and injuries, whether through war experience, dangerous work conditions, or simple poverty. The first episode features a character scarred by shell shock, and other war-injured men are cited or shown, such as the one-armed artist Jack employs for a commercial design task and the shipyard fitter who was doubly unlucky to catch a bullet in conflict and then Spanish flu afterwards, resulting in lifelong pleurisy. As with another, more recently made exploration of masculine pathology, *Peaky Blinders* (2013–), discussed elsewhere in this book by Dan Ward, the programme diagnoses the psychological impact of warfare, not least through the eventual statement by the orphaned Jack Ford that almost all of his true friends died in the war, thus giving a rational explanation for his ruthless business streak, but also his attraction to the Seatons as a compensatory family. His inscrutability may well make sense as a defence mechanism, but there is also room to interpret his 'marra' code of loyalty to his fellow soldiers as a coldly opportunistic performance – as a means, for instance, of asserting dominance over those who did not witness the same level of wartime bloodshed. As the series progresses into the 1920s and then 1930s, his oft-told story about a dying soldier buddy is met with mounting indifference, particularly by the various women around him who are quick to express weariness at the long shadow of the 'damn war'. In the final series, he exposes, with some good humour, the falsehood of a begging war 'veteran', who is wearing medals honouring, impossibly, his involvement in battles that took place simultaneously. Even at this late stage of the series, it is unclear whether this old man is to be regarded as a warped mirror of Jack himself, forever clinging to the past, or a doleful comment on the way the Great War was slipping away from the public consciousness, even as a new storm was gathering across Europe. There are also insinuations about Jack's alcoholism, again diagnosable in relation to his war experiences, but not exactly uncommon within the Gallowshields community; even the upright Seaton matriarch Bella is affectionately portrayed as prone to temptation. Should *When the Boat Come In* ever inspire a drinking game, there should be a special tipple for the many times where Jack, or others, take a swig following a toast to someone's 'good health' – quite the irony, given my analysis here of the show's preoccupation with the body in peril.

Then there are the wretched townsfolk who inspire the Seatons and other characters to acts of charity, like the widowed mothers with malnourished children; Tom takes pity on a child who has been stealing from his vegetable allotment, Jack goes to prison as a result of intervening on behalf of a struggling family, and Bella gives shelter to an orphaned child whose subsequent thieving results in him being sent on an emigration scheme to Australia. On his way to becoming district secretary of the fitters' union, and then in post and after, Jack becomes embroiled in a number of compensation cases involving injuries which convey, like Bill's pit accident, the exploitative treatment of workers, and the complicated strategies required to ensure appropriate pay-outs and medical care. But debilitating health conditions are no respecter of class or wealth either. The self-made businessman Sir Horatio Manners, Jack's former collaborator turned entrepreneurial rival, has lost his only son in the war, and the fact that Jack witnessed his dying moments on the battlefield (or claimed to, anyway) gives a complex quasi-filial element to his relationship with his father. But there is also a strange, hothouse quality to the rooms where Manners holds court with Jack, with allusions in the dialogue to his 'reptilian' requirement for intense heating, presumably a symptom of some sort of debilitating blood-thinning illness. It is never specified, but Manners does at one point issue a splenetic response to a criticism of his harsh treatment of his workforce: 'the diseases of management are ulcers, thrombosis and blood pressure – if I'm risking those, no shop steward's dictating to me when I fire a slacker'.

The implication of what Manners says is clear: that being successful in business and being frail of health are simply incompatible – to succeed is to stay well. The frailties associated with the Seaton family and those in their neighbourhood only serve to accentuate the almost superhuman ability of Ford to survive all that fate – and the scriptwriters – throw at him, which includes: outliving most of his 'marras' on the battlefield, numerous physical attacks upon his person (including by a gang of fascist thugs), a near-death escape when trying to explode a stately home with dynamite, a Mob vendetta, and bankruptcy following the Wall Street Crash that reduces him to near-vagrancy. One of the ultimate ironies of the story is that Jack is ultimately not brought down by any of his more obvious adversaries – Horatio Manners, his rivals in politics in business, the Mob, or even the women he has loved and left – but by a rather unexpected figure from his past: Dr Billy Seaton. Their antagonism emerges slowly over the course of the four series; at first, they are on good terms, despite Billy's repeated campaigning of Jack to turn his organisational acumen to better social use – to become not just a more active citizen, and a committed socialist, but to enter the political arena. As the characters begin to cross swords over time, it becomes clear that the programme is positioning them as opposing points of a political and philosophical spectrum that sees one as an embodiment of material aspiration, the other of a tenacious commitment to the assistance of the poor – with the various other characters occupying fluctuating positions on this spectrum, depending on their circumstance and health. What are we to make of the way, in the final episodes of the series, Jack's violent demise is brought about by the machinations of a supposedly 'good' doctor, albeit in the name of the anti-fascist cause?

In hindsight, the different philosophical positions represented by Jack and Billy – the 'self-made man' versus the altruistic doctor coming to the rescue of the poor – have a loose parallel in the epidemiological debates of the mid-1970s (the time of the programme's first broadcast) around the changing relationship between citizenship and the welfare state (Clark, 2020). Virginia Berridge (2003) has observed that by this time, a new approach to public health was in the ascendant internationally, emphasising the role of the individual to take responsibility for their own health (as demonstrated, for example, by the proposals of the 'Lalonde' report published in Canada in 1974). The idea of the 'risk-avoiding individual' would become enshrined

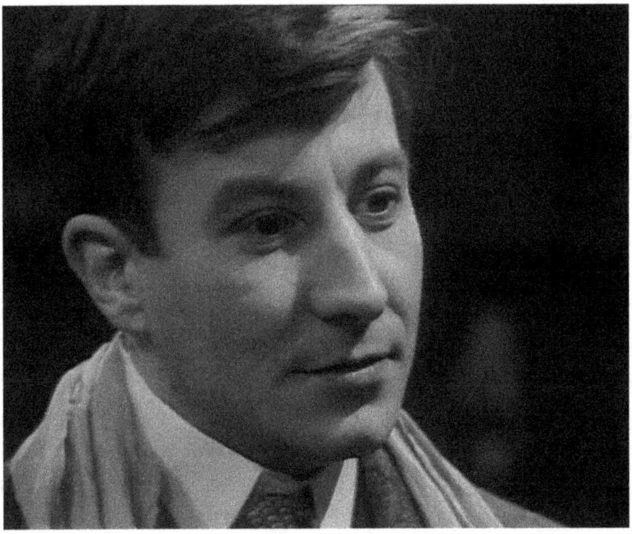

Figure 9.2 Dr Billy Seaton (*When the Boat Comes In*)

in UK public health policy; according to Charles Webster (2002: 137), the 'sick were accused of bringing ill health upon themselves and thereby wasting the resources of the NHS'. Key to this was the idea that 'prevention' was a means of addressing the financial shortfalls of the NHS, which underwent a major reorganisation in 1974. The concept underpinning such thinking is that certain diseases can be understood as caused primarily by an individual's behaviour, be it smoking, alcohol intake, sexual activity, drug-taking, etc. As I will discuss, such thinking is anathema to Dr Billy Seaton, and the broader world of *When the Boat Comes In*, which repeatedly associates illness with living and working conditions that an individual, or their family, have no real power to change. With its polluted air, widespread poverty, and high rate of diseases such as TB, industrial Tyneside is figured as an inherently unhealthy place to live, and a number of Billy's patients, including those with terminal illnesses, observe that they are powerless to follow his suggestions, for example, that they give up work, or even alcohol (Gallowshields has its fair share of alcoholics who convey that there is little else to live for) (see Figure 9.2).

When the Boat Comes In and the TV doctor

Before looking in detail at the shaping of the Billy Seaton story, it is worth considering how *When the Boat Comes In* dovetailed with the generic expectations of contemporary viewers. Even the most positive contemporary reviewers acknowledged that it was working some well-worn televisual seams: most notably the 1920s-set drama (such as *Upstairs Downstairs* [1971–1975]), and the 'gritty northern saga' (Purser, 2002: 26) involving characters struggling to escape or survive harsh industrial environments: examples include the 1975 ITV adaptation of A. J. Cronin's 1935 novel *The Stars Look Down*, the controversial *Days of Hope* (1975), and the Yorkshire-set *Sam* (1973–1975). Given that the first series of *When the Boat Comes In* also coincided with a BBC adaptation of Richard Llewellyn's novel *How Green Was My Valley* (1975–1976) about a Welsh mining community and an ITV adaptation of Arnold Bennett's Potteries-set *Clayhanger* (1976), it was hard to avoid certain clichés of representation and storytelling, particularly where the perils of manual labour were concerned. For example, in a review of an early episode of *When the Boat Comes In*, Clive James praised the overall quality of the programme, but expressed mock sadness about the plot concerning the coal-mine roof falling upon the Seaton family patriarch: 'it is one of the blessings of *Clayhanger*', he went on, 'that the series is set in the Potteries, thus ruling out the possibility that the roof of a coal-mine will fall on the hero's father; there is always the chance, I suppose, that a kiln will instead' (James, 1976: 26). Although *When the Boat Comes In* was of course neither promoted nor received as a medical-based drama, its portrayal of the pre-NHS health care landscape of the interwar years may have evoked viewer memories of the BBC's long-running and relatively cosy *Dr Finlay's Casebook* (1962–1971), set in rural Scotland of the 1920s, and often featuring plotlines about its young titular GP clashing but ultimately compromising with older colleagues about how to best dispense treatment (Clark, n.d.).

However, there was perhaps a more obvious comparison to be made with the BBC's 1970s *Poldark* serial, which was coming to the end of its first series around the time of the debut broadcast of *When the Boat Comes In*. There are indeed some similarities between the dramatic function and philosophies of Billy Seaton and his late-eighteenth-century counterpart Dwight Enys (Richard Morant/Michael Cadman), whose characterisation in the BBC's more recent update is the subject of Barbara Sadler's chapter in this volume. Both men have a strong relationship with the respective central characters of the show, Ross Poldark (Robin Ellis) and Jack Ford, although Billy's unshakeable socialist principles frequently bring him into collision with Jack's schemes. Billy and Dwight are similarly positioned as progressive young medics, rubbing up against the medical establishment and orthodoxy, not least by a willingness to serve the poorest of their communities without taking payment. The characters thus have broadly similar conceptual functions within their respective programmes' evocation of community and hardship in a particular place and time: they are a conscientious foil to the main protagonist. In *When the Boat Comes In*, this could not be spelt out any clearer than by its concluding image of a dying Jack being held by Billy and his sister Jessie, a former romantic partner of Jack and likely true love. Although Billy does not appear for much of the final series, his return in the last few episodes, and his centrality in the final moments, serves to emphasise the structural and thematic importance of this seemingly 'secondary' character to the programme overall. The clearest difference between Billy and Dwight, however, is their vastly different social background, and *When the Boat Comes In* pays attention to the debts and compromises involved when someone of humble origins comes to be educated out of their class.

Billy Seaton: from student to practitioner

At the time of the first series, Billy is a student of medicine at Edinburgh University, returning back home to Gallowshields out of term time, or on the occasions when he comes close to abandoning his studies. Although not the first member of his family to study for a 'professional' vocation – his older sister Jessie is by now working as a school-teacher – Billy is presumably the first Seaton man of many generations not to become a manual worker, and to study away from home, and there is some predictability to his double alienation from, on the one hand, the fellow students who are condescending towards his working-class background or the colleagues who treat him as an 'idiot child', and, on the other, those in his community and family who belittle his passionate socialism as the indulgence of, in his father's words, a 'college boy'. The location of the university is significant: Edinburgh is not only nearer to Tyneside than London, but it was also commonplace for the gentry and bourgeoisie of north-east England to send their sons there (Jackson, 2019: 16), hence the culture shock for Billy among the region's well-to-do. There is a telling confrontation with a former schoolmate, now a policeman, who is criticised by Billy as a class traitor for being prepared to attack strikers; the policeman retorts that 'we can't all escape to fancy jobs', and sends Billy on his way with a cutting 'ha'way, Karl Marx'.[1] It is at this point in his studies that he first expresses his desire to be a 'socialist doctor not a capitalist doctor', and comes close to throwing away his qualification because of what he perceives as the powerlessness of the conscientious doctor to bring about any societal good. As he says:

> There's a ward full of bairns full of rickets in the infirmary, and there's doctors treating them, but what for? They're just sending them back on their feet into the same rotten system that put them there in the first place!

Edward Wilson brings a sympathetic earnestness to the part, but such sentiments are not received well by his family, not least because of the perceived debt he owes to his family for his education (which will become a real bone of contention in the second series onwards). A number of early scenes convey the gauche unworldliness of the character when bumping up against the pragmatism of others, particularly Jack Ford. In the first episode, Billy informally diagnoses the erratic, violent behaviour of a shell-shocked veteran as a nervous breakdown, and is puzzled that Jack has long fathomed this out himself. He tells Billy that it 'doesn't take a genius to work it out': after all, unlike the younger man, he was *there* in the field of battle – not for the first time in the series, experiential knowledge trumps intellectual interpretation and practical charity triumphs over political theory. Furthermore, the character is often framed in ways that suggest his *unmanliness* in the eyes of others; family members frequently bar him from physical tasks, and his contribution to a New Year musical get-together is the appropriately infantilising (and perhaps emasculating) 'Daddy Wouldn't Buy Me a Bow Wow'.[2]

Billy becomes more central to the plotlines of the second series, which sees him returning home as a qualified doctor, deciding to stay in Gallowshields rather than continue his studies as a specialist, and then taking an unsalaried position at a slum clinic that treats the town's poorest inhabitants. Billy's educational achievement is potentially the pride of his family, and his father admits that 'the thought of him becoming a doctor got me through more hard [mining] shifts'. The series plants early the idea that professional training is a ticket out of a town that Billy's sister Jessie describes bluntly as a 'dump'. In the first series, the widowed miner Tom briefly courts a nurse about to relocate to Edinburgh for midwifery training, and she defines the 'Gallowshields sickness' and its limited escape routes. No wonder Billy's father declares the town as 'no place for doctors'. The idea that Billy can be a good socialist doctor on his own doorstep is not just anathema to his family, but perceived as a kind of betrayal of their collective aspirations for social and financial betterment. In a way typical of the show's attention to material specifics, his father takes a moment to calculate as precisely as he can the cost of Billy's education, factoring in his four extra years of school (his brother Tom left at fourteen to work in the mine), his five years of college studies, and other elements such as the piano they sold to support him: the total comes to £1,080, which Billy vows to pay back in instalments. The programme gives a glimpse of the rewards on offer for GPs who only treat affluent paying customers when Billy attends an unsuccessful interview to work alongside a middle-aged doctor based in a wealthy neighbourhood; the doctor confesses to having had socialist ideals in his youth, which have been driven away by a desire for the 'status quo and a nice life', which are only attainable through patients that are less likely to die than those in working-class areas.

However, Billy finds an alternative role model in the free Wellesley Street clinic – described by his sceptical brother Tom as a 'kind of casualty' ward – operated by the ailing Dr Stoker (John Gabriel) in an unsafe, rat-infested slum quarter due for demolition, where the doctors can sleep rent-free. Stoker asks Billy if he is a 'saint or an idiot' for taking a job with no remuneration other than payment in kind (which seems to be mostly a lot of unwanted cod). The programme's juxtaposition of two highly contrasting models of interwar UK health care – that is, private provision for the wealthy versus charity for the neediest – works well thematically, but does not quite convey the complexities of a system that was by this time moving to a 'highly effective mixed economy of mutual payment schemes, local authority services and not-for-profit providers, with little place for commercial medicine' (Doyle and Wall, 2018).[3] The 1911 National Insurance Act had provided compulsory health insurance, and free access to GPs for manual labourers (and some non-manual labourers), although there was no hospital treatment offered, nor any provision offered to the wives and children of workers – who are the ones seen coming to Wellesley Street, along with the unemployed and the elderly, many of whom are reckoned by the doctors to be beyond help. Out of necessity, Billy accepts the role of consultant for the fitters' union presided over by Jack Ford, but this leads to an ethical dilemma that pits Ford's pragmatism against Billy's professional code of honour. A fitter with pleurisy called Stan Mather (Fred Pearson) is fatally injured at work, after having been declared unfit for work by the doctor. Billy is blackmailed by Jack into destroying his case-notes, to ensure that his death is deemed 'murder' rather than 'suicide', and thus gain the highest amount of compensation for the man's family.

'Physician, heal thyself': the sickening doctor

The ancient proverb 'Physician, heal thyself' is uttered numerous times in the show's third series, which throws even more impediments and dilemmas in the way of its struggling doctor. The clinic's founder, Dr Stoker, is now in the advanced stages of stomach cancer, and warns Billy to 'concentrate on the curable', as opposed to the helpless Wellesley Street clientele, for the sake of his own health. Before Stoker passes away, there are lengthy scenes of discussion about whether it is morally wrong for him to express his agnosticism to the altruistic clergyman who helps to run the clinic: Stoker remarks that 'man can't concern himself with eternal damnation while he's suffering from pain and hunger'. Indeed, as a representative of the now declining Christian Social Union movement, the Church of England association of the late nineteenth century that had rallied for the remedy of poverty and social injustice, Father Courtenay (Ralph Michael) seems to have been introduced into the cast to allow for on-screen debates about a GP's political and moral responsibilities. Stoker's prophecy quickly becomes true, when Billy, now the sole doctor at the clinic, becomes himself bed-ridden through nervous exhaustion, a condition met with incredulity by his father – a surrogate for the community at large perhaps – who instructs him to get 'back on his feet the way a man should'.[4] However, Billy's particular form of heroism is belatedly recognised by at least one member of his family, the physically robust Tom, who has survived a spell in the notoriously grim Durham Gaol, but finds a night spent in Billy's quarters in the rat-infested clinic to be a real eye-opener: 'we had it soft compared to our Billy', he says, and expresses shock at the volume of human misery captured in the case-notes piling up there. Another character goes as far as to describe the openly atheistic Billy as a 'real Christian' for his activities.

As the third series progresses, a number of plotlines hinge upon the antagonism between Billy and Jack Ford, and their respective credentials as 'socialists' and also of readers of human psychology. The building housing Billy's clinic is bought by Jack as a part of a complicated bargaining strategy with a tycoon, Colfax (David King), who wants the space for the expansion of his own factory. Whilst Billy is naturally unforgiving of Jack's brute capitalism, which means the closure of the clinic, Jack makes the case that his own actions are just as philanthropic, given that his condition of sale to Colfax was that he allowed the unionisation of his workforce, and thus of significant benefit to the health and wellbeing of the Gallowshields community. Another wealthy industrialist comes to Billy's rescue by providing him free space for a new clinic, an act that is partly conscience-salving in recognition of the way factory pollution has endangered public health, but also a cunning way to push down dividends. A story arc across the three final episodes concerns a patient named Dixon (Morgan Sheppard), whose eccentricities are presumed to stem from an industrial accident at the Lewis Bishop yard, for which he received no compensation. The fact that he was considered fit for work by the bosses generates righteous indignation on the part of Billy's new assistant Isobel (Mary Larkin), a medical student of independent wealth who shares his political views and assumes this is a case of an exploitative industrialist in cahoots with corrupt union officials: 'It shows you what a stinking mess capitalism is; even when they drive a man out of his mind, they don't pay him what they really owe', she says. Unsurprisingly, the prospect of a female doctor garners some hostility in Gallowshields, but Isobel's troublingly progressive credentials also emerge through her espousal of psychoanalytic interpretation; where everyone else just regards the unfortunate Dixon as 'crackers', she refers to Freud's theorising with a diagnosis of 'hypermania', where the patient is subject to uncontrollable fits of rage. And yet, these medical and political interpretations of Dixon's condition prove to be less valuable than the practical detective work that Jack undertakes in relation to Dixon's shady past. Just like the very first episode, where Jack seems to provide more useful, pragmatic help to a shell-shock victim than the medical establishment, here he is able, following an observant visit to Dixon's home, to deduce that the man actually had a kind of personality disorder, and an inclination towards violence, long before his war experience or his accident at work. It transpires that Dixon has been sending threatening letters and killing animals belonging to his perceived enemy, the Duke of Bedlington (William Fox), and it is only through Jack's intervention that he is prevented from further violence. The last encounter in this series between Jack and Billy is predictably tense, particularly as Billy has reason to believe that Jack has been wooing his assistant Isobel, for whom he harbours romantic feelings himself: Jack's last words to him, 'either belt us [hit me] or do a bit of courting', are good-humoured, but put Billy firmly in his place as someone who has not yet attained Jack's levels of adult wisdom and masculine strength.

The fourth and final series of *When the Boat Comes In* is in many ways an outlier. Broadcast after a gap over three years since the previous series, it moves swiftly through the 1930s and focuses almost exclusively on Jack's fall and rise, away from Gallowshields and the Seaton family. The medical plotlines fall completely away, and aside from a brief cameo mid-way through, Billy Seaton only re-appears in the final episodes, as part of a convoluted plot involving Jack being persuaded to smuggle guns to those fighting the Republican government in Spain; Jack dies in the closing moments of the series, not through the attack by members of Franco's Moorish cavalry, but by a gunshot from a communist sympathiser trying to prevent the ammunition reaching the socialists. It's an appropriately muddled ending, but a strong statement nevertheless about the left's 'betrayal of itself', and about Jack's potent life force ultimately sapped by tribal conflicts and the march of history. So where does Billy Seaton, the good doctor, fit into this? Jack's demise is ultimately the result of Billy's involvement with communist agitators, and the subterfuge around the gun-running expedition: Billy does not fire the fatal shot, but he is implicated in the actions that lead to it. As mentioned, the programme ends with a static tableau, viewed from an upwards craning camera, of the dead Ford being held by Billy and Jessie, as the credits roll silently. For Karen McNally, the ending illustrates the 'difference between the coldness of earnest politicians and Jack's form of honourable working-class capitalism' (McNally, 2007: 119). In this reading, Jack is positioned, or at least positions himself, as a class hero, in contrast to men like his murderer and Billy, who consider him to have betrayed his background. Certainly, the final series invites no particular interest in or sympathy with Billy, who is now adopting the clothes, bearing, and accent of the upper class, now he has apparently become a successful specialist in London – although this might be interpreted as a 'trojan horse' manoeuvre to disguise his radical political leanings. In contrast, Jack holds on to his accent, gestures, and worldview throughout, never dropping his habitual 'bonny lads' and 'bonny lasses' patter even among rarefied company; Billy's apparent betrayal of his poorer patients, and comfort with endangering the lives of others, seems like a violation of both the medical code and of his youthful political beliefs.

So, as the series reaches its denouement, Billy Seaton has been abridged to a one-dimensional figure, a conduit for Jack's death, possibly even a working-class traitor. It is hard to know whether this was the series creator James Mitchell's intention all along; that is, that the supposedly 'good doctor' was envisaged early as the nemesis of the apparent 'hero' of the tale. *When the Boat Comes In* has always been Jack's story, but the traducing of the doctor character to a mere cipher is regrettable, given the programme's recognition, in its earlier series anyway, of health and health care as one of the main factors shaping (and limiting) working-class aspiration and quality of life in the early twentieth century. In this way, the series illustrates both the possibilities and pitfalls for a long-running serial drama that dares to incorporate medical concerns into its conceptual and narrative framework.

As conveyed by Katherine Byrne's preceding chapter in this volume about *Call the Midwife* (2011–), the medical period drama gives extraordinary, rich opportunities to describe historical realities and developments, as well as speak to contemporary concerns around health care policy. But even thirty years after *When the Boat Comes In*, the sense remains that the incorporation of medical plotlines into non-medical period drama is an ongoing challenge for writers, and indeed audiences. Towards the end of the sixth and final series of *Downton Abbey*, for example, the narrative takes a slightly unexpected detour to encompass a feud between the Dowager Countess of Grantham (Maggie Smith) and the upper-middle-class Isobel Grey (Penelope Wilton) over the future of Downton's Cottage Hospital; the latter – herself a nurse, and from a family of doctors – is aligned with the forces of modernity through her campaign for it to merge with the larger Royal Yorkshire Hospital. With its cameo appearance from Neville Chamberlain, the Minister of Health in 1925, and its detailed airings of the opinions on all sides of the argument about the future of the hospital, *Downton Abbey* seemed to aspire, like *When the Boat Comes In* before it, towards a multi-faced depiction of the social, cultural, and political forces shaping British identity in the early twentieth century. Whether *Downton*'s sustained engagement with the future of hospitals truly won the hearts and minds of viewers is another question, however. Writing for the *Radio Times*,

Ben Dowell's review (2015) of one episode carried the damning headline 'Is the saga of the Downton Cottage Hospital the dullest plotline in TV history?' A little unfair, perhaps, but a reminder nonetheless that medical characters and concerns are still regarded, by some, as troublingly alien bodies within the bloodstream of period drama.

Notes

1. The expression 'ha'way' is a well-known Geordie exhortation of encouragement, usually understood to mean an approximation of 'come along'; depending on the context, it can be used aggressively or in a familiar and reassuring fashion (see Jackson, 1999: 6).
2. This is an 1892 music hall song by Joseph Tabrar, written for and first performed by Vesta Victoria. Ostensibly a lament by a young girl wishing for a dog as pet, the song, like many others from the music hall, has been decoded for its sexual connotations – prompted by the apparent use of the term 'bow-wow' as slang for penis (Thompson, 2001).
3. For more detail on UK health care in the pre-NHS era see, for example, Hayes (2012), Doyle (2014), and Campbell (2017).
4. As a compassionate, progressive medic with a history of professional self-doubt, Billy has some affinity with the character of Dr Patrick Turner (Stephen McGann), the middle-class and somewhat older doctor of *Call The Midwife* (2012–), who is briefly mentioned in Katherine Byrne's preceding chapter; although Turner's equivalent nervous breakdown (following World War II) predates the events of the programme, it is only gradually revealed in the series.

References

Berridge, V. (2003). 'Post-War Smoking Policy in the UK and the Redefinition of Public Health', *Twentieth Century British History* 14, pp. 61–83.

Clark, A. (n.d.). 'Dr Finlay's Casebook', *Screenonline*, www.screenonline.org.uk/tv/id/481822/index.html (accessed 1 September 2020).

Clark, P. (2020). '"Problems of Today and Tomorrow": Prevention and the National Health Service in the 1970s', *Social History of Medicine* 33: 3, pp. 981–1000.

Dowell, B. (2005). 'Is the Saga of the Downton Cottage Hospital the Dullest Plotline in TV History?', *Radio Times*, 11 October, www.radiotimes.com/news/2015-10-11/is-the-saga-of-the-downton-cottage-hospital-the-dullest-plotline-in-tv-history/ (accessed 1 September 2020).

Doyle, B. (2014). *The Politics of Hospital Provision in Early Twentieth-Century Britain*. London: Pickering and Chatto.

Doyle, B. and R. Wall (2018). 'What Was Healthcare Like before the NHS?', *The Conversation*, 3 July 2018, https://theconversation.com/what-was-healthcare-like-before-the-nhs-99055 (accessed 1 September 2020).

Gosling, G. C. (2017). *Payment and Philanthropy in British Healthcare, 1918–48*. Manchester: Manchester University Press.

Hayes, N. (2012). 'Did We Really Want a National Health Service? Hospitals, Patients and Public Opinions before 1948', *The English Historical Review* CXXVII: 526, pp. 625–651.

Hutchings, P. (1996). '"When the Going Gets Tough…": Representations of the North-East in Film and Television', in T. E. Faulkner, ed., *Northumbrian Panorama: Studies in the History and Culture of North East England*. London: Octavian Press, pp. 273–290.

Jackson, D. (2019). *The Northumbrians: North-East England and Its People*. London: Hurst & Company.

James, C. (1976). 'Unintelligibuhlity', *The Observer*, 15 February 1976, p. 26.

McNally, K. (2007). 'The Geordie and the American Hero: Revisiting Classic Hollywood Masculinity in *When the Boat Comes In*', *Journal of British Cinema and Television* 4: 1, pp. 102–120.

Mitchell, J. (1976). 'I Am Not a Preacher – I Write about People', *The Stage and Television Today*, 1 April, p. 26.

Purser, P. (2002). 'James Mitchell', *The Guardian*, 19 September, p. 24.

Thompson, W. (2001). 'Have a Gay Old Time', *The Guardian*, 9 March, www.theguardian.com/friday_review/story/0,3605,448635,00.html (accessed 1 September 2020).

Webster, C. (2002). *The National Health Service: A Political History*, 2nd edn. Oxford: Oxford University Press.

Part III

Dissecting the body

10

'And when you touched my naked body ... your fingertips running along my flesh ... this was abuse, not science': Victorian medicine in Showtime's *Penny Dreadful*

Julie Anne Taddeo

In the opening episode of Showtime's *Penny Dreadful* (2014–2016), Victor Frankenstein (Harry Treadaway) explains to the adventurer Sir Malcolm (Timothy Dalton) that he is no mere 'medical practitioner' but an explorer much like himself, motivated by the 'elation of discovery': 'there is only one worthy goal for scientific exploration, piercing the tissue that separates life from death ... that is my river, that is my mountain, there I will plant *my* flag' (S1E1; emphasis in original quote). Victor's 'discoveries', of course, rest on 'planting his flag' on the working-class corpses provided by the resurrectionist (grave robbing) trade. Victor's third attempt at literal resurrection, via galvanism, involves the body of a poor Irish woman, who, once reborn, is subjected to his civilising efforts to make her 'the perfect woman', mirroring what scholar Anne McClintock has called the imperialist's mission of 'the transmission of white, male power through control of colonized women' (McClintock, 1995: 2–3).

The appeal to fans of this neo-Victorian mashup of multiple gothic texts has rested, in part, on *Penny Dreadful*'s sexual elements and depiction of fluid identities (Poore, 2016; Strother, 2017), but its storylines around its strong female protagonists who 'smash the patriarchy' – Brona/Lily (Billie Piper) and Vanessa Ives (Eva Green) – have sealed its status on fan sites as 'feminist' period television (Kohlke, 2018). Indeed, *Penny Dreadful* ultimately subverts Victor's mission and instead empowers the character who was, in Shelley's source text, an unnamed, unfinished bride for his first Creature. Victor's attempts in *Penny Dreadful* to transform the prostitute Brona Croft into Lily Frankenstein, the ideal Angel in the House, highlight the tenuous boundaries the Victorians constructed between the angel/whore but also within the medical field in which Victor is seeking to distinguish himself (he asserts he's a 'researcher' not a mere 'practitioner'). Victor's treatment of Brona/Lily is further indicative of how, by the late Victorian period, the fields of psychiatry, gynaecology, and surgery were merging, coalescing around the medicalisation of women's morality, a process to which Vanessa Ives is also subjected during her stay at the Banning Clinic. Thus *Penny Dreadful* exposes the gendered relationship between Victorian upper-class male medical experts and their female patients. While exaggerated for neo-gothic effect, the medical theories and practices espoused by men like Victor seem, as Lily points out in the quote which informs this chapter's title, more like 'abuse' than 'science'.

Penny Dreadful is not the first period drama to equate the male-dominated Victorian medical profession with the subjugation of women. Two decades prior, *Bramwell*'s (1995–1998) opening scene of its inaugural episode introduced viewers to the titular female medical student (Jemma Redgrave) by placing her in the surgical amphitheatre with her male colleagues – all of whom are given the title of 'Doctor' while she is pointedly referred to as 'Miss' – as the arrogant head surgeon Sir Herbert Hamilton (Robert Hardy) prepares to perform an ovariectomy on a working-class woman to cure her post-partum melancholia. Bramwell's tentative admonition that no evidence substantiates the curative effects of such a risky procedure is resoundingly booed by her colleagues, who then clap and cheer as the patient bleeds out on the operating table, a scene so gruesome as to be worthy of inclusion in the sensationalist *Penny Dreadful*. Later in that same episode, Bramwell is admonished by Sir Herbert for revealing a syphilis diagnosis to an upper-class patient for fear it would destroy her husband's reputation. His solution, to prevent the patient from disgracing her husband in future with a 'deformed child' and to 'calm her down', is to 'whip out her ovaries' – a remedy he is denied performing once Bramwell informs the woman of the risks. As the story of a New Woman doctor (who would be a contemporary of *Penny Dreadful*'s Victor in 1890s London), replete with divided skirt and bicycle, forging ahead despite sexist discrimination, *Bramwell* was explicitly marketed as a feminist period drama, the grittier British version of *Dr. Quinn, Medicine Woman* (1993–1998) (discussed in Antonovich's chapter). *Bramwell*, as well as the BBC's 1989 adaptation of *The Yellow Wallpaper* (to be discussed later in this chapter) followed in the wake of Elaine Showalter's highly publicised history, *The Female Malady* (1985), which presented Victorian medicine, psychiatry in particular, as a form of social control of women.[1] Despite multiple attempts by more recent scholars to debunk her thesis – with statistical evidence, for example, that the ratio of male to female inmates in asylums was relatively equal – the premise of Showalter's book still remains largely unchallenged: that Victorian doctors 'persisted in linking mental illness with women' (Goodman, 2015: 151) and diagnoses were gendered, with men's symptoms attributed to 'overwork' but women's to their rejection of their domestic role.

The medical mistreatment of women, in particular but not exclusively poor women, has remained a constant motif of Victorian-themed period dramas. Even for Dr Bramwell, working-class women are sometimes disposable test subjects, for example, when she performs experimental surgery on a sideshow 'freak' to make her 'normal', only to leave her bedridden for the rest of her life. In the period comedy *Quacks* (2017), early Victorian surgeon Robert Lessing (Rory Kinnear) tries to sabotage the career of a woman from his own class – Florence Nightingale (Millie Thomas) – so threatened is he by her efficiency and her challenges to both his masculine authority and lack of hygienic measures in the sickroom. While largely absurdist (in the tradition of *Blackadder*), *Quacks* underscores the misogyny that not only hindered most women's ascendancy in the medical profession but likely hurt female patients as well. In another recent series discussed in this volume by Andrea Wright, *The Frankenstein Chronicles* (2015–2017), a charity hospital doctor deems it his right to rape helpless teen girls in their hospital beds as payment for his medical care. Like *The Frankenstein Chronicles*, *Penny Dreadful* is not a medical period drama per se (often exploiting medicine for horrific effect rather than presenting a history of medicine), and yet, it seems that neo-gothic dramas like these perform a vital function ignored by more recent medical dramas like *The Knick* (2014–2015) in which the male pioneering doctor remains the dramatic focus. While *Penny Dreadful* plays with historical realities and the Victorian timeline (situating Victor at the tail end of the nineteenth century for starters), it does succeed in restoring the voices and agency of the female patient long silenced in medical records and popular culture.

Brona Croft/Lily Frankenstein

In a notable change from Shelley's source text, *Penny Dreadful* imagines what would have happened had Shelley's doctor completed the 'bride' he was ordered by his first Creature, self-named Mr Clare (Rory Kinnear), to create for him (demanding a beautiful woman, not one stitched together and disfigured like himself). Fortuitously, Victor is called to the bedside of Brona Croft by her lover, Ethan Chandler (Josh Hartnett), but it's too late for the Irish prostitute, whose sheets are blood-soaked from the TB that has ravaged her lungs. Brona checks all the boxes for diseased Victorian femininity: Irish, poor, a prostitute, consumptive (and possibly syphilitic, although this disease is curiously never mentioned in a series in which so much sex occurs). Knowing Brona cannot recover, Victor, in an act reminiscent of Burke and Hare, hastens her death by suffocating her with her bloodied pillow and claims her as his own ('I'll take care of the body', he reassures Ethan). Before he kills her, he tells Brona he believes in 'salvation', as she confesses 'I've not been good; hell waits for me on the other side of the door.' In life, such a place likely would have been a Magdalene asylum to reprogramme 'fallen women' like herself through prayer, penitence, and hard work – the type of underpaid work (usually in domestic service) that drove women to the streets in the first place (Logan, 1997). That Brona's 'salvation' is to be resurrection for an arranged marriage reinforces late Victorian feminists' comparison of the institution to a legalised form of prostitution (Forward, 1999): in life and in death Brona is expected to play both whore and angel for men.

The scenes that follow mimic Victorian autopsy art that eroticised the dissection of female corpses (Jordanova, 1989; Holmstrom, 2017). Returning to his apartment laboratory, Victor unveils Brona's lifeless naked body, then takes his surgical knife and cuts as the Creature/Mr Clare watches in awe; it is an erotically charged moment that pays homage to Hasselhorst's lithograph, 'Dissection of a young, beautiful woman', in which 'the woman not only appears to accept this assault [upon her body] but turns her head to invite the masculine perusal of her body' (Holmstrom, 2017: 37). In nineteenth-century medical drawings, the anatomist's grisly work is never shown in detail; instead the anatomist is depicted gazing at his female subject on the surgical table, often in the company of male colleagues, and the corpse appears more lifelike than dead, adorned with flowing locks of hair, her breasts often bared, reflecting what Holmstrom describes as a 'transgressive relationship between the clothed anatomist and the young beautiful and exposed female corpse' (ii).

As Brona's lifeless body soaks in the tub of amniotic fluid, Victor talks to her, strokes her chest scar, tentatively caresses her breasts. As he thinks aloud about all he will teach her, his hand wanders towards her pubic area just as someone knocks at the door and he guiltily withdraws it, caught, as Lily later reminds him, 'like a child, cramming his hand in the sweets jar', in an act that had nothing to do with science but was in fact abuse. When Brona is reanimated on a stormy night via electricity, she rises naked from the tub, standing before Victor and his first Creature, like an Anatomical Venus revealing her mysteries to them. Even the location of Brona's V-shaped scar resembles that from Victorian medical art in which the anatomist stares pointedly at the incision below the corpse's breasts (Holmstrom, 2017: 46). Such drawings indicated that the corpse's heart had been or was about to be removed. Unlike Victor's first Creature, this one is not comprised of various body parts stitched together, so the chest scar suggests that only Brona's whore's heart has been removed, much like the beautiful young prostitute depicted in Simonet's 1890 painting *Anatomy of the Heart* (Holmstrom, 2017: 46). Presumably, Brona has been given a better one that will aid in her resurrection as the purer Lily, 'the flower of rebirth', as Victor anoints her.

The female cadaver was 'by far the most popular subject of artistic engagements with post mortem dissections' (Holmstrom, 2017: 38) as well as part of Victorian popular entertainment that was marketed to the general public as 'scientific' and 'educational' (Ebenstein, 2016). For a small price, the curious layperson could observe, outside the privileged arena of the surgical amphitheatre and medical school, a wax model (a.k.a. an 'Anatomical Venus') of such a female corpse (see Figure 10.1). Typically adorned with a long pearl necklace that drew attention to the bared breasts and long tresses, the wax model essentialised femininity and bore the traits of 'calm, poise, serenity' that Victor says define 'the perfect woman'. Of course, the *Penny Dreadful* viewer, like the Victorian voyeur, is just as complicit in this enjoyment of the nude female corpse as we are invited by the camera to join Victor and Clare's perusal of Lily's body on multiple occasions (Figure 10.2).

While awaiting the completion of his bride, Clare becomes a creator himself, obtaining employment at Putney's Wax Works, a subplot that raises a grisly connection between medicine, crime, and entertainment via the eroticisation of the female corpse. The wax figures that comprise Putney's Chamber of Crimes are a telling indictment of the profession that has both made Mr Clare an outcast and in which, by his demand for a bride, complicit. The Jack the Ripper tableau, with victim Annie Chapman sprawled

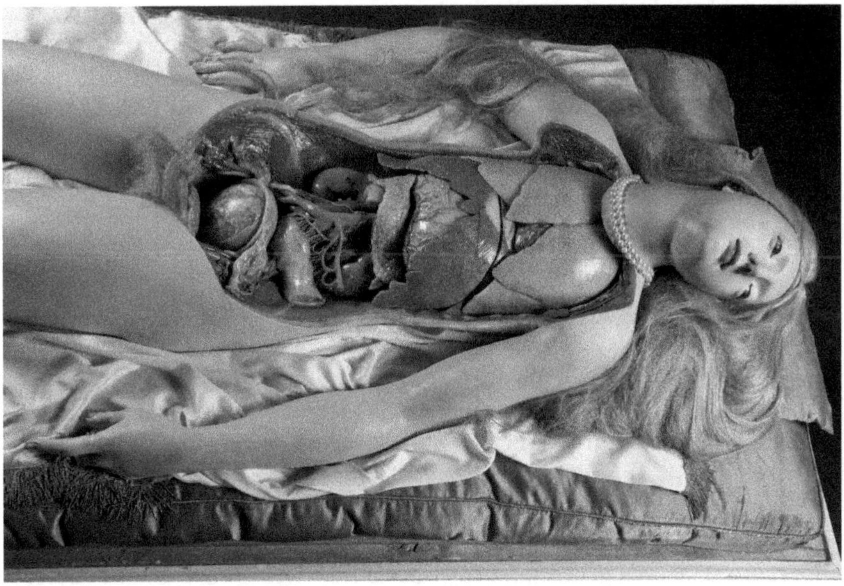

Figure 10.1 Anatomical Venus (Ablogin/Josephinum, Ethics, Collections and History of Medicine, MedUni Vienna)

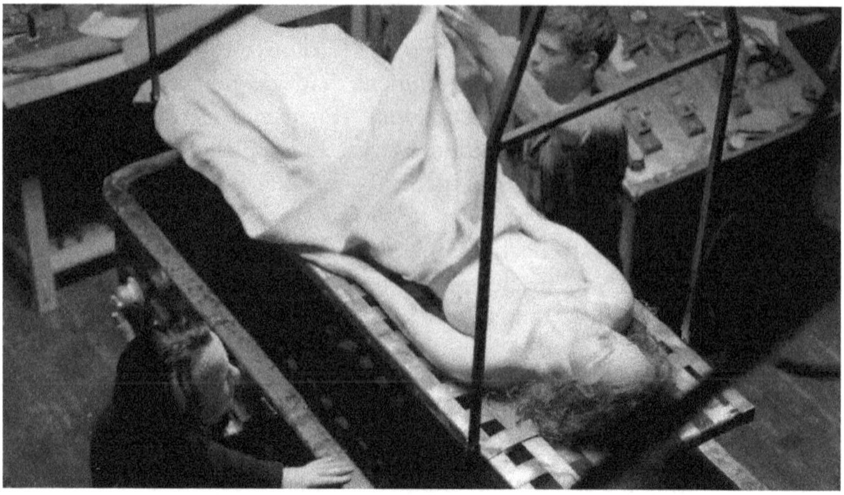

Figure 10.2 Brona on the table (*Penny Dreadful*)

on the ground, looks much like Brona on Victor's operating table – her hair spread out, her insides open to the gaze of the killer standing above her, knife in hand. The many theories about the identity of the Ripper (butcher, physician, a patient deranged by syphilis) further stress the connection between medicine and crime. The daring men of medicine don their blood-spattered black leather aprons – the garb of butchers and doctors alike, worn by Victor in the opening episode and of course suggestive of one of the many nicknames for the Ripper: 'Leather Apron'. The obvious conclusion is that medical research is not possible without crime, and even the well-intentioned Anatomy Act failed to stop the illegal trade in bodies decades after its passage in 1832. As Ruth Richardson (1987) has documented, that law was in part a response to the notorious Burke and Hare murder spree (crimes prompted by the demand for corpses by doctors like Victor), which is also showcased at Putney's. Because of Clare's demand for a bride, Victor too has become a murderer, grave robber, and anatomist in this scenario, and Brona is his Mary Paterson: the eighteen-year-old prostitute suffocated by Burke and Hare and sold to Dr Robert Knox who was so taken with her beauty that he had the artist John Oliphant sketch her naked corpse, posed like Borghese's sculpture Hermaphroditus, before preserving her in a tub of whiskey for three months (MacDonald, 2002: 34–37).

Dissected, like Mary Patmore, of her whore's heart, Brona is also deprived of all remnants of her past life so that even her Irish brogue has been replaced with a genteel, more pleasing (to Victor's ears) English accent. Victor insists on dying her brown hair blond, like a 'fair-haired angel', and buys her a corset, white dress, and heels – garments she complains constrict her breathing and movement. Lily echoes the views of late Victorian dress reformers (as well as contemporary critics) who condemned the corset as an unhealthy garment that deformed a woman's spine and hindered her social emancipation (Summers, 2001). Even as Lily bemoans its limitations, she's aware of its erotic appeal as Victor observes it 'flatter(s) the figure'. Neo-Victorian texts and subcultures often repurpose the corset as a garment of empowerment, worn on the outside, for example, by female steampunks, while at the same time critiquing the Victorian corset as a 'straitjacket of femininity' (Taddeo, 2012: 45), and *Penny Dreadful* (as neo-Victorian period drama) likewise interrogates how the corset marked the female body as 'a political object par excellence' (Summers, 2001: 129). Victor and Lily's conversation is worth repeating in full since it lays bare all of these tensions. Lily asks if 'women wear corsets so they don't exert themselves … what would be the danger if they did?' to which Victor replies, partly in jest, 'they'd take over the world. Anyway, we men prevent that by keeping women corseted, in theory and in practice.' Victor tells her she needn't wear one, but Lily understands at that moment that 'all we do is for men, isn't it? Keep their houses, raise their children, flatter them with our pain?' (S2E4). And yet, once Lily recognises her immortality and strength, she sheds the white frilly dresses Victor has chosen for her, favouring low-cut, red and black gowns with tightly laced bodices – she may be wearing a corset, but on her terms, not to please a man. It is not just a cosmetic transformation Victor attempts to work on Lily as he plays Higgins to her Eliza: teaching her to dance, how to comport herself so that she doesn't embarrass herself (or him) when they have tea with Vanessa or attend her first ball, prompting her to ask, 'Did I do right, Victor?' But more significantly, he feeds her new memories – 'reminding' her that they are cousins reunited after several years apart. In their youth, he tells her, they shared a bed when Lily was frightened by thunderstorms. Hence, one night, a storm drives her to his bed, and the inevitable happens – his Creature's intended has become his own – and as she cooks his breakfast the next morning, he beams with pride amid his newly manufactured domestic bliss.

Unfortunately, for Victor, their brief honeymoon ends when Lily meets and moves in with Dorian Gray, having discovered their shared immortality. Memories of her previous life resurface, and she soon develops a predilection for killing men who try to solicit her on the street – her old life melding with her new. As she drinks tea one afternoon with Justine, a teen she has rescued from prostitution, the two observe several respectably dressed women being arrested by the police. Justine observes, 'they think as you do, the Suffragettes'. 'No', responds Lily, 'our enemies are the same, but they seek equality.' 'And we?' 'Mastery', Lily declares. Marie-Luise Kohlke (2018) faults *Penny Dreadful* for trivialising the feminist gains of the late Victorian era and favouring a violent resolution to gender inequality. But, even though they may be living in Dorian's mansion, Lily and Justine acknowledge their shared working-class origins which would set them apart from the protesters who were, for the most part, comprised of middle- and upper-class women (many of whom engaged in philanthropic efforts to 'rescue' women and girls that they regarded not as 'sisters' but as 'fallen'). Still, Lily's comment erases the efforts of certain middle-class feminists like Josephine Butler who protested the Contagious Diseases Acts (1864–1886) that just a few years before *Penny Dreadful*'s setting would likely have resulted in Brona's arrest. These laws gave the police in port cities the authority to arrest any woman or girl they suspected of prostitution, forcibly submitting them to medical examination for signs of venereal disease (in what Butler called an act of 'instrumental rape'); those deemed diseased were then incarcerated in 'lock hospitals' until 'cured' (which in the nineteenth century simply meant an absence of chancres). As historian Judith Walkowitz (1982) has shown, the Acts, which amounted to a form of medical colonisation of working-class women's bodies, ultimately failed to curb syphilis rates (since men were exempt from the law), but a secondary goal was the 'remoralisation' of patients: just like in the Magdalene asylums, while incarcerated in the hospitals, patients were forced to read their Bible and perform menial domestic tasks, a process similar to Victor's efforts to transform working-class Brona into his middle-class ideal through surgery and re-education. Thus, having tired of a society that never ceases to bring poor women 'to their knees' (either through prayer or prostitution), Lily devises her own solution – one that mimics a medical act: she orders her newly organised 'army' of former prostitutes to go forth and bring back the severed arms of men until Dorian's expensive dining room table, covered with bloody limbs, resembles the mortuary in which Victor toiled away in the series' opening episode.

Determined to rescue Lily from what he regards as her descent into madness, Victor plots with an old schoolmate, Dr Henry Jekyll (Shazad Latif), to kidnap and, as the latter says, 'domesticate her'. Jekyll is himself an outcast in England: the illegitimate son of 'an exotic whore' and an aristocratic British father who abandoned them both, he is subjected to taunts and stares when walking London's streets. Despite a Cambridge education, he can only find employment as Bedlam's 'resident somnalist', keeping the most violent lunatics sedated in return for a lab and 'no end of diverting subjects'. Bedlam occupies a special place in our twenty-first-century neo-gothic imagination – the stand-in for all Victorian asylums which we rarely see portrayed as spaces of treatment or kindness, when in fact, as Thomas Knowles reminds us, many Victorian asylums were 'built upon the principles of moral treatment' (2015: 51), introducing a regimen of fresh air and activity (albeit gendered, with sports for men, sewing for women). Nevertheless, it's to that sensationalist Bedlam that *Penny Dreadful* resorts and to which Lily is sent against her will (she's chloroformed by Dorian who hands her over to Victor and Henry in an act that resembles a gang rape; Henry even says leeringly, 'she'll be yours, old boy, to do with as you will').

At the centre of Jekyll's subterranean lab (which Lily aptly compares to a dungeon) is a barber's chair 'with my [Jekyll's] own modifications'. Into this contraption, the two doctors have planned to strap Lily, gag her, and inject into her brain Jekyll's 'calming serum' via Victor's electrified needle to maximise the serum's success. The goal of the procedure, Victor says, is to make Lily 'more calm, render the beast dormant' – to return her to that 'perfect' state he enjoyed when she was first 'born' in his lab. When he tells Lily that he will make her 'calm, serene, we're going to make you ... into a proper woman', his words echo those of other terrifying Victorian doctors like gynaecologist Isaac Baker Brown whose clitoridectomy procedure on hundreds of female patients he diagnosed as hysterical also promised to make them 'calm', 'pink', and 'modest'.[2] Victor reminds her that they were happy, to which Lily replies, 'No Victor, you were happy ... I would rather die who I am than live as your demure little wife ... even if you keep me locked in the attic' (a nod to Mr Rochester, who himself played psychiatrist to his first wife). In the end, Lily persuades Victor to let her go – but only after she tells him she needs her scars and her memories of her dead child Sarah – that last remnant of her human life – which she would not give up to be 'perfect': 'Monstrous I may be in your eyes but I am the sum part of one woman's days ... that woman has known pain, let her be who she is.' Moved by her tears and her personal account of motherhood – the semblance of femininity he so longed for – he relents. As Elaine Showalter (1985: 87) has argued, exhibiting such signs of 'appropriate' gendered behaviour indicated to Victorian doctors that their female patients were 'cured' of their mental illness. Perhaps, though, some patients learned to perform femininity to escape further treatment at the hands of doctors, and so Lily's tears may be less genuine than her captor wants to believe.

Vanessa Ives

It is her refusal to 'counterfeit normality well enough' (S1E7) that prompts Vanessa Ives's stay at Dr Banning's clinic, a repressed memory which she recalls while under hypnosis by Dr Seward in S3E4. Sent there after a mental breakdown following the death of her friend Mina (for which she feels complicit, having seduced Mina's fiancé), Vanessa equates her prolonged patient status at the clinic with her inability to adequately perform femininity: 'I spoke lowly. I bent my head. I was a submissive dog. I was the woman he [Banning] wanted me to be. I almost succeeded.' Her choice of words recalls an earlier conversation with Victor – called to treat her depression in S1E7 – in which she compared the sexual urges that marked her as diseased to 'an animal scratching to get out'.

While not the subterranean asylum in which Jekyll chains and experiments on his 'diverting subjects', this private clinic, as Vanessa's nameless attendant (Mr Clare in his previous life) increasingly recognises, uses treatments that increasingly border on 'torture'. The relationship that develops between the working-class Clare (his status is made clear when he comments on his poor reading skills and his insistence on calling her 'Miss') and his upper-class charge is reflective of how asylum staff 'occupied the middle ground between doctors and patients', functioning as 'controller, observer, general nurse, disciplinarian and labourer' (Chatterton, 2015: 85). The 1890 Lunacy Act, passed around the time of Vanessa's incarceration, recognised the hands-on and potentially intimate nature of this relationship, and thus made ill-treatment or neglect of patients or aiding in a patient's escape punishable offences (Chatterton, 2015: 92). Indeed, this episode is as much about Clare's transformation as it is about Vanessa's illness; initially stern and a stickler for the rules, by the episode's end he is desperate to save Vanessa from Banning's increasingly harsh treatments. His character arc challenges historians' and popular culture's stereotype of the lazy, cruel attendant; even Victorian psychiatrists at the time recorded the difficult balance of being 'firm but gentle' that was required by staff in the care of patients diagnosed with mental illness (Chatterton, 2015: 97). Clare admits he has taken on such work only because 'jobs are scarce' but by the time of Vanessa's scheduled neurosurgery he has given his notice, reflecting further the high staff turnover rate in asylums likely due to the physical and emotional difficulty of the job. Perhaps he is also escaping his own sexual attraction to Vanessa, who at one point bares herself to him; in drawing the viewer's gaze to yet another vulnerable, naked patient, the series makes us uncomfortably aware of the easy access to her body which the padded, sound-proofed room affords the medical staff in charge of her care.

Vanessa's isolation in that padded cell seems an extreme form of punishment, used no doubt for dramatic effect. Private asylum patients obviously tended to be middle- or upper-class like Vanessa but were not typically secluded since social activities were part of the treatment to rehabilitate a sense of normalcy (Wiles, 2015). Even the straitjacket which she's forced to wear, though now so imbued by gothic and neo-gothic literature and film as a symbol of punishment (Wiles, 2015: 179), was originally intended to allow the patient to move about and enjoy the asylum's landscaped grounds without causing harm to herself or others (Wiles, 2015: 170) – mobility which for some reason is never afforded to Vanessa. Instead, to modern viewers, her straitjacketed body reinforces 'the cultural myth of the asylum as a place of threat rather than cure' (Knowles and Trowbridge, 2015: 1). And when Vanessa continues to refuse food despite Clare's warning that 'there will be consequences', she reviles his efforts 'to make me normal ... like all the other women you know ... compliant, obedient' until she is force-fed by a reluctant Clare in a scene that evokes the force-feeding of imprisoned suffragists.

In humanising the role of the attendant, *Penny Dreadful* also highlights the gendered cultural assumptions behind Victorian theories and treatments of mental illness which trickled down from doctor to staff. For example, in his attempts to secure Vanessa's release, Clare smuggles in his wife's hairbrush and rouge, to make over her dishevelled appearance into a more feminine version of herself (mirroring Victor's attempts to transform Brona into the more ladylike Lily) (Figure 10.3). Clare advises Vanessa that in order to avoid surgery, she must 'pretend to be cured', play the role of woman Dr Banning expects of her. In her examination of late-nineteenth-century asylums, Anne Shepherd observes that female patients were 'expected to conform to ideas of socially acceptable behavior' while 'expectations within the asylum reflected those of society outside' (Shepherd, 2004: 225).

The episodes involving Vanessa's mental health have echoes of the BBC's 1989 adaptation of *The Yellow Wallpaper*, which transplanted Charlotte Perkins Gilman's story to 1890s England. When Victor examines Vanessa in S1E7, she submits to his stethoscope but after admitting she sometimes 'goes away' (in her mind), the camera turns its focus to the faded yellowish paper that covers her walls – perhaps a nod to Gilman's fictional Charlotte

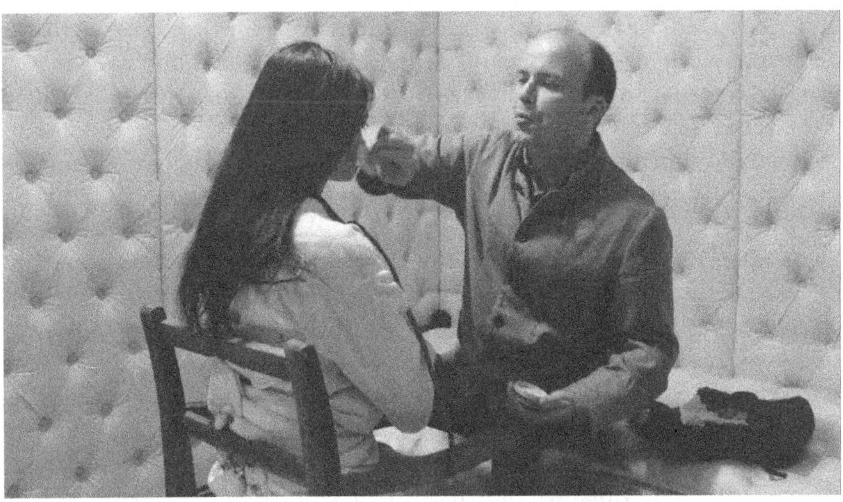

Figure 10.3 Clare makes up Vanessa's face (*Penny Dreadful*)

whose confinement to a similar-papered nursery and treatment at the hands of her physician (modelled after rest cure inventor, Silas Weir Mitchell) only furthered her descent into madness. In the BBC version, Charlotte (Julia Watson), in response to praise about her improving appearance, counters, 'so that's *better*, to be calm and pink?' In another scene (not in the original short story), Charlotte's husband John (Stephan Dillane) and her physician Charles Stark (James Faulkner), over cigars and whiskey, gaze almost erotically at photographs of actual female asylum patients in various poses: from those with dishevelled looks or in provocatively draped nightdresses (signifying insanity) to the properly attired and composed (signifying they're cured).[3] When he examines Charlotte, Dr Stark comments on her 'charming earrings' and urges her to put on weight: 'Surely I can appeal to your vanity if nothing else', concluding that 'there's nothing seriously wrong with her' that taking more interest in her appearance and domestic duties wouldn't cure. Unfortunately, like Charlotte, feigning colour in one's cheeks isn't sufficient to secure her release and thus Vanessa is subjected to hydrotherapy, force-feeding, and straitjacket restraints, culminating in an unspecified type of neurosurgery, which Clare says leaves patients 'a broken thing'. The objective of Dr Banning's surgery is no different from the intended results of Dr Stark's rest cure, Victor's electrified injection on the unruly Lily, or Sir Herbert's ovariectomy on female hysterics, of which the latter boasts, 'we can restore her [the female patient's] equilibrium with one decisive and radical operation ... to calm her hysteria and temper her moods' (*Bramwell*, S1E1).

Outside of the asylum, Vanessa has consistently rejected the dictates of her sex (in addition to giving in to those 'animal urges', she smokes, moves about the city unchaperoned, and lives alone with Sir Malcolm, the father of her deceased friend). She also has a curious power which some Victorian doctors associated with a type of mental illness to which the 'weaker sex' were susceptible. Since women were 'receptive vessels for other spirits' they were deemed 'particularly apt for mediumship because they were weak in the masculine attributes of will and intelligence, yet strong in the feminine qualities of passivity ... and impressionability' (Walkowitz, 1992: 176–177). In S2E1, Vanessa brings the séance held at Egyptologist Ferdinand Lyle's home to an abrupt halt as the spirits of Sir Malcolm's deceased children speak through her; she even levitates, as her fellow partygoers look on in horror. While Vanessa's abilities are assumed to signify demonic possession, real Victorian mediums were in great demand for private séances, thus proving a form of power and authority for women excluded from traditionally male areas of expertise. This power came with a caveat since doctors warned that 'women under the influence' of spirits behaved in a manner lacking decorum, violating the rules of modesty (indeed Vanessa shouts profanities and leaves the party to have sex with a random man on the street, and Victor attributes her behaviour to a 'deep psychosexual responsiveness'). Thus, female mediums ran the risk of accusations of insanity, as the newspaper-headlining case of Georgina Weldon illustrates. Weldon, a middle-class woman who dabbled in spiritualism, narrowly escaped certification in 1878 by a psychiatrist (hired by her husband who wished to lock her away); the doctor identified 'mediomania' as a manifestation of hysteria – the main symptom of which was the unwomanly urge to 'make a spectacle' of oneself (Walkowitz, 1992: 189). With the media on her side, Weldon ultimately won her case in court against her husband and achieved fame for her lecture 'How I Escaped the Mad Doctors' (Walkowitz, 1992: 180). The sympathy her case generated among other women, who were familiar with the trope of false confinement from the sensationalist fiction of the period, had the added effect of demonising in the public's eyes the psychiatric profession as misogynistic. According to Walkowitz, the Weldon case put 'mad doctors on the defensive' and perpetuated an 'iconography of medical evil' (Walkowitz, 1992: 188) that persists to this day in popular culture. In placing Vanessa in the care of the off-screen Dr Banning, the series underscores how a profession dominated by upper-class male professionals could prove quite detrimental to its female patients. Indeed, the only doctor who helps Vanessa is Dr Seward (Patti Lupone); as Amanda Howell and Lucy Baker point out, by changing Dr Seward's gender from its source text in *Dracula* (1897), 'the series undertakes an explicitly feminist intervention into the all-male environment of the Victorian medical establishment' as well as 'alter[ing] the gendered dynamic of early experiments with the talking cure like those recorded by Breuer and Freud in *Studies in Hysteria*' (Howell and Baker, 2017). Unlike Banning, who wants to silence her, or Victor, whose first instinct is to ask, 'is she intact?', echoing Victorian gynaecologist Dr William Acton's diagnosis of 'nymphomania' for women who did not conform to the 'natural' 'passionless' state of womanhood (Tosh, 2007: 45), Dr Seward urges Vanessa to talk until she gets to the source of her trauma.

Conclusion

Despite the reality that women (albeit in small numbers) were finally making their way into medical practice in the 1890s in which *Penny Dreadful* is set – and which *Bramwell* previously chronicled – they remain (Patti Lupone's Dr Seward aside) curiously absent as doctors in Victorian-themed period dramas, appearing instead as nurses and patients. Likewise, the male mental patient remains a rarity, used only in storylines of war and trauma, as seen in *Peaky Blinders* (2013–) and *Downton Abbey* (2010–2015). *Poldark*'s

(2015–2019) fifth season (as discussed in Sadler's chapter), however, sees not only medical experiments performed on non-consenting male prison inmates, but its main villain George Warleggan (Jack Farthing), suffering from severe depression over the loss of his wife Elizabeth; subjected to the horrors of bleeding, purging, ice water baths, and restraints, George's treatment reflects the pre-Victorian notion that a man who'd lost his reason had lost his claim to humanity, a beast who needed to be tamed (Scull, 2015). Dr Enys (Luke Norris) successfully counters his medical colleague's cruel and ineffective remedies with empathy, fresh air, and exercise, foreshadowing the shift toward 'moral treatment' pioneered by French physician Philippe Pinel that Victorian psychiatrists would later apply to their asylum patients (Finelli, 2015: 120), but which *Penny Dreadful* conveniently ignores.

Like the sensationalist novels and penny weeklies that inform *Penny Dreadful*, this TV series reflects the distrust and fears many Victorians themselves held toward a profession whose power reached beyond the medical college and teaching hospital and which often shaped social policy. Not only did experts in gynaecology like Dr Acton advocate for the Contagious Diseases Acts, but he, along with colleagues specialising in psychiatry and reproductive medicine, warned against women's access to higher education and the vote on medical grounds and equated female desire with perversion. While *Penny Dreadful* grossly exaggerates the 'tools of the trade' (doctors of course did not use giant electrified needles or even perform lobotomies at this time), it captures how some of the most vocal opponents of Victorian women's emancipation were doctors who themselves employed sensationalist imagery as a warning. As Aude Fauvel notes, 'would-be reformers were warned [by doctors]: to enable women to become more like men would lead, at best, to a society of "sexless" individuals, similar to that of ants, and at worst to a generalised degeneration of humanity, dragged down by female "vampires"' (Fauvel, 2013). In Vanessa's case, the 'animal' within her ultimately brings on the vampiric 'end of days' until she's killed by Ethan Chandler, perhaps, as Kohlke suggests, undermining the feminism of this drama, or, as I'd counter, further highlighting the anxieties Victorians had about women's sexuality and which doctors like Acton and Baker Brown sought to tame.

The professional arrogance of Victor in *Penny Dreadful*'s opening episode resembles that of his real historical contemporaries like those noted above, but by the series' end, he's transformed by his new awareness that ambition has indeed made *him* the 'monster' that Lily spurns. While Victor's first creature, Mr Clare, has also rebuked Victor for never thinking of the consequences of his actions ('a young man's ambitions'), Clare is not subjected to the sexual manipulations of his body or mind that Lily endures. Victor's electrified needle, like Dr Banning's brain surgery, is a stand-in for actual treatments, from the rest cure to the more invasive procedures of ovariectomy and clitoridectomy, used to re-make Victorian women diagnosed as 'hysterical' into the 'calm' or 'demure little wife' that Lily and Vanessa refuse to be. Described in medical literature as an 'amputation' of 'diseased' organs (Baker Brown in Jeffreys, 1987: 27) such surgeries revealed how Victorian gynaecology and psychiatry had become inseparable, reinforcing that not only were a woman's reproductive organs different from a man's but so were her brain and social function (Fauvel, 2013).

This indictment of the male medical professional, who in *The Frankenstein Chronicles* is referred to as 'the beast with the face of a man', obviously ignores all of the good that medical research and treatments have accomplished and from which we benefit today. Many of those Victorian asylums, as recent studies argue, were places of healing and Shepherd even suggests that women's longer periods of confinement were not indicative of a policy of female oppression but instead possibly hinted at women's enjoyment of the freedom from childcare or dangerous employment – or more likely the lack of relatives campaigning for their release (Shepherd, 2004: 244). Nevertheless, as Goodman concludes, Victorian psychiatry persisted in linking mental collapse with women's biological predisposition, while contemporary popular culture still closely entwines madness with femininity (2015: 149). *Penny Dreadful*, as this chapter has tried to argue, however, does not reinforce the victimisation of women at the hands of doctors so much as it allows Lily and Vanessa, in critiquing and resisting such treatments, to rewrite this narrative.

Perhaps, on another level, these medical horror stories in *Penny Dreadful* speak to our own awareness of and fears of medical abuses that of late have been much in the British and American news. Katherine Byrne sees *The Frankenstein Chronicles* as an 'anti-establishment parable' that challenges a still largely male-dominated medical establishment for its corrupt and predatory practices against women and the poor (2018: 160). Similarly, when Brona accuses Victor of stroking her naked body for his unscientific pleasure, it brings to mind such recent scandals as the sexual assault of comatose hospital patients;[4] the crimes of the US Olympics doctor Larry Nassar who performed his specially designed treatment of 'pelvic massages' on hundreds of teen athletes;[5] and British broadcaster Jimmy Savile ('Saint Jimmy') whose fame and charitable work both aided and shielded him for decades as he molested hundreds of children in over fourteen medical establishments, including psychiatric hospitals, in the UK.[6] Victor's desire to transform a prostitute into a virgin even has hints of vaginal rejuvenation surgery and other products that promise twenty-first-century women to make them 'Like a Virgin' or '18 Again' (Saint Thomas, 2017), while drug testing, like Jekyll's, on non-consenting, or at least poorly compensated, subjects persists to this day. Even the Anatomical Venus and wax models of seductively posed victims of Jack the Ripper or Burke and Hare have their equivalent in sex dolls and robots (indeed, there is a 'frigid setting' on female sex robots to let their owners simulate rape [Baynes, 2017]).

Lastly, Brona/Lily and Vanessa, in their refusal to 'counterfeit normality well enough' and submit to the probings by 'expert' hands, are supported by historical precedent. Prostitutes protested their treatment by doctors authorised by the Contagious Diseases Acts, and joining forces with Victorian female reformers led by Josephine Butler, they helped secure the repeal of these Acts in 1886 (Walkowitz, 1982). Other women, inspired by Georgina Weldon's case, formed lunacy reform societies, countering that social factors, not physiology, caused mental illness in women (Walkowitz, 1992), while Gilman's short story, *The Yellow Wallpaper* (published at the same time as *Penny Dreadful*'s setting), rebuked psychiatrists whose female-specific cures were in fact punishments (Showalter, 1985). Dr Seward's compassion toward her patient suggests the healing possibilities when women's voices like Vanessa's are heard. *Penny Dreadful* therefore ends with a message, not for women to 'seek mastery' as Lily first charges her all-female army, but for those entrusted with the care of their minds and bodies to be, as Victor finally realises, 'more human'.

Notes

1 As a scholar who has also been a contributor to popular magazines *People* and *Vogue*, Showalter helped shape the historical narrative about female hysteria and the male-dominated psychiatric profession which continues to inform pop culture. See, for example, Elaine Showalter, 'What it really means when you call a woman "hysterical"', *Vogue*, 10 March 2017, www.vogue.com/article/trump-women-hysteria-and-history (accessed 25 September 2019).

2 See excerpts from Dr Baker Brown's records documenting his 'cure' in Sheila Jeffreys, ed., *The Sexuality Debates*, Routledge, 1987, pp. 11–41.

3 The photographs in this scene are reproduced in Elaine Showalter's *The Female Malady* (1985), which discusses the use of photography as cure in asylums; Showalter also discusses Gilman's short story and Weir Mitchell's use of the rest cure as more 'punishment' than cure.

4 The story of the comatose patient raped and impregnated by her male nurse at an Arizona nursing home made international headlines in 2019. See, for example, www.nytimes.com/2019/01/23/us/nathan-sutherland-vegetative-arizona.html (accessed 5 October 2021). Such real-life accounts of vulnerable patients raped by their caregivers have long been the stuff of pop culture horror, such as the film, *Brimstone and Treacle* (1982).

5 For details of the Nassar abuse cases, see www.theguardian.com/us-news/2017/nov/22/usa-gymnastics-doctor-larry-nassar-plea-deal-25-years (accessed 5 October 2021).

6 'Profile: Jimmy Savile', www.bbc.com/news/entertainment-arts-19984684?intlink_from_url=https://www.bbc.com/news/topics/cz8596rk269t/jimmy-savile-sexual-abuse-scandal&link_location=live-reporting-story (accessed 12 September 2019).

References

Baynes, C. (2017). 'Sex robots with "resistance setting" let men simulate rape and should be outlawed, say campaigners'. *Independent*, www.independent.co.uk/life-style/gadgets-and-tech/news/sex-robots-that-let-men-simulate-rape-should-be-outlawed-says-campaigner-a7959071.html (accessed 23 September 2019).

BBC News (2016). 'Profile: Jimmy Savile'. www.bbc.com/news/entertainment-arts-19984684?intlink_from_url=https://www.bbc.com/news/topics/cz8596rk269t/jimmy-savile-sexual-abuse-scandal&link_location=live-reporting-story (accessed 12 September 2019).

Byrne, K. (2018). 'Pathological masculinities: Syphilis and the medical profession in *The Frankenstein Chronicles*', in K. Byrne, J. Leggott, and J. A. Taddeo, eds, *Conflicting Masculinities: Men in Television Period Drama*. London: I.B. Tauris.

Chatterton, C. (2015). '"Always bear in mind that you are in your senses": Insanity and the lunatic asylum in the nineteenth century – from keeper to attendant to nurse', in T. Knowles and S. Trowbridge, eds, *Insanity and the Lunatic Asylum in the Nineteenth Century*. London: Pickering & Chatto, pp. 85–97.

Ebenstein, J. (2016). *The Anatomical Venus: Wax, God, Death & the Ecstatic*. New York: Distributed Art Publishers.

Fauvel, A. (2013). 'Crazy brains and the weaker sex: the British case (1860–1900)', trans. by Jane Yeoman. *Clio: Women, Gender, History*, 37, pp. 41–64, https://journals.openedition.org/cliowgh/352#ftn36 (accessed 13 September 2019).

Finelli, A. (2015). '"Attitudes Passionelles": The pornographic spaces of the Salpêtrière', in T. Knowles and S. Trowbridge, eds, *Insanity and the Lunatic Asylum in the Nineteenth Century*. London: Pickering & Chatto, pp. 115–133.

Forward, S. (1999). 'Attitudes to marriage and prostitution in the writings of Olive Schreiner, Mona Caird, Sarah Grand and George Egerton'. *Women's History Review*, 8:1, pp. 53–80.

Goodman, H. (2015). '"Madness and masculinity": Male patients in London asylums and Victorian culture', in T. Knowles and S. Trowbridge, eds, *Insanity and the Lunatic Asylum in the Nineteenth Century*. London: Pickering & Chatto, pp. 149–165.

Holmstrom, N. (2017). *Beautiful, Dead, Dissected: The Dismembered Female Body in Artistic Representation*. PhD thesis, University of Tasmania.

Howell, A. and L. Baker (2017). 'Mapping the demimonde: Space, place, and the narrational role of the flâneur, explorer, spiritualist medium and alienist in Penny Dreadful'. *Refractory*, http://refractory.unimelb.edu.au/2017/06/12/howell-baker/ (accessed 23 September 2019).

Jeffreys, S. (1987). *The Sexuality Debates*. Milton Park: Routledge.

Jordanova, L. (1989). *Sexual Visions: Images of Gender in Science and Medicine between the Eighteenth and Twentieth Centuries*. New York: Harvester Wheatsheaf.

Knowles, T. (2015). 'The Legacy of Victorian Asylums in the landscape of contemporary British literature', in T. Knowles and S. Trowbridge, eds, *Insanity and the Lunatic Asylum in the Nineteenth Century*. London: Pickering & Chatto, pp. 41–55.

Knowles, T. and S. Trowbridge (eds) (2015). 'Introduction', in *Insanity and the Lunatic Asylum in the Nineteenth Century*. London: Pickering & Chatto, pp. 1–10.

Kohlke, M. (2018). 'The lures of neo-Victorian presentism (with a feminist case study of *Penny Dreadful*)'. *Literature Compass*, 15(6):e12463, pp. 1–14.

Logan, D. (1997). 'An "outstretched hand to the fallen": The Magdalen's friend and the Victorian reclamation movement: Part I. "Much more sinned against than sinning"'. *Victorian Periodicals Review*, 30:4, pp. 368–387.

MacDonald, H. (2006). *Human Remains: Dissection and Its Histories*. New Haven: Yale University Press.

McClintock, A. (1995). *Imperial Leather: Race, Gender and Sexuality in the Colonial Contest*. New York: Routledge.

Poore, B. (2016). 'The transformed beast: *Penny Dreadful*, adaptation, and the Gothic'. *Victoriographies* 6:1, pp. 62–81.

Richardson, R. (1987). *Death, dissection and the destitute*. London: Routledge and Kegan Paul.

Saint Thomas, S. (2017). 'The truth about whether 5 "vaginal tightening treatments" actually work'. *Allure*, www.allure.com/story/vaginal-tightening-treatments-surgery (accessed 9 September 2019).

Scull, A. (2015). *Madness in Civilization: A Cultural History of Insanity, from the Bible to Freud, from the Madhouse to Modern Medicine*. Princeton: Princeton University Press.

Shepherd, A. (2004). 'The female patient experience in two late nineteenth-century Surrey asylums', in J. Andrews and A. Digby, eds, *Sex and Seclusion: Perspectives on Gender and Class in the History of British and Irish Psychiatry*. New York: Rodopi, pp. 223–248.

Showalter, E. (1985). *The Female Malady: Women, Madness, and English Culture, 1830–1980*. New York: Pantheon Books.

Showalter, E. (2017). 'What it really means when you call a woman "hysterical"'. *Vogue*, 10 March 2017, www.vogue.com/article/trump-women-hysteria-and-history (accessed 25 September 2019).

Strother, A. (2017). '"Monsters all, are we not?": Sex and the human connection in *Penny Dreadful*', in L. Coleman and C. Siegel, eds, *Intercourse in Television and Film: The Presentation of Explicit Sex Acts*. London: Lexington Books, pp. 133–156.

Summers, L. (2001). *Bound to Please: A History of the Victorian Corset*. Oxford: Berg.

Taddeo, J. A. (2012). 'Corsets of steel: Steampunk's reimagining of Victorian femininity', in J. A.. Taddeo and C. J. Miller, eds, *Steaming into a Victorian Future: A Steampunk Anthology*. Lanham, MD: Scarecrow.

Tosh, J. (2007). *A Man's Place: Masculinity and the Middle-Class Home in Victorian England*. New Haven: Yale University Press.

Walkowitz, J. (1982). *Prostitution and Victorian Women: Women, Class, and the State*. Cambridge: Cambridge University Press.

Walkowitz, J. (1992). *City of Dreadful Delight: Narratives of sexual danger in late-Victorian London*. Chicago: University of Chicago Press.

Wiles, W. (2015). '"Straitjacket": A confined history', in T. Knowles, and S. Trowbridge, eds, *Insanity and the Lunatic Asylum in the Nineteenth Century*. London: Pickering & Chatto, pp. 167–181.

11

The surgical gaze in the operating theatre: early twentieth-century surgery on screen

Marie Allitt

In an early episode of *The Knick* (2014–2015), Dr Algernon Edwards (André Holland), who has been forced to perform surgery in secret in the hospital basement after hours, records details of the process with photographs. Later, we see him, and eventually his colleagues, consult these images through a stereoscope. Edwards makes these photographs partly for patient case notes, and partly to track the progress and provide visual evidence of his developing experimental procedure for an inguinal hernia. In these visual depictions of medical records, we begin to see how 'the emergence of [new visual] technologies in the early twentieth century entailed a reconceptualization of the role of the surgeon as image-maker' (Palfreyman and Rabier, 2018: 289). The camera and stereoscopic viewer are just some of the examples of new visual technologies in medical practice that are depicted in the historical medical dramas discussed here. With a focus on two twenty-first-century shows set in the first decade of the twentieth century, the BBC's *Casualty 1900s* (2006–2009) and HBO/Cinemax's *The Knick*, I explore the representation of surgery and how these ideas play out on screen, specifically through period drama.

A considerable amount of medical knowledge is constituted by the visual, from the Foucauldian clinical gaze to anatomical atlases. This is especially the case for surgical knowledge, such as the illustrations by Vesalius and Charles Bell, which have been vital for learning and instruction in anatomy and surgery. In this chapter, I seek to build upon recent efforts to refocus the significance of the visual as key to the construction of surgical knowledge by considering how surgery and a surgical gaze are represented on screen. The visual medium opens up the surgical, clinical gaze in new, representative, ways, which is further complicated by the different surgical spaces themselves, such as the theatre or auditorium. The depiction of surgery in historical drama conveys a sense of risk, wonder, and shock that is different to contemporary medical shows. Discovery and experimentation are often central, so it becomes a case of simultaneous discovery for both the surgeon and the audience. I explore the representations of growing medical knowledge, framed by acts of surgical intervention, in a space of shared, innovative surgical developments.

The period medical drama

The Knick ran for two seasons between 2014 and 2015, directed by Steven Soderbergh, depicting a fictionalised version of the Knickerbocker Hospital in New York City in 1900 and 1901. The hospital staff are the focus of the show, centring primarily on the surgeons, but including storylines involving the ambulance drivers, nuns, nurses, hospital superintendent, and hospital owners. The beginning of the first episode immediately sets up the central crux of surgery at this time: the unsuccessful procedure on a *placenta previa* patient. Mother and baby cannot be saved, and it is clear to the viewer that this is just one of dozens of attempts with this procedure; the surgeons know they need to get the baby out and limit the loss of blood as quickly as possible. The surgeons are more than disappointed, and the Chief of Surgery, J. M. Christiansen (Matt Frewer), returns to his office, where he kills himself. In response, Dr John Thackery (Clive Owen) is made the new Chief of Surgery and he is able to choose his second in command. Without his consultation, the heads of the hospital hire their first and only African American member of medical staff, Dr Algernon Edwards (André Holland), fresh from surgical success in Paris and London. Thus, the scene is set for professional rivalries, grounded not only in competition and jealousy, but also racism, which underpins much of the show's narrative (and which is discussed in more depth in McQueeney's chapter).

Across the two seasons (twenty episodes overall), medical experimentation, exploration, and ambition are set against the backdrop of key technological and medical concerns of the period, such as electricity, x-rays, blood transfusions, eugenics, animal experimentation, and cocaine addiction. In a review of the show published in *The Lancet*, Jason Socrates Bardi describes Soderbergh's style as 'a fresh approach to surgical cinematography, filming operating room sequences in sharp focus with bright lighting to distinguish them from scenes outside … Such artistic elements help establish the world Soderbergh has created as both dreamy and dismal: a gritty dawn of modern surgery in a brutal New York city' (2014: 2016). The show is certainly gritty and does not shy away from either graphic scenes of injury or sex, or highlighting racism, criminality, gang violence, and blackmail. The centre point of the show is the operating amphitheatre, which is no reprieve from the brutality. Inspired by the New York Presbyterian Hospital (Adams, 2018: 264), it is a gleaming white surgical space, which is in sharp contrast with the dark brown of the gallery seating and wall panels.

Casualty 1900s focuses on three years at the Royal London Hospital, Whitechapel, in the East End of London. It is similarly set against a backdrop of key innovations, such as the introduction of x-rays, light therapy, galvanic baths, psychoanalysis, and developments in anaesthesia. The show grounds itself in true stories. Its central characters are real people, and some of the patients and events are drawn from medical records of the time. Each episode's opening credits include the remit that 'All cases, characters and events in this film are based on hospital records, newspapers and personal memoirs' – although it is not entirely clear what sources have been used, or which parts of the narrative have been fabricated or embellished: the show inevitably takes some liberties with the truth. The show ran for three seasons, with potentially confusing labelling: the first episode, *Casualty 1906*, was a pilot in 2006 and did not pick up again until 2008, with three episodes of *Casualty 1907*, and then six episodes of *Casualty 1909* in 2009. For the avoidance of confusion, I treat each as a season within the *Casualty 1900s* show.

While the series was released as *London Hospital* for North American audiences, it was known as *Casualty 1900s* in the UK – which carries a certain popular cultural association for UK audiences. The name suggests itself as a spin-off from the long-running British continuing series, *Casualty*, which began in 1986, set in contemporary time. This titling seems a deliberate choice to appeal to long-faithful viewers and set the show within the context of British health care. The actual similarities are few: the setting is not the same, but it is possible to see in *Casualty 1900s* some of the same ideology and motivations behind this precursor. *Casualty* 'tended to understand itself as part of a campaign against UK government cuts to the health service', and 'was strongly bound to contemporary issues of UK healthcare and part of its integration of medico-political news stories into its drama' (Jacobs, 2003: 22, 23). The show employed a style of realism, drawing upon contemporary news stories and health care issues. *Casualty 1900s* similarly highlights social welfare problems; it acknowledges in every episode the poverty of London's East End and the lack of health care and welfare support for the poor. The opening credits also establish the focus of the show in relation to current, twenty-first-century understandings of medicine and health care, that all too often we take for granted: 'Antibiotics, and public funding by the NHS, were still 40 years away.' Framed in this way, the show consciously encourages viewers to reflect on their own relationship with the medical service, in turn destroying any nostalgic impulse one might assume from a period drama. Instead, all sense of nostalgia is undermined by an awareness that in this relatively recent past many would not survive. In a way that seems to turn back the clock, the audience is taken back in time to the early twentieth century, where we had even less than we have now.

This specific framing and mention of the NHS are significant and certainly deliberate. The UK's National Health Service, founded in 1948, with free health care for all, is one of the unique assets of the British welfare system – a health care system that does not exist anywhere else. Since its inception, it has been an idealistic system that has been increasingly hard to manage, but it has survived nevertheless. Yet it has repeatedly come under criticism, with increased attacks over the past few decades, with welfare cuts and attempts at increased privatisation. *Casualty 1900s*, then, explicitly frames itself in relation to the NHS, on the one hand showing us that we have it so much better than before, while also showing us what we risk without it. Such an agenda is also seen in *Call the Midwife* (2012–) (also discussed in this collection); set in London's East End in the 1960s, it too offers an 'unapologetic defence of the National Health Service' (Taddeo, 2019: 52). Of course, medical advances and knowledge have changed life expectancy, but *Casualty 1900s* strives to remind us that welfare is intrinsically tied to health and wellbeing of all kinds, and our lives depend on universal access to free health care.

Such a celebration and support for universal health care is markedly different in *The Knick*, which is created and set in the US, where they are yet to experience free health care. Consequently, the Knickerbocker Hospital is infected with a general cynicism and greed that compromises the provision of charitable health care. The airing of the show in 2014 and 2015 coincided with the Obama administration, and the roll-out of the Patient Protection and Affordable Care Act, or Obamacare, from 2010, which is the closest the US has come to providing affordable health care. In the show, there is a background theme of charity, with the adjoining orphanage run by Catholic nuns, and an underlying desire to provide care for the poor, which mainly stems from Cornelia Robertson (Juliet Rylance). In fact, one of the storylines throughout the first season is resisting the move of the hospital uptown, to 'where the money is', to attract wealthy patients.

While it seems clear that *Casualty 1900s* inherits a commitment to a message of social welfare from its namesake, the styles of the shows vary substantially. *Casualty 1900s* has an unusual style as part-reconstruction, part-documentary, while also striving to be a medical drama in its own right – which descends most often into sensationalism, sentimentality, and melodrama. The documentary style is no surprise when its writers and director have a strong background in documentary filmmaking. The descent into melodrama and cliché is one of the pitfalls of trying to create stories of real people – where there are necessary narrative gaps that must be filled and shaped. Unfortunately, giving multidimensionality to many of these characters (based on real people) often generates a romantic storyline. Despite this, the series as a whole becomes far stronger and manages to balance the documentary roots with drama more successfully by its final, 1909, season.

It may seem unfair to place these two shows alongside one another and compare them, given their vastly different production values and star attraction. They differ in many respects – not only because the former is from the US and the latter from the UK. What they do have in common is a focus on medicine in the first decade of the twentieth century, depicting key medical innovations and technologies introduced during this period. Both shows put a spotlight upon the American and British medical scene between 1900 to 1909, with particular inclusions of surgery, and grasp the opportunity to educate viewers and rework aspects of the period drama genre.

Without a doubt, these shows are period dramas that both challenge and fulfil fundamental generic expectations. The distinct focus on a specific time period in both shows offers particular insight into events and attitudes of the past. Period dramas cleverly play on imbalances between what the audience already knows and what the characters do not, and it is no exception in these shows. For example, when Thackery is finally admitted to a rehabilitation facility for treatment for his cocaine addiction, the camera focuses on the doctor's new drug as it sits on the bedside table, with the label, 'heroin'. Without explicitly saying so, the viewer knows that Thackery will now become addicted to heroin. The power of the period drama genre does not solely rely on what an audience already knows, but also on what they might learn. The historical topic and engagement with the past, as Jerome de Groot suggests, has the potential 'to educate the viewer' (2009: 184). When it comes to medical history and the less mainstream focus on turn-of-the-century medicine, there is certainly a potential in both of these shows to educate viewers in the developments of medicine and surgery, but more importantly, the audience can realise how recent such developments have been. This is especially important in light of previous comments on access to free health care, and the intention of these shows to demonstrate how recent basic medical welfare has been achieved, and how fragile such access is.

Yet both *The Knick* and *Casualty 1900s* have been influenced by other television genres and more recent trends in visual storytelling. *The Knick*, in particular, inherits much of its style from the popularity of medical dramas (especially in the US), from the 1990s onward:

> The new forms of television realism that emerged in the early 1990s were indicative of a voyeuristic interest in everyday life – television's 'ambition to see everything' exemplified in 'reality TV' and workplace documentaries. Many of these shows used rapid transitions between different spaces, stories and people within an overall stylistic umbrella that stressed immediacy and authenticity. What made such shows appealing was a combination of voyeurism and reactive immediacy to contingent events – the crime, crash, emergency, argument – so that the camera seemed as if taken by surprise. (Jacobs, 2003: 13)

Shots of the hospital and procedures in *The Knick* are rapidly paced, with frequent jumps in time and cuts to different scenes and perspectives. Very little time is given to exposition: it does not pause to explain, so the viewer is thrown into the room, and sometimes left wondering what is happening. These shows uniquely benefit from a blending of contemporary medical shows with the genre of period drama: in seeking to capture 'immediacy and authenticity' that ensures realism, both shows bring alive specific moments in medicine that are not regularly seen on screen, with aesthetics and tone which feel distinctly modern. *The Knick* specifically, in its embrace of grit and seediness, seems to be a relative of other contemporary and violent shows such as *Boardwalk Empire* (2010–2014) and *Peaky Blinders* (2013–), both of which have a period setting, but adopt a contemporary and more 'immediate' feel. Given that '[G]raphic depictions of serious injury became the norm [in contemporary medical drama] with bleeding wounds, screaming patients and fast-talking medical staff key elements in the *mise en scéne*' (Jacobs, 2003: 54), both shows embrace the opportunity to produce often shocking visuals of injuries and procedures. In blending the period drama genre with features of contemporary medical drama, as well as challenging subliminal medical knowledge, both of these shows develop the tone, style, and possible subject matter of period dramas.

A history of surgery

Surgery of the early twentieth century has received comparatively less attention than surgery of other periods, but current research is serving to fill in these gaps and bring significant surgical developments to light. In fact, the early decades of the twentieth century experienced influential medical, clinical, and technological innovations, radically influencing surgical practice, some of which are introduced in these shows, such as x-rays and radiology. In the early episodes of *The Knick*, an x-ray machine is purchased, and we see it occasionally in use. There is giddy excitement for the appliance, whereas *Casualty 1900s* demonstrates from the start the damage that experimentation with unstable radiation poses, and its unknown long-term effects – consequences not realised for many decades. In the first episode of *Casualty 1900s*, set in December 1906, the x-ray's power is explicitly articulated. Ernest Wilson (Jason Watkins), the radiographic technician, is introduced as having worked with x-rays for a long time; his hands are dramatically damaged by radiation burns and he has subsequently lost several of his fingers. At the end of the first episode, he undergoes surgery to remove a further two fingers.

Interestingly, neither show gives much focus to the radiographic images themselves, instead indicating the early mechanics of the technology and the underestimated dangers. In the very final episode of *The Knick*, corrupt hospital superintendent Herman Barrow (Jeremy Bobb) comments on the mysterious marks appearing on his hands. To the suggestion that he get an x-ray, he responds 'oh, I've had hundreds': the camera closes in on his hands, and the audience realises these are radiation spots – playing on the dramatic irony of what the audience knows, and they can diagnose what will happen to him. The desire to see inside the human body is there, but in these shows, it is a bloodlust that is sated. The peripheral glimpse of the body's interior without cut or incision runs counter to the impulse of both dramas to show us the butchery and precision, the experimentation and exceptionalism of surgical actions, which in turn satisfy the intellectual hunger that 'to cut was to see, to see was to know' (Palfreyman and Rabier, 2018: 285). These shows offer us a focus that goes beyond the clinical gaze to introduce a distinct 'surgical gaze'.

The surgical gaze

This concept of a 'surgical gaze' is a form of the 'clinical gaze', but one more grounded in both the aesthetics of anatomical and surgical illustrations and the embodied act of viewing surgery. Not entirely dissimilar to what Christopher Lawrence terms the 'surgical point of view' (1992: 23), this concept articulates a distinctive viewpoint of surgeons, surgical students, and an audience (both gallery observers and TV viewers). In this 'surgical gaze', we have the perspective of the surgeons as they look upon their patients, and as they navigate the developing surgical field, but we also have the complex extension of the students, audience, and TV viewers observing both the surgeon and the surgery. These multiple layers of looking and learning are further advanced by the depiction of surgical spaces, especially the surgical amphitheatre, as seen in *The Knick*. At the same time, we witness further layers of this through the depictions of surgical teaching. Medical dramas tend to rely upon a teacher–student structure as a way to 'teach' the audience how things work – as well as itself being a source of drama (Jacobs, 2003: 14); not only are the characters looking in order to learn, the TV audience is learning from looking. More often than not, in both of these dramas, the audience witnesses the medical procedures, not through the eyes of the patients, but either through the eyes of the medical students or separate from any personal viewpoint. Consequently, the imbalance of power orchestrated by this kind of gaze is less about the dehumanising and objectification of the patient (although that is certainly still present) and more about the relationship between teacher and student. The act of teaching through surgical demonstration relies upon a kind of performance, and so the operating table becomes the surgeon's stage.

Seemingly intentionally, neither of these shows offers the point of view of the patients. Although we gain some insight into the patient experience through certain storylines, for the most part, and especially in surgical scenes, the patient's gaze is not explored. However, while the viewer relies solely on the clinician and care provider's perspective, there is an opportunity here to re-consider power dynamics in relation to multiple types of gaze. In her extensive re-examination of the clinical gaze, Johanna Shapiro outlines different versions, such as 'the voyeuristic gaze', 'the avoidant gaze', and 'the scientific gaze', which, crucially, does not isolate the 'clinical gaze' to the examining physician (2002: 164–165). By taking inspiration from Shapiro, we can explore 'the surgical gaze' and precisely how its complexities are demonstrated, taught, and ingrained in medical culture, through the prism of these dramas.

How we see and what we see of the surgeries varies throughout these shows. At times the viewer is given an unnatural view of the surgery and the surgeons, other times it is a realistic viewpoint from the gallery – but this is never consistent. It is significant that throughout the first episode of *The Knick*, 'Method and Madness', the view of the surgery is never from the perspective of the gallery. The camera shot is unnatural, at waist height, just above the operating table. We see the belly and the incision, and the camera cuts to repeated images of bloody sponges thrown into a bowl. The camera remains at waist height, but tilts upwards occasionally to see the surgeons' faces with close-ups on instruments and materials. There are no views from the amphitheatre gallery: we do not see the operation as it would be seen by the observers. It is only once the

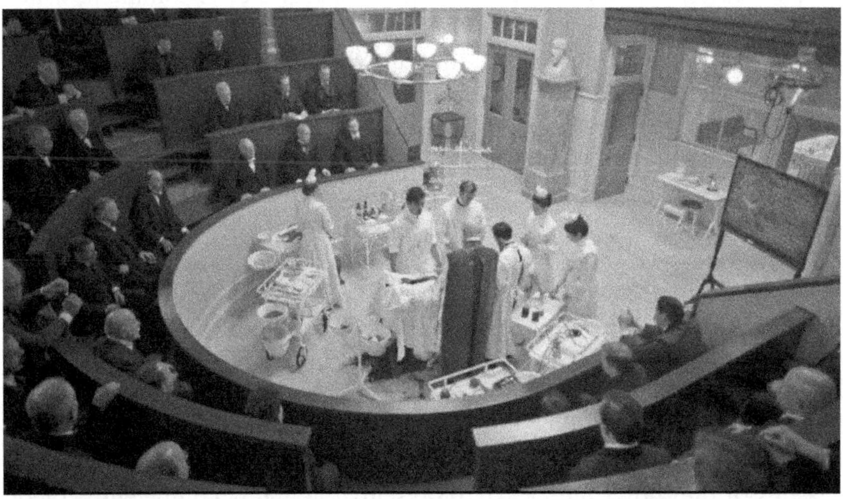

Figure 11.1 *The Knick* (dir. Steven Soderbergh), S1E1 'Method and Madness', 2014

mother and baby have died that the camera moves higher and further back, to view the scene from the back of the gallery, looking down. The unnatural angles serve to demonstrate the embodied aspects of surgical practice. By watching the surgeons' faces from a position at the same level as the table, we can get a sense of their posture; of the distance and tactile connection they have with the patient. More than anything, we gain an insight into the embodied relationship that the surgeon has in the surgical field and the nature of the surgical space itself (Figure 11.1).

The surgeon is his field

> *Mr Fenwick (carving meat):* 'In another life I would have made a damned good butcher.'
> *Dr Lawes:* 'Or a murderer.'
> *Fenwick:* 'Some would say I already am.' (*Casualty 1900s*, S2E2)

A focus on the figure of the surgeon is central to this discussion and, fitting all the stereotypes, the surgeon is made central in these shows. In order for this surgical gaze to become explicit to an audience, the shows must play upon the stereotypes of the surgeon, and it is then that the different manifestations of the visual can begin to break down our assumptions about surgeons. The above scene offers an overt reference to the perceptions of surgeons as butchers, and as careless and violent individuals whose slaughter and cruelty are equivalent to murder. It is only a brief comment, which is not overtly revisited, but takes on new power when considered in relation to events in the final season. In the 1909 season, dominant storylines include accidental death from dangerous anaesthesia (ether), as well as the controversy surrounding the use of stovaine as spinal anaesthesia. These narrative strands draw out the contrasts between surgical practitioners and emphasise the different styles of medical innovation and degrees of clinical ethics.

There are two main surgeons throughout *Casualty 1900s*, who, although dramatisations of real figures, are intentionally contrasted with one another. One of the recurring surgeons is Mr Edwin Hurry Fenwick (David Troughton), a senior surgeon, based upon the real-life surgeon of the same name who worked at the London Hospital from 1890–1910 and was a significant and influential urologist and proponent of radiology. We do not learn much about Fenwick, but he features throughout the three seasons of the show, and clearly represents the highly competent surgeon and teacher, who, though traditional, is not afraid of gradual change. In the 1909 series, we are introduced to Mr Henry Percy Dean (Paul Hilton), who was influential in the introduction of spinal analgesia, but who is presented as cocaine-addicted, brash, unreliable, arrogant, and rude to the nurses. Dean has far more in common with the protagonist of *The Knick*, Dr John Thackery, who is a deeply flawed yet highly skilled surgeon. Thackery is loosely based on Dr William Halsted, who was similarly a highly successful and skilled surgeon but also addicted to cocaine throughout his lifetime.

The surgical amphitheatre of *The Knick* is central – there is not an episode where we do not go inside the operating theatre – and more often than not, the scenes taking place here are narratively essential. One of the subtleties of the show is how, although the surgical scenes are dramatic and tense, they are not always given equal weight. Although the events of the operating theatre seep out to other spaces, the narrative importance of the scenes varies, keeping the viewer on their toes. The surgical amphitheatre has more similarity to the surgical spaces we see in *Charité* (2017), the first episode of *Bramwell* (1995–1998), and several episodes in *The Frankenstein Chronicles* (2015, 2017), all set during the mid to late nineteenth century. In contrast, the surgical spaces in *Casualty 1900s* are of a smaller and less spectacle-inducing scale. The operating room has a small set of free-standing tiered steps to one side, where the students stand to observe. There is specifically no space allocated for public or general observers. In *Casualty 1900s*' third season, set in 1909, the programme not only takes on a slightly different tone, but the operating rooms are completely different. The operating room is an octagonal, high-ceilinged, fully tiled room, with an upper, in-built balcony gallery, where students stand and look down on the operating table. The style of surgical space depicted in these dramas has a direct impact upon how the surgery is viewed, and thus on the connotations of such a representation of surgery and the surgeon. Is the operating room a classroom, a laboratory, a lecture theatre, an entertainment venue, or a carnival sideshow? At various times it is all these things, and more.

'Welcome to our circus'

In the February 1904 edition of the *London Hospital Gazette* (run by medical students), the presumably pseudonymous 'A. B. Lighter' offers 'An Everyday Occurrence', a scene from 'The Operating Theatre of the Great Firm, Slaughter & Scrag', and depicts the popularity and curiosity of watching surgery in action:

> the galleries are filling. Word has gone round that Mr. Slaughter means to surpass himself this afternoon, and accordingly the eagles have gathered … These would-be spectators … have the stolid *blasé* air with which the *habitués* of the

> Roman amphitheatre might have waited to see whether a lion could demolish a martyr who had proved incombustible. (Lighter, 1904: 128)

The scene is a satire of surgical attitudes, outlining the unabashed intrigue for seeing a body brutally opened and 'slaughtered'. The audience is likened to bloodthirsty and hungry spectators, desiring to see 'blood spurt above the heads of the dressers' (1904: 128) and bodies opened (a scenario parodied in BBC's *Quacks* [2017] about early Victorian surgery). But the scene is cut short: a curtain descends to a note that 'Whatever surgeons may do in theatres, Medea must not slay her child before the eyes of the crowd' (1904: 129). It is a poignant ending, which draws attention to the fact that the appetite for spectating has been quashed. It is no longer to be a spectacle; it is not Greek tragedy; it is not a theatrical scene – except in direct teaching moments, it is not to be observed.

During the nineteenth century, surgery 'was often a public event, and showmanship was part of the business' (Schlich, 2015: 385), and thus the hospital became a site of spectacle. This eagerness to witness rapidly diminished in the latter part of the century, and into the twentieth: it is generally accepted that 'as surgery became increasingly successful it was losing its tension and drama and thus no longer satisfied the innate craving for sensation' (Morgeli, 1999: 180), but the fundamental style of the operating room also changed. Towards the end of the nineteenth century, the operating theatre design changed from an amphitheatre to smaller operating rooms, due to concerns over germ control and the self-containment of the overall space (Schlich, 2007: 243). *The Knick* demonstrates, in part, the transitions around the appetite and interest to view surgeries: to an extent, there is still spectacle, but for the most part, it is about learning and teaching from mentors and peers.

There is the recurrent analogy (which is not subtle) throughout *The Knick* that the Knickerbocker is a 'circus', and the operating theatre, in Edwards's words, is the 'Big Top', reinforcing the image of showmanship and performance. This is a central stage, for performance, and the star attraction is Thackery, who is one of the surgeon celebrities (Schlich, 2015: 384). The appetite to see Thackery perform surgical 'miracles' becomes blurred and complicated by the introduction, in the second season, of bodies that are themselves objects of attraction. The comparison with the 'freak show' is explicit in the second season, where events in the hospital are intercut with the characters socially visiting the carnival sideshow, which hosts biological mysteries. The sideshow becomes an extension of the hospital; the circus. Thackery uses this space to procure specimens, specifically drug addicts in order to research the cause of addiction. This 'use' of the sideshow seems to be a deliberate echo of Dr Frederick Treves's 1884 encounter with 'The

Elephant Man', Joseph Merrick, at a freak show: in the name of science, Treves took Merrick across the road to the London Hospital to take clinical photographs of his body (and later admitted Merrick to the hospital for further study in 1887 where he stayed until his death three years later) (Durbach, 2009: 36). In both Treves's and Thackery's actions we see successive layers of voyeuristic looking and viewing in the name of benevolent scientific research that quickly blurs the line between curiosity and exploitation.

What Thackery sees at the sideshow awakens and re-energises his medical experimentation imagination – specifically, conjoined twin girls, who are attached at the liver. This leads to a core surgical episode, with his attempt to separate the conjoined twins. What at times seemed to be benevolent motivations and genuine care for the twins' welfare clearly becomes more about Thackery's reputation. He is searching for the next big thing, the next big experiment for his career, and a buzz that only risk and danger gives him. Thackery performs for the crowd, compelling his audience to look at these strange objects: 'This is their last day as a sideshow attraction, and you their last audience. This is no magic trick, no illusion, no sleight of hand, this is scientific knowledge and rigorous experimentation.' His speech mirrors the way the girls' owner had introduced them at the sideshow: the girls are spoken about; they are objects to be stared at. He adopts the language of the conjurer or magician, hypnotising his audience into the spell that his presence, and surgical skill, cast.

But this encouraged desire to see the girls' bodies is undone by the sudden cut to after the surgery. The viewer does not see the surgery take place; after the initial incision, it cuts to the recording of the surgery, with Thackery's voiceover, talking us through the procedure. The viewer only sees a mediated version of the landmark surgery, so our complicit voyeurism is undercut. The recent technology of the video camera (moving-picture camera) adds complexity to the visuality taking place in these scenes. Thackery's interest in separating the conjoined twins offers parallels with real-life French surgeon Eugène-Louis Doyen, who, in 1902, attempted the separation of 'the Orissa Twins', Radica and Doodica. More significantly, as Nadja Durbach notes, Doyen 'was known for filming his procedures so that he would be able to evaluate his performance and use the films for teaching purposes' (2009: 66), in precisely the same way Thackery records the operation. Doyen's film 'was shown not only in medical contexts, however, but also on the fairgrounds', so we can only imagine how far afield Thackery's film would travel (Durbach, 2009: 67). The juxtaposition of viewing bodies and body parts is further highlighted by the fact that we have already seen Henry Robertson (Charles Aitken) use this same camera to create pornography. The camera begins to tread a thin line between knowledge resource and voyeurism. Thackery is an overt 'image-maker', but of a new, excitingly modern, age of surgery. By recording the surgery, Thackery both proves himself as an unsurpassable surgical star, and as someone who has successfully traversed previously untouched lands. Consequently, the image of the surgeon-as-performer overlaps with that of the surgeon-as-explorer.

Exploration and experimentalism

The medical authority of the physician has often been discussed in relation to colonisation and exploration (Frank, 1995: 10). This extends to the surgeon, especially the ambition-, research-, and solution-driven character of the surgeons depicted here. There is a reason that collections of anatomical illustrations are known as atlases, which are 'concerned with the "mapping" of the body' (Petherbridge and Jordanova, 1997: 63). We see this specifically in Thackery, whose persona as a performer is connected with his thirst for adventure. Thackery seeks to traverse every aspect of the surgical landscape, but he only has a partial map.

Thackery is the lone, intrepid explorer, who continuously attempts to expand his surgical terrain. It is especially in the second season, where arguably his fight to solve everything that faces him becomes, itself, pathological and symptomatic of his increasingly dangerous cocaine addiction, that his hunger to conquer becomes most oblique. He successfully cures Abigail Alford's (Jennifer Ferrin) syphilis, but the realisation that he cannot solve everything hits him hard, especially with her sudden death. This downfall, or failure, comes to represent the danger of the lone surgeon, in contrast to collaborative teamwork. The introduction of Dr Levi Zinberg (Michael Nathanson) in the latter part of the first season, and recurring in the second, serves to emphasise the different research and teaching styles of the eminent surgeons. By the end of its run, *The Knick* has shown the importance of laboratory research as much as the 'heroic', lone explorer at the operating table. While Thackery is still the rebellious maverick, careless and selfish, by the end (and his own end), his colleagues and the audience are convinced of the importance of medical exploration and experimentation which is slower, more cautious, and not about one-upmanship. Although slower, the more cautious and collaborative approach to innovation succeeds, where the single maverick star-surgeon fails.

Surgical pedagogy – 'see one, do one, teach one'

Underpinning this whole discussion has been the topic of knowledge production, teaching, and learning. In his research into evolving styles of surgery, Thomas Schlich has articulated the distinctiveness of surgical teaching: 'surgical styles were passed on through imitation between practitioners because in many respects surgical training follows an apprenticeship model, as is typical for crafts' (2015: 381). We can see some of the ways the apprenticeship model plays out, specifically in the relationship between Thackery and his apprentice Dr Bertie Chickering Jr (Michael Angarano). It is especially in the friction, failings, and eventual reconciliation that the dynamics of their teacher–student relationship comes through. Their inequalities in power are evident early on when Thackery persuades Bertie to join him in experimenting on prostitutes, and yet this is complicated by Bertie's effective amendment to what becomes their successful device to help with the *placenta previa* cases – so much so that Thackery acknowledges Bertie's contribution by naming it the 'Christiansen-Thackery-Chickering placental repair'. Potential tensions between the surgeon and apprentice are articulated by Bertie's father's insistence that he move out of Thackery's service to a more suitable mentor. Dr Chickering Sr's wishes are eventually met when Bertie moves, however briefly, to the service of Dr Zinberg at Mount Sinai Hospital. In *Casualty 1900s*, we see glimpses of the British 'firm' system, where students work specifically with a consultant surgeon – not very different to the working relationships in *The Knick*.

First-hand observation of surgery is fundamental in surgical teaching. What is perhaps less recognised, certainly in this early twentieth-century context, is how much can be learned from the surgeon's specific performance: not just watching what the surgery entails, but how the surgeon's body is positioned and moves. Much of the learning from watching is about witnessing the surgeon's performance (in every sense of the word), and their embodied practice of surgery. In these instances, our established understanding of the clinical gaze which objectifies the patient is complicated: in viewing the surgery, the patient is somewhat sidelined for the preferential focus on the surgeon's actions and movements. The student learns from witnessing and identifying how the working surgeon's body moves in certain ways in order to perfect the procedure: 'surgical techniques become ingrained in the body – in its movements and even in its sinews and muscles' (Schlich, 2015: 380). Thus, there is no straightforward imbalance of power through the gaze. The surgeon does not lose his power by being watched, but instead maintains, and even strengthens, his authority and agency through his physical presence. Furthermore, 'surgical skill can be seen as embodied material practice that becomes manifest in series of gestures surgeons perform in a particular way' (Schlich, 2015: 380), and so the surgeon-in-training not only learns by doing, but firstly by seeing: the 'see one, do one, teach one' in action.

In exploring contemporary, twenty-first-century surgical teaching and learning, Rachel Prentice recognises 'training as a fully embodied activity, one based on the intertwining of learning and treatment, action and response, thought and feeling' (2007: 7). Retrospectively, in these period dramatisations, we can begin to appreciate how this has been critical in medical education for a long time. As Prentice argues in her anthropological study of surgical learning, mastery is learned as much through 'physical skill, socialization, situated knowledge, and intuition together as nonformalizable knowledge' (2007: 536) – and learning to ride a bicycle is often cited as an example of this. Riding a bicycle is 'a physical skill that can be explained but cannot be learned except by riding' (Prentice, 2007: 536). Coincidentally, both shows include scenes where the central characters learn to ride a bike or help others to learn. Not only is the bicycle a symbol of modernity and independence (and especially female emancipation and independence, as it is cast here), the bicycle also symbolises the combined theoretical and embodied learning by doing. In seemingly innocuous scenes, with brief interludes into a more carefree aspect of their personal lives, the image of riding a bicycle reiterates the importance of embodied and experiential learning. Thus, the 'see one, do one, teach one' becomes clearer still. The student begins as the spectator, before then embodying the position of the surgeon and enacting the procedure, and teaching cements the mastery, by a combination of seeing and understanding the phenomenology of the action.

Conclusion

While it is easy to see how important the visual is in medicine, the shows discussed make a convincing case for the specific visuality of surgery and surgical teaching. The focus on early twentieth-century operations, in particular, helps to promote the significance of surgical developments at this time: although attitudes to both surgery and surgical knowledge significantly altered in the late nineteenth century, *The Knick* and *Casualty 1900s* demonstrate how developments in surgical understanding retained an important relationship with what can and cannot be seen, and the desire to cut in order to know. Surgery and the observation of surgery rely on multiple layers of looking. The visual medium of television helps in this respect, enabling a language, style, and form that can show as much it can tell about medical and surgical culture, while simultaneously challenging viewers' assumptions about medicine and health.

In the 'surgical gaze', we can recognise how the predication of surgical knowledge on vision is heavily tied to the surgical spaces. The observational viewpoint is key, and thus we can recognise that viewing galleries, in their multiple forms, are directly linked to the production and acquisition of knowledge. Furthermore, in the act of observing surgery, the assumption of power imbalances is challenged: it is still certainly present, but takes on a new character in light of observing not just the patient, but the surgeon. The student must learn by looking and by doing: before they can ride the bicycle, they need to see how it works. Learning is as much about knowledge as it is about skill, and the acquisition of those precise skills is something particular to surgery, especially in early clinical surgery and in the transitional period of the twentieth century.

Many film and television scholars have noted that period drama is never only one thing: it comprises many styles, aesthetics, themes, and subgenres (Leggott and Taddeo, 2014; Monk and Sargeant, 2002: 2). Both *Casualty 1900s* and *The Knick* offer examples for the directions of future period drama, showing that there are a great many opportunities for challenging subject matter in the blending and merging of genres and subgenres. For these shows, the blending of the period drama with the contemporary medical drama brings a reality and immediacy to the history of medicine – it breathes life into aspects of history hitherto underexplored in historical drama on stage, text, and screen. Both of these shows recognise the potential for surgery, and medicine more broadly, to be explored through a visual mode that captures shock, intrigue, risk, and which comes most alive when it is amalgamated with a contemporary style of rapid editing and makes the most of opportunities to depict graphic, realistic scenes.

The subject matter of modern medicine and early twentieth-century surgery gains new life with developments in visual language and style. Such shows, to an extent, play upon the viewers' knowledge and present facets of modern medicine with dramatic irony – but this can only work with the delicate use of visual cues that remove the need for words: a longer pause on a medicine bottle; an ironic glimpse of a skin blemish; the presence of a specific medical instrument. That we, as viewers, can recognise and interpret these signs plays to existing and newly acquired knowledge. It is almost as if the audience has been allowed to become diagnosticians, inhabiting the exact position of students observing the procedure: looking at bodies and drawing on received knowledge to identify what might be wrong with the patient.

Historical drama can be a vehicle for medical education, putting medical developments into a context that can be compared and contrasted with the contemporary climate. These shows challenge possible audience naiveties about medical innovation and work to educate viewers in both medical history and ethics. Lastly, these shows, with their emphasis on bodies opened, show that period drama is not solely about comfort or nostalgia, but can be about gaining perspective, and especially in these instances, thankfulness for current medical practice.

References

Adams, A. (2018). 'Surgery and Architecture: Spaces for Operating', *The Palgrave Handbook of the History of Surgery*, ed. T. Schlich, London: Palgrave Macmillan, pp. 261–281.

Bardi, J. S. (2014). 'The Gritty Dawn of Modern Surgery', *The Lancet*, 384.9959, p. 2016.

Cartwright, L. (1995). *Screening the Body: Tracing Medicine's Visual* Culture, Minneapolis: University of Minnesota Press.

De Groot, J. (2009). *Consuming History: Historians and Heritage in Contemporary Popular Culture*, London: Routledge.

Durbach, N. (2009). *The Spectacle of Deformity: Freak Shows and Modern British Culture*, Berkeley: University of California Press.

Foucault, M. (1963). *The Birth of the Clinic*, translated by A. M. Sheridan, Abingdon: Routledge, 2005.

Frank, A. (1995). *The Wounded Storyteller: Body, Illness, and Ethics*, Chicago: The University of Chicago Press, 2013.

Jacobs, J. (2003). *Body Trauma TV: The New Hospital Dramas*, London: British Film Institute.

Lawrence, C. (1992). *Medical Theory, Surgical Practice: Studies in the History of Surgery*, London and New York: Routledge.

Leggott, J. and J. A. Taddeo (eds) (2014). *Upstairs and Downstairs: British Costume Drama Television from* The Forsyte Saga *to* Downton Abbey, Lanham: Rowman & Littlefield.

Lighter, A. B. (1904). 'An Everyday Occurrence', *London Hospital Gazette*, pp. 128–129.

Monk, C. and A. Sargeant (2002). *British Historical Cinema: The History, Heritage, and Costume Film*, London and New York: Routledge.

Morgeli, C. (1999). *The Surgeon's Stage: A History of the Operating Room*, Basel: Editiones Roche.

Palfreyman, H. and R. Christelle (2018). 'Visualizing Surgery: Surgeons' Use of Images, 1600–Present', *The Palgrave Handbook of the History of Surgery*, ed. T. Schlich, London: Palgrave Macmillan, pp. 283–300.

Petherbridge, D. and L. Jordanova (1997). *The Quick and the Dead: Artists and Anatomy*, Manchester: Cornerhouse.

Prentice, R. (2007). 'Drilling Surgeons: The Social Lessons of Embodied Surgical Learning', *Science, Technology, & Human Values*, 32.5, pp. 534–553.

Schlich, T. (2007). 'Surgery, Science and Modernity: Operating Rooms and Laboratories as Spaces of Control', *History of Science*, 45.3, pp. 231–256.

Schlich, T. (2015). '"The Days of Brilliancy are Past": Skill, Styles and the Changing Rules of Surgical Performance, ca. 1820–1920', *Medical History* 59.3, pp. 379–403.

Shapiro, J. (2002). '(Re)Examining the Clinical Gaze Through the Prism of Literature', *Families, Systems & Health*, 20.2, pp. 161–170.

Taddeo, J. A. (2019). 'Let's Talk about Sex: Period Drama Histories for the Twenty-First Century', *Journal of British Cinema and Television*, 16.1, pp. 42–60.

12

Of gods, monsters, and men: science, faith, the law, and the contested body and mind in *The Frankenstein Chronicles* and *The Alienist*

Andrea Wright

Since 2012 there has been a noticeable trend in nineteenth-century-set gothic mysteries that take inspiration from history, myth, and fiction. These include *Ripper Street* (2012–2017), *Dracula* (2013–2014), *Penny Dreadful* (2014–2016), *The Frankenstein Chronicles* (2015–2017), and *The Alienist* (2018–). Often bringing together international casts, locations, and production companies, the shows offer dark, graphically violent narratives and themes associated with mortality, morality, class, and gender, especially masculine crisis. Each, to varying degrees, also connect to advancements in science, which situates them in relation to nineteenth-century progress. *The Frankenstein Chronicles* and *The Alienist*, in particular, engage with medical science, social reform (including the Metropolitan Police Act of 1829 and the Anatomy Act of 1832 in Britain and Theodore Roosevelt's term as President of the New York City Board of Police Commissioners [1895–1897] in the United States), and the position of religion. Consequently, the body and mind are contested by powerful influences in changing times. *The Frankenstein Chronicles* was described in *The Telegraph* by Michael Hogan as 'rather like a Frankenstein's monster itself, constructed from stitched-together elements of *Sharpe*, *Sherlock*, *Oliver Twist*, *Ripper Street* and *Penny Dreadful*' (2015), but this belies its complexity. As well as drawing upon established tropes, recognisable characters, and hyperbolic Victoriana, it deals with social tensions, and therefore its 'stitching' goes beyond simple intertextual references. Like Mary Shelley's *Frankenstein, or the Modern Prometheus* (1818), it, and *The Alienist*, question the nature of monstrosity and the pre-eminence of science, but they also explore and critique dominant societal forces through representations of faith, politicians, and agents of law and order. By skilfully interweaving historical figures, legal and civil change, medical practices, especially those pertaining to the human cadaver, with fiction, myth, and, in *The Frankenstein Chronicles*, the supernatural, they suture quite innovative forms. There is, perhaps, not just a fear of scientific progress expressed, but also a preoccupation with morbid spectacle that speaks to deep-seated human attraction to its own mortality and vulnerability. Sarah Artt astutely points out that '*Penny Dreadful* and *Black Mirror* confirm that we are still very much living in the age of Frankenstein: a period of fascination with the body, gender and scientific innovation' (2018: 258), and *The Frankenstein Chronicles* and *The Alienist* reinforce this notion. This chapter will explore how these two series address these multifarious tensions, with a specific focus on the representation of emerging medical practices and experimentation. Furthermore, it will consider how the body and mind are pivotal in the struggle for dominance between these forces.

'There is no God. Once you grasp that, anything is possible'

The Frankenstein Chronicles, created by Barry Langford and Benjamin Ross, was first screened on the British television drama channel ITV Encore between 2015 and 2017, and consists of twelve episodes split over two series. The story opens in 1827 London against a backdrop of social change explicitly connected to Robert Peel's (played by Tom Ward) term as Home Secretary (January 1822–April 1827 and again from January 1828–November 1830). The central character is the troubled former soldier and widower, John Marlott (Sean Bean), a river policeman tasked with tracking down a murderer when the body of a child pieced together from several cadavers is found at the waterside. Marlott is drawn into a shadowy world of child prostitution and illegal experimentation, and, with reference to Shelley's *Frankenstein*, is reanimated after death. In the second series, he exists outside his previous life and the law, but persists in trying to track down his creator, who continues to manipulate the natural processes of life and death.

1827 is a particularly interesting date for the series to begin. Sarah Wise, in a vivid account of murder and grave robbery in London informed by archival records and contemporary accounts, writes that the pre-Victorian era was turbulent:

> There is no mistaking the flavour, the dominant mood, of the later 1820s/early 1830s in the writings that have survived. Everywhere is heard an insistent, articulate call for change in every aspect of British life: parliament, the judiciary, the church, medicine, gaols, schooling, public and private manners and mores, architecture, street planning – all were loudly condemned for being outmoded, inefficient, unworkable, 'old'. Britain was felt to be teetering to the point of collapse because of an inability to embrace and implement change. (2005: xvi)

The first episode, 'World Without God', visually and thematically exudes the sense of a society and place torn between the vestiges of the past and advancement. Marlott's insistence on using the leading surgeon in the country, Sir William Chester (Samuel West), rather than the local coroner attracts the attention of Peel, a key advocate of modernisation. The Home Secretary fears that attempts to reform the 'antiquated medical profession' via legislation are being deliberately sabotaged by whoever created the 'abomination'. In the mortuary where Marlott first meets Peel, he is accosted by an aggressive man who states that he 'supplies the subjects around here', and moments later the audience witnesses him taking payment for a body. The clash between progress and existing macabre customs is immediately established. Marlott is also personally caught between the past and present. Remnants of his former life as a soldier and memories of his dead family (which are conveyed to the viewer in hazy dream-like sequences) further enhance the evident turmoil.

For contemporary audiences, the period probably maintains a hold on popular imagination because of morbid fascination with body snatching. Accounts of the eighteenth-century Edinburgh anatomist Robert Knox and the murderous William Burke and William Hare have impacted history and subsequent re-presentation and fiction. Accordingly, the sinister world of the so-called 'resurrectionists' is recreated in the series, and the body becomes central to shifts in legislation that would alter from where cadavers could be sourced. Since 1752, the Murder Act had allowed the bodies of executed murderers to be used in medical experimentation, but increased demand for raw materials, the illegal activities of body snatchers, and the Edinburgh murders and the exploits of the London Burkers in the capital amplified pressure for reform. The controversial Anatomy Act permitted the use of unclaimed corpses (principally from workhouses, prisons, and hospitals) in anatomical studies, thus having the most significant impact on the bodies of the poor. It also made it a legal requirement to obtain a licence from the Home Secretary to practise anatomy. The Bill and subsequent Act were designed to end the criminal activity as well as introduce regulation that would aid the legitimacy and respectability of human dissection for scientific purposes. A key proponent of dissection was Jeremy Bentham, who bequeathed his own body for dissection and preservation. His death in June 1832 occurred when the Anatomy Bill was between its first and second reading in the House of Lords, thus positioning his body firmly within the debate.

In *The Frankenstein Chronicles*, the body is tied to medical science, politics, and crime, and is consistently employed as a spectacle. Indeed, the series opens with a gruesome discovery on the banks of the Thames, which sets the tone. In a palette of muddy greys, a child's pale body stands out against the black silt and trailing weeds. As Marlott inspects the corpse the camera slowly moves from the feet to the head, exposing grotesque wounds and crude stitching. When he looks closely, the cadaver appears to twitch, which causes him to recoil, thus adding to the visceral horror of the scene. Marlott's own body is also repulsive and mutilated. Initially he bears the physical mark of syphilis on his hand which he conceals in a black glove, but which constantly draws others' and the viewers' gaze to it. Later he is scarred by execution and reanimation. Further monstrous exhibition can be seen in Lord Daniel Hervey's (Ed Stoppard) laboratories and cold storage facility. The icehouse featured in the second season is a particularly ghastly display of human organs frozen for preservation. The viewer is encouraged to gaze at the candlelit underground space lined with shelves of individually illuminated ice blocks containing specimens.

Perhaps the most disfigured body, though, is Shelley's original text. Its continued presence in popular culture has led to multiple adaptations and retellings that have obscured significant elements of the story. Victor Frankenstein and the monster have proved mutable according to concurrent themes and fears and each adaptation has taken on meanings appropriate to the time of production. As Jude Wright argues, '[t]he complicated web of adaptations often overtakes the originary text so that it is ultimately unclear what belongs to the text itself and what belongs to an adaptation' (2015: 250). Jeffrey Allen Johnson's (2018) fascinating attempt to reclaim Shelley's *Frankenstein* debunks common misrepresentations, and, in turn, perhaps offers an insight into the representation of scientific and medical practices found in *The Frankenstein Chronicles*. As Johnson emphatically states, Victor is not a medical student and his transformation into the mad doctor is a horror trope introduced by twentieth-century filmmakers (2018: 288). The German and Swiss contexts of the novel, especially a tradition of German medical chemistry originating from the work of Paracelsus, who combined chemistry and alchemy, as well as the author's own exposure to the work of Benjamin Franklin, Erasmus Darwin, Humphry Davy, and others, Johnson argues, distance Victor from medical studies (2018: 291–293). Significantly, 'Shelley's portrayal of Victor as someone who uses modern means to achieve ancient goals makes him a central figure in the transition from mad alchemist to mad scientist' (Johnson 2018: 293).

The 'mad scientist' at the centre of *The Frankenstein Chronicles*, Hervey, is similarly distanced from legitimate medicine and surgical practices. When Chester examines the components of the body, he categorically assures Marlott that this is not the work of a surgeon. The images of jointed slabs of flesh support Chester's conclusion that this was the hand of a butcher or a barber. Creating a distance between barbers and surgeons was a part of the ongoing distinction between the professions. The Company of Surgeons became independent of the Company of Barber Surgeons in the mid-eighteenth century and only as recently as 1800 gained a Royal Charter to form the Royal College of Surgeons in London (Royal College of Surgeons of

England from 1843). Hervey is introduced to Marlott after a parliamentary debate about the Anatomy Bill and he declares that he is not a supporter of Peel's legislation, which he calls an abuse of the rights of the poor. He purports to find surgery, and more specifically, dissecting the dead, distasteful, and dismisses experimental techniques such as galvanism as fraudulent. His determination to disrupt the passing of the Bill, although veiled by outwardly benevolent intentions, is a self-serving attempt to secure his continued access to 'patients' for his research. But, despite Hervey being disassociated from respectable medicine, the show, more broadly, seems ambivalent in its message about the impact of medical advancement, and there is a sense that the profession and its practitioners are flawed and dangerous.

The 'respectable' face of medicine is marred by the early life of one of its key advocates, Chester, who is revealed to have dabbled in unethical experiments which resulted in tragedy. The unfortunate incident also implicates Mary Shelley (Anna Maxwell-Martin), who recalls the event in a flashback. What is fascinating about the memory is that it evokes cinematic misinterpretations of Shelley's novel. In a shadowy laboratory, Mary, Percy Shelley (Richard Clements), Chester, and James Hogg (a historical figure connected with the Shelleys, but here inaccurately and fictionally deployed and played by Hugh O'Connor) excitedly drink to the 'unflinching eye of the intellectual soul' before drawing straws to determine who will be the subject of the experiment. Hogg draws the short straw and is smothered to death by his companions so that he can be reanimated, and here the scene makes use of numerous popular cultural references. The premise of young medical students covertly experimenting with life and death is comparable to Peter Filardi's *Flatliners* (Schumacher, 1990; Arden Oplev, 2017), while the suitably intricate electricity generator complete with bulbous knobs, wires, and conductors is dramatically hand-turned to create lightning-like blue streams of electricity, recalling James Whales's 1931 *Frankenstein*. The charge itself is administered in a manner reminiscent of defibrillation, likely to be familiar to viewers from innumerable medical dramas. Despite the performance and spectacle, the experiment fails and Hogg dies. Crucially, the use of electricity in the process of reanimation so often, as Johnson observes, present in screen adaptations of the novel proves ineffective. Not only that, although Chester is certainly guilty of misadventure in the past and the murder of his cousin in the present in order to remove a threat to the passing of the Anatomy Act, he can be discounted as a 'real' Victor because he is unsuccessful and has turned to more conventional surgery. Authentic medicine is absolved, at least in part, and the madman is revealed to be Hervey, but there is perhaps an underlying suspicion lingering. As Katherine Byrne argues, it seems to 'reflect and reinforce an underlying distrust of medical professionals which persists today' (2018: 148) (see Figure 12.1).

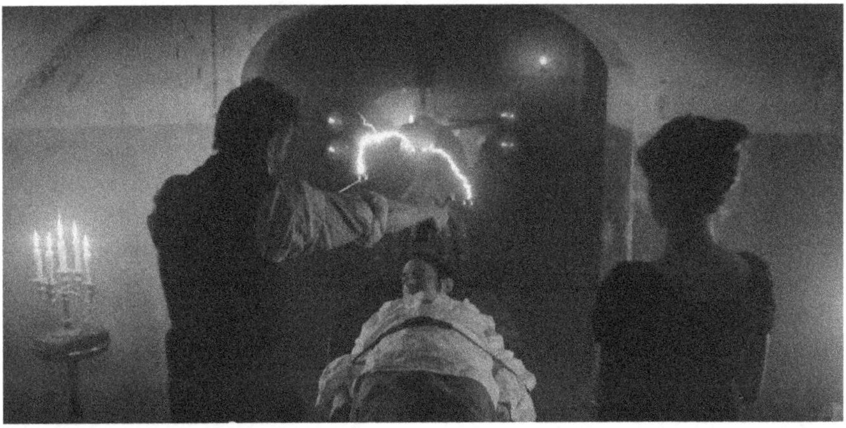

Figure 12.1 *The Frankenstein Chronicles*, S1E5: Chester and Shelley attempt to bring Hogg back to life

The climactic episode of the first season aligns Hervey closely with Shelley's protagonist. Hervey's method of resurrection is chemical rather than electrical and is inspired by alchemy and natural science, not surgery and established medicine. There is also direct mention of a supposed inspiration for Shelley's story, Johann Conrad Dippel, who reputedly created an elixir of life. Dippel, Hervey tells the newly 'reborn' Marlott, was his teacher and from his approach, which shunned the work of surgeons, Hervey developed his own tincture infused with cells from foetuses. The process, like Shelley's description of Victor's experiments, remains vague and is suggestive of, as Johnson notes about the novel, 'a biochemical or physiological-chemical process' (2018: 300). In the second season, the distinction between legitimate medicine and dangerous, unethical research is enhanced by Hervey's even more mysterious experiments. Hervey, who has been able to continue his 'work' because he is believed to have died, is assisting Dippel's son, Frederick Dipple (Laurence Fox). Dipple has a potion that has suspended the ageing process, but, and evoking popular culture's sequels to *Frankenstein*, he wants a 'bride'. Hervey is employed to deliver this woman, and, in return, Dipple will pass on his father's formula. Dipple's own fascination with automatons and the unveiling of a life-like clockwork woman that he has created with scientist and mathematician Ada Byron (Lily Besser) adds another dimension to the series' engagement with the uncanny nature of artificial life. It also potentially evokes contemporary anxieties about the rise of artificial intelligence and automation, thus extending Byrne's assertion that the series reinforces a suspicion of the medical profession to incorporate scientific advancement more generally.

These aspects are concerned primarily with the corporal, but the complex interaction between body and mind are also frequently explored. After his execution by hanging, the physical frame that exists may be recognisably Marlott, but his consciousness is detached, and he occupies a liminal space somewhere between life and death where he frequently wrangles with his identity and lives under an assumed name. Ownership of the body and the mind is thus obscured for the characters and the audience through Marlott's contested form. Moreover, and directly connected to the programme's intertextuality, Bean's casting makes it difficult to extract Marlott from the actor's other famous roles, most notably Richard Sharpe. Siân Harris comments that *Sharpe* (1993–2008) was instrumental in 'not only bringing the actor to wider attention but in continuing to shape, and more problematically, to sometimes limit his star persona' (2016: 247). Utilising this powerful legacy, and perhaps drawing on more recent parts as Boromir and Ned Stark, makes Marlott at once sympathetic and pathetic, familiar and unfamiliar. As Byrne points out,

> [i]n keeping with the gritty theme of the series, his clothes look scruffy and grubby, and when he is viewed without them, his slightly flabby body is far from the toned physique he displays in other roles. And, of course, his desirability is further compromised by the disease which makes his sexuality so pathological, and which is empathised [and emphasised] rather than disguised by the stained bandage on his hand. If he is a version of Sharpe, it is Sharpe ravaged by time, illness and grief. (2018: 156)

By the opening of the second season, Marlott has lost his faith and feels abandoned by God, which is perhaps amplified because his body is a creation of experimental science. After his reanimation, Marlott's malady and internal struggle, which previously allowed him to see his dead wife and child in warmed-toned dream sequences, is displaced by a cold, harsh, grey-coloured shore where he finds disjointed fragments of his former life. Distant voices and pained howls intermingle with graphic snippets of past violence and his current semi-conscious state in an asylum cell. It is an especially cruel limbo as Marlott can see ghosts, but his own family have disappeared. These aural and visual sensations seem to confirm that it is a world without God. The comfort of faith and a belief in an afterlife that reunites loved ones is not available to a man whose body has been claimed for medical research. The role of established institutions of faith is further challenged in the second season as the murders are directly connected to the Church: the Dean of Westminster (Guy Henry) is portrayed as corrupt and driven by greed, and the parish wardens impede the progress of the police investigation in a territorial and juridical conflict. Additionally, Marlott's virtuous and incorruptible former partner, Nightingale (Richie Campbell), is killed in the line of duty, thus confirming that even the righteous cannot be saved. In this world without God, it is men who have control over life and death, the body and the mind, and science, legitimate or otherwise, is an especially powerful force.

'People aren't ready for this new, high-falutin' form of investigation'

The Alienist, based on Caleb Carr's 1994 novel of the same name, is a ten-part series produced by Anonymous Content and distributed in North America by TNT and by Netflix in the UK and most of Europe. Set in 1896 New York, it focuses on a team of unlikely and unofficial investigators, led by the titular alienist, Laszlo Kreizler (Daniel Brühl), society cartoonist and illustrator John Schuyler Moore (Luke Evans), and New York Police Department secretary Sara Howard (Dakota Fanning), as they seek the serial killer behind the grisly murders of young male prostitutes. Set in the later years of the nineteenth century, it engages with similar, but also distinct, challenges concerning the tensions between faith, the law, and medicine. It explores the emergence and processes of criminal profiling and forensic science and paints a vivid picture of a turbulent society that has the potential to create monsters. As Annalee Newitz notes in relation to Carr's novel, the story is not about serial killers, but instead 'the social apparatus that detects them' and the history of the society that creates them (2006: 14). Furthermore, it highlights resistance to changing approaches to mental illness and criminality. Andrew Scull has argued that the history of psychiatry is beset with questions about its legitimacy. In the Victorian era, although it is often celebrated as progressive in terms of the care and handling of mental illness, there were public and professional doubts expressed about treatments, institutions, and the capability of psychiatrists to effectively treat patients. Scull contends that more contemporary enquiries about legitimacy stem from historical debates about boundaries between 'insanity and criminal responsibility', the 'wording and implementation of commitment laws' that impacted public perceptions, and disputes within the profession itself about 'whether to account for mental illness in physical or psychological terms' and how to treat patients according to gender (1981: 2–3). Similarly, the development of forensic psychiatry, or 'alienism', has been plagued by questions of effectiveness and legitimacy. Kenneth J. Weiss observes in his short history of American forensic psychiatry that there is a persistent uneasiness caused by 'the natural tension between the aims of medicine and the law, the degree to which medicine can improve jurisprudence, the ethics of practice, and the ambiguity present in psychiatric concepts' (2015: 3).

Accordingly, the respectability and validity of alienists and innovative detection techniques are consistently foregrounded in the series, alongside significant changes in urban policing and a backdrop of rising tension caused by class inequalities despite the progress and economic growth of the so-called Gilded Age.

The setting is essential in creating a sense of shifts and upheaval and the contrasts between spaces are consistently emphasised. Where in *The Frankenstein Chronicles* there is a distinction between rich and poor, the environments they inhabit have in common a sparseness and gloomy quality; in *The Alienist* the division between wealth and poverty is sharply defined. There is a bright opulence in the places inhabited by the privileged; production designer Mara Lepere-Schloop explains that Kreizler's house 'was designed to represent the worldly and intellectually zealous character that he embodied. The set was dripping in Gilded Age decadence' (2018: 86). Conversely, there is a shabby, sinister feel to the streets, brothels, and lodgings. In a particularly poignant scene where Kreizler walks through the city streets, the camera lingers on ragged children sleeping in doorways and stairwells. Kreizler, seemingly unaware of or unaffected by the display of abject poverty, moves swiftly back to his more customary luxury. It is also noteworthy that the urban space provides an impression of the past making way for the future, but at the same time, it is plagued by crime and haunted by the past. The setting and the murders are intrinsically linked, as Lepere-Schloop observes; '[t]he killer leaves the bodies of young boys in a series of locations that comprise a Who's Who of turn-of-the-century landmarks in New York', including the construction site of the Williamsburg Bridge, the Statue of Liberty, and Croton Reservoir (2018: 86). This historically 'authenticates' the series by making the environment recognisable, and assists the spectacle associated with the beleaguered bodies and minds of the characters.

Each of the protagonists has their own torments that manifest variously. Kreizler has lost the use of one arm, which causes him to struggle with simple tasks. He angrily refers to himself as a 'cripple' and describes his disability as a congenital birth defect. Eventually it is revealed that it was caused by an injury inflicted by his father when he was a child. Part of Kreizler's journey is acknowledging his father's actions, but also forgiving the now frail old man. Whilst he is adept in diagnosing and exploring the afflictions of others through proto-Freudian psychoanalysis, he is less able to acknowledge his own trauma. He appears to derive a sense of power, that, in turn, masks his own weaknesses, from exposing the secrets of other people's minds. Moore, despite his wealth and position in society, is drawn to an underworld of excessive drinking and prostitution because he is unable to get over a broken engagement. This also makes him the closest character to the netherworld of New York and its depravity, and thus he appears to have the most empathy with the victims. Importantly, it is through Moore's perspective that the audience first glimpses the horror of the child with its eyes gouged out at the first murder scene. The full ghastly spectacle is revealed as Moore shakily sketches a record for Kreizler. Dissatisfied with the image, which he calls 'idealised', Kreizler forces the visibly disturbed artist to verbally recount the full dreadfulness of the mutilated corpse. Moore's role has been altered in the television adaptation from a writer to an illustrator, and, unlike in the book, he is not the first-person narrator. He remains, though, central to the viewer's perception and Petra Clark argues that:

> Moore's opportunities to illustrate what he observes are limited, but the choice to switch his medium from a written to a visual one perhaps aligns with the transition from book to screen. In this context, Moore's attempts to visualize his findings are legible to the viewer and thus partly make up for the loss of Moore's interiority, but they are also broadly representative of the team's collective progress of piecing together a complete picture of the killer. (2019: 63)

Howard's demons are connected to the suicide of her father. Whilst he made her strong and resilient and taught her how to survive in a man's world, he also made her complicit in his death, which led to a period in a sanatorium. Consequently, her outward appearance denotes a fascinating paradox. Smooth, fair skin, prominent blue eyes, and severely styled blonde hair make her somewhat doll-like, a look accentuated by her fine, tailored clothes. When she is introduced, she is wearing a long, heavy green and brown striped silk gown with dramatic puffed sleeves, a cameo brooch at the neck and a cinched waist. Conversely, the cut and colour are austere and a man's pocket watch hangs from her belt, and hint at the tenacity and independence of this seemingly delicate woman. She is also regularly seen smoking, which sets her apart from upper-class women of her social circle. Howard is a fictional character, but it is likely she is based on pioneering women who entered police forces in the United States in the early twentieth century. Robert L. Snow documents the increased calls from groups such as the Suffrage Movement and the Women's Christian Temperance Movement for female police offers to help to protect women in custody (2010: 13–15). The first official appointment was Lola Baldwin in Portland in 1908, and by 1912, New York City employed Isabelle Goodwin, a policeman's widow who had previously assisted with undercover work, as a detective (2010: 16). The contested position of women, therefore, was instrumental in changes to law enforcement, and the inclusion of Howard as secretary to Roosevelt (Brian Geraghty), but also keen amateur detective, in *The Alienist* acknowledges this history in its fiction. Furthermore, Howard is subject to sexual harassment and discrimination, and she has to defend herself against unwanted advances and crude jokes from police officers, as well as battling her associates' misplaced, but well-meaning, desire to protect her, as the 'gentler sex', from the gruesome nature of the crimes they are investigating.

Howard is not alone in finding the police force resistant to change. Roosevelt is consistently hampered by attempts to undermine his authority as commissioner. The recently retired Chief Burns (Ted Levine) is held in high esteem by his officers and the wider community, and openly scorns Roosevelt's reforms. The police, especially Captain Connor (David Wilmot), are deeply suspicious of Kreizler and the new methods he endorses, thus foregrounding yet another tension between past and present, but also medical practices and the established tools of the law. In addition, the friction seems to be heightened by underlying ethnic, cultural, and class differences. Roosevelt (like Moore and Howard) is a society New Yorker; Kreizler is the son of wealthy German immigrants; Burns, Connor, and most of the male police offers are Irish; while the forward-thinking detective sergeants and budding forensic scientists, Marcus (Douglas Smith) and Lucius Isaacson (Matthew Shear), are Jewish. The enthusiastic brothers state that their secondment to Kreizler is because they will not be missed in the police department. The alienist comments: 'I imagine your modern methods don't make you very popular.' Lucius flatly replies: 'that, and the fact we're Jews'. The body that prompts the investigation is that of a poor Italian immigrant, sneeringly referred to by Connor as a 'boy whore'. His tearful mother, translated by the dead child's older brother, says that 'nobody cares'. Howard's discovery of two unsolved murders of young boys hidden in the police archives confirms the failings and apathy of the police. Moreover, the reluctance of the law to solve the murders is connected to class, but also sexual identity, which leads to further deaths. In the brothels where they work at night, the boys perform femininity, and by day, on the streets, they dress in traditionally masculine attire. Their fluid gender identities and performance make them vulnerable and exploited; indeed, one tells Kreizler 'we do things real girls don't do'. In dark and grimy rooms and underground clubs, they are controlled by bordello owners and used and abused by the men, especially the rich 'swells', who frequent them. Their bodies become central to a power struggle within their society and the key to unlocking the mind of the killer.

The viewers, and the protagonists, are misled as to the identity of the murderer on several occasions, and each time the suspect is found to be physically marked and perceived to be mentally incapacitated and/or driven by debauched sexual desire. The first man arrested for the crimes is an adult male prostitute suffering from advanced syphilis. The half-light of the asylum cell where he is being held highlights the red, angry lesions that obscure his facial features, thus rendering him monstrous. Such grotesque representation is not uncommon and is reminiscent of Marlott's nightmare of his face eaten away by the disease in *The Frankenstein Chronicles*. While the man admits to the murder of a former friend in an altercation, he is not the child's killer, simply a convenient 'deviant' to accuse. The second suspect, Willem Van Bergen (Josef Altin), is from a privileged family and is known to frequent brothels. The audience is encouraged to assume his guilt because he is introduced as a fragmented, shadowy figure in the third episode 'Silver Smile'. In a bathhouse, young boys, silhouetted by a golden glow through a large semi-circular window, frolic carefree in the water. On the soundtrack, the high, solo voice of a choir boy sings Mendelssohn's 'O for the wings of a dove' to denote their innocence. The scene cuts to a tight close-up of a man's eye, and the intensity of his gaze is emphasised by the reflected image of the boys on the shiny surface of his iris. His obvious pleasure is further accentuated by the hint of a smile on his pursed lips and an inhalation of breath with closed eyes. Van Bergen is made monstrous by his 'silver smile', a side effect of taking mercury salts, which was a treatment for syphilis. Despite a warning to Roosevelt from the upper echelons of society not to betray his own kind, Van Bergen becomes the prime suspect as the slaying continues. In the meantime, Kreizler's psychological profiling of the killer takes his investigation in another direction. Ultimately, Van Bergen, who is about to board a boat out of New York, is dispatched by an enraged Connor, who calls him a 'dirty sodomite' twice before shooting him in cold blood. Regarding both suspects, the series upholds established stereotypical links between sexuality, disease, and monstrosity. As Harry Benshoff observes, such derogatory representations are endemic in horror cinema and help to circulate the notion that 'homosexuals are violent, degraded monsters and their evil agenda is to destroy the very fabric of American society' (1997: 1).

The use of modern methods of evidence-based forensic science, rather than Connor's instinctive police work, leads to new avenues of inquiry, which also connects *The Alienist* to similar representations of the evolution of policing based on pathological investigation. The body, in both series, is observed, dissected, and mined for clues, thus facilitating creative deduction as well as supplying material substantiation. On the third body, as well as the removal of an eye and damage to the genitalia, Roosevelt recognises a scalping wound from his time ranching in the West. Kreizler and Moore's visit to the Natural History Museum confirms that while the method of disfigurement may have taken inspiration from Native Americans, it is a defilement of customs that could only have been practised by someone who has seen and misunderstood their purpose. The subsequent scrutiny of

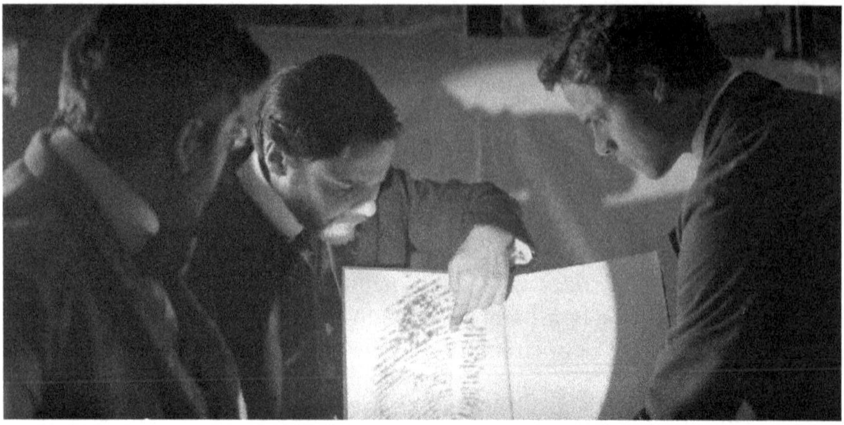

Figure 12.2 *The Alienist*, S1E3: Kreizler and Marcus and Lucius Isaacson study a fingerprint

documents and visits to asylums takes the characters and the viewers to the darkest recesses of the human mind through vivid descriptions and visual spectacles of degradation. Clark argues that the horrific themes of the novel are taken to 'new extremes' in the series (2019: 64). The viewers are forced to look and see, and 'by encouraging this voyeurism, the audience too is implicated' (2019: 65) (Figure 12.2).

Eventually, the monster they are seeking is unveiled and, in keeping with Clark's observations, much is made of describing and showing to compel the audience to look and hear. Japheth Dury/John Beecham (Bill Heck) has been shaped by his ostracisation as a child due to a severe facial twitch and turbulent family life. His father, described as a 'hellfire and damnation' preacher, worked as a missionary on the plains and brought back a collection of photographs showing white victims of the 1862 Minnesota Massacre. He used them to encourage local children to be God-fearing, thus elucidating his son's later obsession with using dates on the Christian calendar for his murders. Death and religion are inextricably intertwined. Dury's brother, Adam (David Meunier), describes the mental torture inflicted on his younger sibling by their mother, 'a woman with no heart'. He was also raped by a man, Joseph Beecham, who befriended him. His revenge on his parents and Beecham was brutal. The team surmise that Dury later took part of Beecham's name to transform himself from victim to aggressor and to re-enact, with his own victims, a trusted figure becoming an abuser.

Throughout the series, Kreizler is driven by a determination to understand the mind, insanity, and how it influences behaviours, which aligns him with accounts of early forensic psychiatry. Weiss explores the impact and influence of Isaac Ray's 1838 *A Treatise on the Medical Jurisprudence of Insanity*, which, he argues, forms the basis of contemporary forensic psychiatry (2015: 3–4). Importantly, Weiss notes that Ray's approach 'melded his trust in science to discover the medical bases of mental disease with the European idea that any "organ" of the mind could become deranged, thereby producing insanity. If insanity could take various forms, it might best explain otherwise culpable behaviours to juries and judges' (2015: 4). Where the blunt investigative methods of the police force, as represented by Connor in *The Alienist*, intended to catch and punish the murderer, the bourgeoning forensic psychiatry, represented by Kreizler, sought to comprehend and rationalise. Frustratingly, for Kreizler, though, the tantalising hints as to the workings of the killer's mind remain speculative because Dury (after being shot by Connor) dies as Kreizler frantically attempts to ascertain why he killed the boys. Even more vexing to the alienist is that the murderer's brain (dissected in close-up) is 'perfectly normal and healthy' and thus proves 'we don't know anything'. In the final scenes, therefore, the narrative seems to demonstrate surprising ambivalence towards the value of psychiatry.

Conclusion

The Frankenstein Chronicles and *The Alienist* are intertextual bodies, and they have a sense of familiarity because they fit into a milieu of contemporary, but nineteenth-century-set television drama that presents a dark vision of the decade. Their focus on the damaged and contested body and mind draws upon landmarks in legal, social, and medical progress, the success and pitfalls of scientific experimentation, and the difficulties inherent in making change when faced with resistance. They blend history and fiction, especially that pertaining to the body and science, visually and narratively, as well as drawing upon a range of popular cultural references and representations. As adaptations, they are an intricate web of borrowings and homage. Linda Hutcheon, writing about repeatedly adapted works such as Bram Stoker's *Dracula* (1897), refers to the audience's 'palimpsestuous intertextuality' which makes certain adaptations 'multilaminated', 'directly and openly connected to recognisable other works, and that connection is part of their formal identity, but also of what we might call their hermeneutic identity' (2013: 21).

The notion of texts constructed of texts and received by an audience aware of their extensive linage is particularly pertinent here. *The Frankenstein Chronicles* uses social unrest and a momentous shift in the history of anatomy and dissection as a backdrop for a re-imagining of Shelley's story and the narrative is littered with historical figures including the author, members of her circle, and William Blake. There are also frequent allusions to other adaptations and misinterpretations in order to foreground the exhibition of scientific experimentation. *The Alienist* takes core themes from Carr's novel, itself influenced by existing history and fiction, and makes reference to public figures such as financier J. P. Morgan and the crimes of Jack the Ripper and child-murderer Jesse Pomeroy. It is also propelled by popular culture's fascination with serial killers. For instance, the method and motivation for killing the young boys, especially the cannibalistic intentions described, recall Hannibal Lecter's predilection for preparing human flesh as part of a meal. Importantly, the prominence of graphic murder and burgeoning forensic science facilitates spectacles of mutilation and autopsy, while the analysis of the mind employs popular psychoanalysis.

Both series explore tensions between tradition and progress, faith, the law, and medical advancement. Consequently, the bodies and minds of the protagonists, victims, and murderers are contested and conflicted. Gods and monsters are indistinct. Power is frequently abused, the pursuit of scientific advancement is prone to corruption, social reform is divisive, and the good and virtuous are susceptible morally and corporeally. These are deliberately sinister worlds that invite the viewer to immerse themselves in macabre spectacle, doubt established institutions, and confront the vulnerability of the body and the mind.

References

Artt, S. (2018). '"An Otherness That Cannot Be Sublimated": Shades of Frankenstein in Penny Dreadful and Black Mirror', *Science Fiction Film and Television* 11.2, 257–275.

Benshoff, H. M. (1997). *Monsters in the Closet: Homosexuality and the Horror Film*. Manchester and New York: Manchester University Press.

Byrne, K. (2018). 'Pathological Masculinities: Syphilis and the Medical Profession in The Frankenstein Chronicles', pp. 146–162 in K. Byrne, J. Leggott and J. A. Taddeo (eds), *Conflicting Masculinities: Men in Television Period Drama*. London: I.B. Taurus.

Clark, P. (2019). 'Sight and Spectacle in *The Alienist*', *Adaptation* 12.2, 61–65.

Harris, S. (2016). 'Sharper, better, faster, stronger: Performing Northern masculinity and the legacy of Sean Bean's *Sharpe*', *Journal of Popular Television* 4.2, 239–251.

Hogan, M. (2015). 'The Frankenstein Chronicles, Review: "Eerily Effective"', *The Times*, 11 November, www.telegraph.co.uk/culture/tvandradio/tv-and-radio-reviews/11989543/The-Frankenstein-Chronicles-review-eerily-effective.html. Accessed 6 August 2019.

Hutcheon, L. A. (2013). *Theory of Adaptation*, 2nd Edition. London and New York: Routledge.

Johnson, J.A. (2018). 'Dr. Frankenstein, I Presume? Revising the Popular Image of Frankenstein', *Literature and Medicine* 36.2, 287–311.

Lepere-Schloop, M. (2018). 'Building 1890s New York in Budapest: The Alienist', *Perspective* May/June, 80–89.

Newitz, A. (2006). *Pretend We're Dead: Capitalist Monsters in American Pop Culture*. Durham, NC, and London: Duke Press.

Scull, A. (1981). 'Introduction', pp. 1–4 in A. Scull (ed.), *Madhouses, Mad-Doctors and Mad Men: A Social History of Psychiatry in the Victorian Era*. Philadelphia: University of Pennsylvania Press.

Snow, R.L. (2010). *Policewomen Who Made History: Breaking Through the Ranks*. Plymouth, UK: Rowman & Littlefield.

Weiss, K. J. (2015). 'American Forensic Psychiatry Begins: Setting Standards', pp. 3–20 in R. L. Sadoff (ed.), *The Evolution of Forensic Psychiatry: History, Current Developments, Future Directions*. New York: Oxford University Press.

Wise, S. (2005). *The Italian Boy: Murder and Grave Robbery in 1930s London*. London: Pimlico.

Wright, J. (2015). 'Listening to the Monster: Eliding and Restoring the Creature's Voice in Adaptations of Frankenstein', *Journal of Adaptation in Film and Performance* 18.3, 249–266.

Part IV

‘Treating’ the mind

13

Bad or mad? Branwell Brontë, mental health, and alcoholism in Sally Wainwright's *To Walk Invisible*

Sarah E. Fanning and Claire O'Callaghan

In December 2016, Sally Wainwright's much-anticipated biopic of the famous Brontë family, *To Walk Invisible*, aired to audiences around the globe. Concluding the bicentenary celebrations of Charlotte Brontë's birth in 1816, the two-hour series, subtitled *The Brontë Sisters* – the first representation of the Brontë family onscreen since the 1970s – tells the inspiring story of the three legendary sisters, Charlotte, Emily, and Anne, between 1845 and 1848, the period in which they wrote and published their now-canonical novels, *Jane Eyre* (Charlotte, 1847), *Wuthering Heights* (Emily, 1847), and *Agnes Grey* (Anne, 1847). Although *To Walk Invisible*'s subtitle suggests a primary focus on the sisters, it juxtaposes a nostalgic rendering of their literary success with the more depressing tale of their brother Branwell's troubles: his successive mishaps, deteriorating health, and alcohol dependency during the same period prior to his tragic death in 1848 aged just thirty-one. Such a biographical parallel between the siblings is one that Branwell's acquaintance, Francis A. Leyland, cautioned against. As he put it, Branwell's 'life should be treated independently of the theories and necessities of his sisters' biographies, and in a spirit not unfriendly to him' (Leyland, 1886, vol. 1: 162). For Leyland, such an artificial divide situates Branwell in a punitive manner. Taking Leyland's concern as a starting point, this chapter considers the ways Wainwright's approach to Branwell aligns with the myths that have carried a negative public image of an addict, failure, and profligate across centuries.

To Walk Invisible was acclaimed by reviewers far and wide who both applauded Wainwright's emphasis on the arduous circumstances under which the revered sisters established their literary careers and welcomed her depiction of the effects of alcohol abuse in a domestic family unit. *The Guardian*, for instance, noted that 'As *To Walk Invisible* makes plain, Emily, Anne and Charlotte channelled their thwarted feelings, unrequited loves and endless frustrations with life into their art; Branwell sought solace in a bottle' (Mangan, 2016: n.p.). *The New Yorker* was more pointed, stating that 'Branwell fails everyone, most of all himself, but his perennial self-pity contrasts sharply with his sisters' preternatural focus and determination' (Fan, 2018: n.p.). *The Atlantic* was even less tolerant of the series' presentation of the troubled brother, lamenting that 'the sisters are so intriguing [and that] is what makes *To Walk Invisible*'s heavy focus on Branwell so frustrating … [actor Adam] Nagaitis allows Branwell flashes of sympathy, but he is, from the beginning, a lost cause, enabled by his father as he terrorizes his household' (Gilbert, 2017: n.p.).

Wainwright's biopic, then, validates a long-standing and popular image of Branwell: that he was not simply a family failure, but a reprobate bent on wreaking havoc and misery on everything and everyone he touched. Wainwright thus replicates a Gaskellian narrative, a shorthand term in Brontë scholarship used to describe the disparaging views of the Victorian novelist, Elizabeth Gaskell, who was the family's first biographer. In *The Life of Charlotte Brontë* (1857), she depicts Branwell as a 'cunning' (Gaskell, 1857: 226) addict who not only would drink excessively but 'steal out while the family were at church – to which he has professed himself too ill to go – and manage to cajole the village druggist out of a lump [of opium]' (Gaskell, 1857: 227). Because of Gaskell, Branwell has been remembered as The Black Bull's most famous resident, from which he had purportedly been dragged home by Emily, on at least one occasion, because he was too inebriated to walk himself, neglecting to extinguish his candle and, thus, setting fire to his bedclothes because of drunkenness; and as the alleged inspiration for his sisters' most repulsive male characters, Anne's Arthur Huntingdon (*Tenant of Wildfell Hall*, 1848) and Emily's Hindley Earnshaw (*Wuthering Heights*, 1847), a point which the series articulates. A focus on these tales and the persistent myth that Branwell sought 'solace in a bottle' means that *To Walk Invisible* offers limited insight into this troubled Brontë's behaviour, especially in ways that restrict a greater understanding of addiction and (his) mental health (Fan, 2018: n.p.).

Despite its prevalence in society, alcohol dependency is a subject rarely explored in period drama. There are exceptions such as the BBC's 1996 adaptation of Anne Brontë's *The Tenant of Wildfell Hall* and ITV's 2009 adaptation of Emily Brontë's *Wuthering Heights*. The BBC's *Tenant* boldly asserts that Arthur Huntingdon's (Rupert Graves) physical and sexual abuse of his wife (Tara Fitzgerald) is the result of his alcoholism while ITV's *Wuthering Heights* makes clear that Hindley Earnshaw (Burn Gorman) uses alcohol to self-medicate. While both adaptations explore the negative effects of problem drinking with respect to dysfunctional relationships and domestic disturbance, neither acknowledges that alcohol addiction is a medical condition. Thus the framing of alcohol abuse around mental health disorder has yet to be fully represented in period drama. While *To Walk Invisible* is one of the first period dramas to centralise alcohol addiction, it circumvents mental health discourse, adopting instead a narrative of shame that heavily points the finger of blame at this troubled Brontë. This chapter, therefore, presents a critique of the moralising stance depicted in *To Walk Invisible*. While recognising the value of dramatising the sociological effects of alcohol dependency onscreen, Wainwright constructs a narrow portrayal of Branwell, one that reduces his habitual drinking to a bad moral choice and overlooks how drink dependency is, in twenty-first-century medical discourse, constituted in more nuanced terms relating to addiction and mental health disorder. While the *Diagnostic and Statistical Manual of Mental Disorders* (DSM-5) (the standard and received classification of mental disorders worldwide) recognises alcoholism (as it is known colloquially today) as 'alcohol use disorder' (AUD) caused by a 'brain disease' (DSM-5, 2013: n.p.), *To Walk Invisible* instead renders addiction as an entwined moral and masculine failing on the individual's part.[1] In this light, Branwell is a 'mad' and 'bad' brother, a weak man who makes poor personal choices rather than an individual suffering from a mental disease, which historical documentation combined with twenty-first-century diagnostic criteria suggests is probable. As a result, while Wainwright's drama sheds some light on the complexity of domestic and corporeal trauma produced by problem drinking, it does little to seek empathy for those who suffer from alcoholism or register and/or reduce the stigma of addiction more broadly. Moreover, rather than considering that Branwell may have had a pre-existing mental health condition that led to self-medicating behaviours, the series suggests, instead, that his addiction is *the result of* his character flaws. Here, *To Walk Invisible* misses the crucial opportunity of reimagining Branwell's problem behaviours and ill-health through a twenty-first-century medical lens and, thus, becomes mired in the very myths it seeks, to use Wainwright's term, to 'debunk' (*To Walk Invisible*, DVD Featurette).

In approaching our argument, we begin first by reviewing the way the series presents a limited diagnostic focus and often conflicting view of Branwell's symptoms, behaviour, and health before moving on to discuss the period drama in relation to medical discourse from the past and present that has conceived of alcoholism in relation to mental illness.

'Solace in a bottle'

From the outset, Wainwright emphasises the idea that *the* problem in the Brontë household in the 1840s was Branwell's 'choice' to abuse alcohol. Although the drama opens with an imaginary flashback, where the four Brontë children are creating stories together with their infamous toy soldiers, the series' first main scene focuses on Charlotte's (Finn Atkins) return home to a commotion at the Parsonage. As she walks into the house, not only can her father and brother's 'raised voices' be heard in the backdrop (a diegetic sound deployed repeatedly throughout the drama), but she is stopped by her youngest sister, Anne (Charlie Murphy) (Wainwright, 2016: 4). In a low voice, Anne whispers to Charlotte: 'Branwell. He's been drinking. He had a letter. From Mr. Robinson. This last Thursday. He's been dismissed' (Wainwright, 2016: 4). The unfolding discussion between the sisters relays (for the benefit of the audience) the story of Branwell's suspected romance with Mrs Lydia Robinson of Thorp Green, the wife of his employer, and how the sisters – Emily (Chloe Pirrie) and Anne – have concealed news of the alleged scandal from their father. Although scholars are divided on the credibility of Branwell's affair with Lydia Robinson, the series takes the position that this single event spurred his decline into addiction. By emphasising Branwell's romantic liaison as *the* cause of his dismissal, Wainwright thus indicates from the outset that it is Branwell's poor moral choices that are the underlying cause of his problem behaviour.

As the scene unfolds, Wainwright accentuates the social effects of Branwell's habitual drinking. When Charlotte walks into the room, a '68-year-old PATRICK' (Jonathan Pryce) is 'doing his utmost to keep calm', while Branwell (Adam Nagaitis) is:

> Livid; angry and emotional. He has tears streaming down his face. He's very drunk, there's an upturned dining chair in evidence of his violent mood. It looks like PATRICK and EMILY are dealing with an injured, dangerous, volatile animal. (Wainwright, 2016: 6)

As the notes to the script suggest, a drunken Branwell is shown in a volatile and heightened emotional state (something reinforced onscreen through Nagaitis's sweaty face and dishevelled demeanour), while Patrick and Emily are handling a decidedly violent and dangerous 'animal' (Wainwright, 2016: 6). The emphasis, therefore, is on the socio-domestic destructiveness of Branwell's drunkenness. His drunken state and inappropriate behaviour are intentionally designed to invite judgement from the audience while guiding sympathy towards Patrick and Emily (as the notes to the script suggest), thus creating a binary 'Branwell' versus 'the family' effect, something which, as indicated in the opening to this chapter, his friend, Leyland, cautioned against. Further, the tension between father and son is centralised, but interestingly, Wainwright, in keeping with recent scholarly analysis concerned with Brontë mythology, refuses to reproduce Gaskell's conception of Patrick as a stern and neglectful parent, opting instead to reflect the contemporary view developed by biographer Juliet Barker that he was a kind and engaged father in his children's life. Here Patrick asks Branwell provocative questions about his dismissal which, in keeping with Wainwright's anti-Gaskellian approach to Patrick, open up the opportunity to re-evaluate the idea that Patrick himself was a – if not *the* – cause of Branwell's decline. Patrick's questions, however, are not answered; they merely ignite Branwell's raging defence:

> BRANWELL
> Just – !
> (he lets out a crazy kind of
> animal roar and kicks
> the upturned dining chair
> into the wall)
> **GOD!** This **HOUSE!** Does it matter? Go
> to bed! Stop asking fucking
> questions! (Wainwright, 2016: 7, emphasis in bold as per the original)

The viewer's first introduction to Branwell Brontë, then, is a negative one; he is an angry and explosive individual. His inability to complete the sentence coupled with a descent into physical violence symbolically connote his physical, emotional, and moral danger. Despite his obvious distress, the scene is constructed to garner little sympathy for Branwell; he is merely a dangerous problem, not a man suffering. Moreover, by situating news of Branwell's affair within a domestic scene notable for its anger and the suggestion of threat (indicated both by Branwell's profanity and his indignant instruction for his family to 'Go to bed!'), *To Walk Invisible* couples Branwell's problem drinking with his 'bad' behaviour, thus constructing a moralistic narrative that reinforces a medical disorder as the mere result of poor choices (Wainwright, 2016: 7).

In reality, Branwell had periods of 'calm' where his 'thoughts' were 'clear and logical' (Leyland, 1886, vol. 2: 58–59); however, despite claims of historical authenticity, there are only three short scenes in the drama that depict Branwell in states of sobriety and composure. These occur when he joins a family friend, John Brown, on a trip to Liverpool (albeit he is being sent away by Patrick as a form of 'punishment' for his transgressions at Thorp Green); when he visits his friend, Joseph 'Joe' Leyland; and when Lydia's groomsman comes to deliver the news of Mr Robinson's death. Apart from these few moments, Branwell is persistently shown in various stages of drunkenness or hungover and attempting to obtain more alcohol. The sustained focus might be said to reflect the plight of an addicted individual but, in fact, they merely interpret Branwell in distorted, simplified, and myth-supporting terms to a twenty-first-century audience and demonise him in favour of a nostalgic, sympathetic, and somewhat self-righteous image of his sisters.

At the same time, Wainwright intersperses sustained images of Branwell in varying stages of inebriation with a debate about addiction and sympathy. Such a discussion is staged between Emily and Anne. During an afternoon walk on the moors, the sisters discuss Branwell's failed attempt to enter the Royal Academy of Arts in London, resulting in him refusing to get on the train because of fear and insecurity. Instead, Emily explains, he spent 'four days in Bradford. Drunk and miserable' because he realised his paintings simply 'weren't that good' (Wainwright, 2016: 20). Emily admits that she has always 'felt sorry for him' because:

> EMILY
> [...] They always
> expected so much of him. More –
> probably – than he was ever capable
> of. And I just thought 'Thank God
> I'm not you' [...]
>
> ANNE
> It's disappointing. I know [...] But we shouldn't give up
> on him. Should we?
>
> EMILY
> No. We shouldn't give up on him.
> But we should see him for what he
> is. Not what he isn't. It's not
> fair on him. (Wainwright, 2016: 21)

At face value, this scene uses Emily to instruct the audience to have sympathy for Branwell, but a closer analysis reveals that the discussion is really concerned with how Branwell's troubled behaviour impacts and victimises them, and how one should perceive an addict, rather than enabling empathy with Branwell. Indeed, Emily's comment encourages Anne to sympathise with Branwell, but this is merely a response to Anne's loaded question that again positions the sisters as victims and centres on the 'problem' of Branwell. It also suggests we should 'see him for what he is', which, by the drama's standards, is merely a habitual drunkard. By framing this discussion around the emotional endurance of those living with problem drinkers, Wainwright implicitly opens a debate on the question of empathy and addiction by creating a reductive binary choice (to sympathise with Branwell or not). Here the script implies that the family (and by extension the audience) should accept his limitations and acknowledge the pressures placed on him as the only son and in an era where unmarried sisters had little alternative but to rely on their nearest male relative for their livelihood. However, in discussions about the drama, Wainwright's position undermines this view and reinforces the idea that Branwell was merely a waster. In conversation with writer Tracy Chevalier, Wainwright proclaimed Branwell was 'an ever-present problem [the family] had to deal with and live with' (Cocozza, 2016: n.p.). Despite this claim, Wainwright cannot help but victimise Patrick and the sisters by looking almost exclusively at how Branwell's illness impacted them.

'Does he *want* to abstain?': inebriation, psychology, and medicine

Admittedly, Wainwright's drama offers some (albeit sparing) psychological acknowledgement that alcoholism is now a widely established medical condition.[2] In one of the drama's few ingresses into modern discourse, Charlotte draws attention to this idea. She enters Branwell's room 'and shuts the door. And what comes out is sadness, not anger or judgment': 'If you don't get on top. Of this habit', she counsels grudgingly, 'When things don't go right for you. If you can't exercise some restraint. It'll take over your life. Branwell, and [...] it'll destroy you' (Wainwright, 2016: 26; full stops as per original). The use of language, here, and specifically the term 'habit', evokes both modern psychological thought through reference to abstinence and choice *and* discourses of self-help, namely acknowledgement of the disorder followed by steps to overcome the illness. This is repeated after a doctor has visited Branwell following an episode of *delirium tremens*, a Victorian medical term referring to tremors caused by alcohol withdrawal, and recommends abstention:

> CHARLOTTE
> Does he *want* to abstain?
>
> PATRICK
> He has to. He has to abstain.
> [...]
>
> CHARLOTTE
> Have you talked to him? About abstention [...] It'll only work if he's determined to do it himself. (Wainwright, 2016: 73)

Here, the drama's dialogue undoubtedly evokes modern approaches to alcoholism, and particularly the rhetoric of Alcoholics Anonymous (AA), an organisation that stresses an individual's 'desire to stop drinking' and admission of a problem, or, in other words, a committed intent to practise self-control.[3] But whereas Patrick's words are hopeful and optimistic towards Branwell's recovery, Charlotte's response is decidedly sceptical and pejorative. Her words, 'to do it himself', while logical, further isolate Branwell in his suffering and ignore contemporary notions of supportive recovery. It is conceivable that the sisters and Patrick would have intervened in helping Branwell take steps towards improving his life, but the drama insists upon a narrative of isolation and atonement. Further, the scene assumes our allegiance with Charlotte's point of view and, therefore, while her words evoke modern notions of addiction and recovery, they do so only to remind the viewer of the moral implications of choice and willpower to sobriety.

Consequently, *To Walk Invisible*'s conception of alcoholism as a psychiatric and medical disease is grudging and complex. Branwell *is* described as 'ill' at times, but illness is, when used by Charlotte or Emily, largely a euphemism for drunkenness. Charlotte's first words reference 'illness' through a voiceover reading of an extract from an actual letter sent to her friend, Ellen Nussey, in 1845: 'Dear Ellen, It was ten o'clock when I got home. I found Branwell ill. He is so very often these days owing to his own fault' (Wainwright, 2016: 3). As Charlotte makes clear through her later attribution of blame, 'ill' is not deployed in a medical way here; it merely means 'drunk'. Similarly, Emily writes that she hopes that Branwell will 'be better and do better' (*TWI*, Part 1). The language of illness and recovery, then, is used to avoid the stigma of publicly acknowledging Branwell's problem drinking.

Such rhetorical ambiguity belies the way in which nineteenth-century medical discourse clearly constituted habitual drunkenness as a disease. Writing as early as 1804, the British physician Thomas Trotter defined drunkenness as a physiological disorder. In *An Essay* [...] *on Drunkenness, and Its Effects on the Human Body*, Trotter wrote that, 'In Medical language, I consider drunkenness, strictly speaking to be a disease; produced by a remote cause, and giving birth to actions and movements in the living body, that disorder the functions of health' (Trotter, 1804: 8). Similarly, in a renowned essay on intemperance, Ralph Grindrod argued that '*Apoplexy, Palsy, Epilepsy, and Hysteria*, are among those diseases of the brain, which are not unfrequently [*sic*] brought on by intemperate indulgence ... *Madness and Idiocy* are, in the present day especially, familiar and deplorable consequences of intemperate drinking' (Grindrod, 1839: 356–359). These views were echoed by Robert Macnish who, in his *Anatomy of Drunkenness* (1828) published in *Blackwood's Edinburgh Magazine* (a journal favoured by Branwell), indicated that, according to reports from various 'institutions for the insane', drunkenness was 'the most common causes of lunacy' such that 'one-half owe their madness to drinking' (Macnish, 1828: 481).

Although Trotter, Grindrod, and Macnish viewed excessive alcohol consumption as *the* underlying cause of a range of bodily and mental diseases, including epilepsy, idiocy, and madness, other medical professionals insisted that habitual drunkenness was not only a cause of madness, but an effect of it. In *The Use and Abuse of Alcoholic Liquors in Health and Disease* (1876), for instance, William Benjamin Carpenter writes that:

> There is no class of aberrant Mental phenomena which is more deserving of careful scientific study, than that which is produced by the introduction into the Blood of substances which are foreign to its composition, and which have the special property of perverting its normal action on the Brain. (Carpenter, 1876: 636)

Although written some years after Branwell's demise, Carpenter's point reminds us that Victorian medicine recognised how alcohol consumption affected both the body *and* the mind.

Patrick's own awareness of how medical science viewed alcohol dependency in relation to insanity is evident from his annotated copy of Dr Thomas John Graham's *Modern Domestic Medicine* (1826).[4] As its title suggests, Graham's book 'present[s] the unprofessional reader with a clear and correct description of the nature, symptoms, causes, distinction, and most approved treatment of the diseases to which the human frame is liable' (Graham, 1826: vii). Significantly, in his copy of the book, Patrick made two annotations to the entry 'Of Insanity'. Firstly, he added a cross next to the word 'intoxication' that points to a later section on 'Delirium Tremens'. Secondly, he underlined the term 'hereditary disposition' in the same section, a reference that conceivably relates to Branwell.[5]

Curiously, in *To Walk Invisible*, Patrick's understanding of alcohol abuse as a medical disorder is obscured and, quite literally, relegated to the background. In a scene situated on 7 July 1846, Charlotte is shown passing through the house to open a door to greet the postman and in the background 'we can hear Branwell shouting at Patrick' (Wainwright, 2016: 60). The exchange between father and son not only centres on Branwell's attempts to get money (willingly or otherwise) from his father, but Patrick's efforts to rationalise with Branwell, telling him that 'You need. To get a situation. You need. To pull yourself together! [...] I beg you to recognise that you are ill' (Wainwright, 2016: 61). The suggestion that Patrick viewed Branwell as 'ill' is recognised here, but it is barely audible.[6] Again, Branwell's 'illness' is reduced to troublesome behaviour: a failure to exercise self-control and gain employment coupled with reckless spending.

The only scene where Branwell's 'illness' *is* acknowledged clearly in medical terms takes place towards the end of the drama, in the final stages of his life. In a scene dated 21 November 1846, Branwell is shown to return home and collapse unconscious outside of the Parsonage. He is carried to bed by Patrick and Emily and attended to by Dr Wheelhouse.[7] Patrick enters the parlour to give the sisters news following Dr Wheelhouse's visit. This is followed by a second scene the next day in which Branwell is shown struggling for breath, shaking and incoherent. This time we learn from Dr Wheelhouse that this is an episode of *delirium tremens*, something that, as noted, Patrick acknowledged in his edition of *Modern Domestic Medicine*. What is significant about these scenes, though, is that it is only when Dr Wheelhouse diagnoses *delirium tremens* does it become clear that Branwell was not, in fact, drunk in either his moment of collapse *or* during the seizure, but sober and his body was craving alcohol. In other words, when *To Walk Invisible does* underline the corporeal effects of alcohol addiction, it bypasses any medical understanding of Branwell's symptoms either by way of Victorian notions of insanity *or* the DSM-5's diagnostic criteria for AUD. Instead, by foregrounding the stereotypical effects of chronic end-stage alcohol abuse, the drama reinforces the morally loaded notion that Branwell is solely to blame for his own condition and is facing the consequences of his poor choices.

While *To Walk Invisible* elides the way in which medical science in the past and present has viewed problem drinking in relation to mental health, it is significant that, even in the nineteenth century, commentators on the Brontës were looking to medical discourse to explain Branwell's behaviour more fully. Indeed, Leyland, in particular, conceived of Branwell's behaviour in relation to Victorian medicine. Although not medically trained, for Leyland, Branwell suffered from 'monomania' (Leyland, 1886, vol. 2: 55). He cites Carpenter on this matter, noting that 'the condition to which Branwell fell at this period [1845] is one very well known to mental physiologists' (Leyland, 1886, vol. 2: 57). 'Monomania', as defined by Carpenter, is a form of 'impulsive insanity' and 'its existence is of peculiar importance in a juridical point of view', for the 'Law of England only recognizes as irresponsible, those who are incapable of distinguishing right from wrong', and those suffering from 'monomania', he suggests, lack such capacity (Carpenter, 1876: 658).

In its portrayal of *delirium tremens*, *To Walk Invisible* inadvertently gestures to some of the symptoms that Carpenter identifies in monomania:

> It is singular how closely the ordinary history of the access of Monomania corresponds with that of intoxication by Hachisch. A man who has been for some time under the strain of severe mental labour, perhaps with the addition of emotional excitement, breaks down in mental and bodily health; and becomes subject to morbid ideas, of whose abnormal character he is in the first instance quite unaware. He may see spectral illusions, but he knows that they are illusive. He may hear imaginary conversations, but is conscious they are empty words. He feels an extreme depression of spirits [...] He has strange thoughts respecting those who are most dear to him, suspects his wife of infidelity, his children of willful disobedience, his most intimate friends of injurious designs, but he has still intelligence enough to question the validity of these suspicions, and shrinks from giving them permanent lodgment in his breast. Dark visions of future ruin and disgrace flit before him. (Carpenter, 1876: 673)

To Walk Invisible partially reflects Carpenter's commentary on the symptoms of monomania during a scene entitled 'Branwell's nightmare' (Wainwright, 2016: 74). The script direction tells us that Branwell is 'fully dressed' as he walks towards Lydia Robinson who 'is draped along a chaise longue, naked, and surrounded by men. All of whom look ready to fuck her ... Suddenly a load of water lands on BRANWELL from above, like God just dropped a bucket load of water on him' (Wainwright, 2016: 74). Wainwright's construction of Branwell's nightmare evokes Carpenter's 'spectral illusions' (Carpenter, 1876: 673). Not only does the transition from realism to dream mimic the psychosis of which Carpenter speaks, but the images that Branwell visualises recall Carpenter's reflections on the visual and auditory hallucinations experienced during monomania, especially those regarding 'infidelity' and 'the injurious design of his friends' (Carpenter, 1876: 673). Nagaitis's physical rendering of Branwell's vulnerability and confusion through slow, short movements coupled with his ever-whitening pallor denote Branwell's instability. However, whereas Carpenter argues for the subject's realisation of the irrationality of the imagined spectrality, *To Walk Invisible* denies Branwell such agency. The very fact that this is a nightmare and not a waking hallucinatory experience renders the moment as the rambling imaginings of an intoxicated cognition.

However, seen through a modern lens, what the Victorians called 'monomania' correlates, in some respects, with twenty-first-century understandings of bipolar disorder. Dr John J. Ross, Assistant Professor of Medicine at Harvard Medical School and author of *Shakespeare's Tremor and Orwell's Cough: The Medical Lives of Famous Writers* (2012), makes this diagnostic claim, arguing that 'Branwell likely had bipolar disorder' (Ross, 2012: 95), an opinion he bases on historical documents that cite Branwell's severe and fluctuating moods. What's more, Leyland records that as a child Branwell possessed 'a sprightly disposition, tinged at times with great melancholy' (Leyland, 1886, vol. 1: 82) and by adulthood could 'pass suddenly from gaiety to moody disquietude' with a rapidity that 'alarmed' his sisters (Leyland, 1886, vol. 2: 44). Yet Branwell's impulsivity, lack of self-control, inability to complete tasks, and overwhelming sense of failure could also point to other potential disorders, including Attention Deficit Hyperactivity Disorder (ADHD) (DSM-5: n.p.), which has been suggested by Nagaitis himself.[8] Despite historical evidence that points to a probable mental health disorder *and* the availability of diagnostic criteria to help examine the possibility of a potential mental health condition, *To Walk Invisible* nonetheless overlooks this in favour of rendering Branwell as a mere drunk in order to amplify the sisters' tormented struggles and emphasise the *female* narrative at the heart of the drama.

Although Wainwright suggested in a commentary on the drama that she 'really didn't want [the Brontës] to be defined by their deaths', her statement clearly only extends to the three sisters, since *To Walk Invisible* offers persistent reminders that Branwell's drinking both equates with death and that it was *the* cause, above all else, of his early demise.[9] In reality, we do not know if Branwell died from liver failure, which historical documentation suggests may have been possible, or from tuberculosis, which was cited on his death

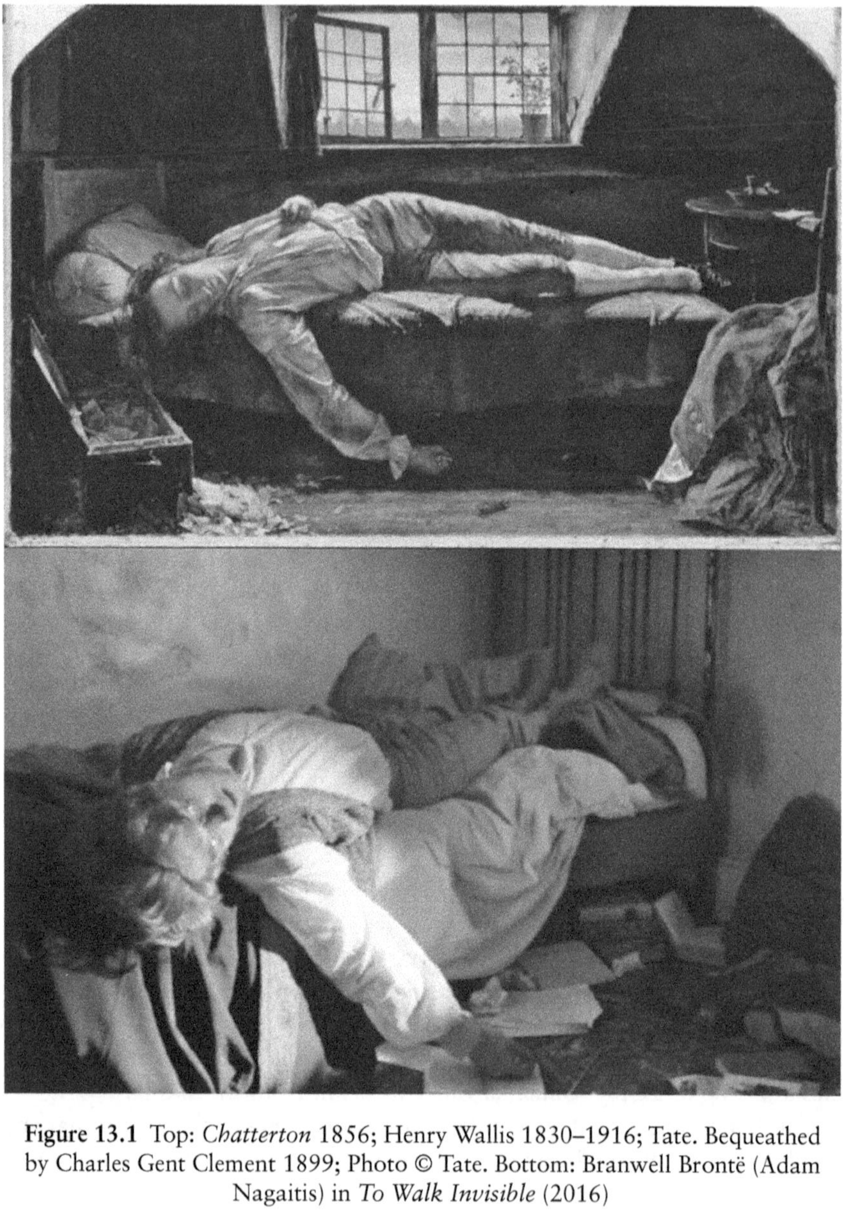

Figure 13.1 Top: *Chatterton* 1856; Henry Wallis 1830–1916; Tate. Bequeathed by Charles Gent Clement 1899; Photo © Tate. Bottom: Branwell Brontë (Adam Nagaitis) in *To Walk Invisible* (2016)

certificate as 'Chronic bronchitis – Marasmus' (severe malnutrition). Yet, through repeated scenes portraying Branwell in an isolated state of disarray, Wainwright nonetheless emphasises that alcohol abuse was *the* cause of his demise. In one particular scene, Branwell is stylised so as to imitate Henry Wallis's *The Death of Chatterton* (1856). Wallis's oil portrait, which is on display at the Tate Museum in London, portrays the Romantic poet Thomas Chatterton's (1752–1770) suicide from arsenic poisoning following artistic failure and financial precarity. Wallis portrays Chatterton's lifeless body lying in sleep-like repose on a bed beneath a small open window from which a ray of light glows. His right arm is touching the floor, and crumpled paper lies ripped by his side. A small bowl – presumably a tincture of arsenic – lies on a table nearby. *To Walk Invisible* reworks Branwell as Chatterton in a morning-after-the-drunken-night-before scenario. United by their flame-red hair and laid-back repose, Branwell also lies asleep beneath his bedroom window (off screen), with his right arm touching the floor. Where Chatterton is surrounded by fragments of his half-written poems, Wainwright provides a close-up of Branwell's unfinished novel *And the Weary Are at Rest* (c. 1845). And in place of Chatterton's poison-filled bowl is an empty bottle of whisky, a parallel which invites the audience to see Branwell's whisky in equivalent terms to Chatterton's arsenic. Wallis's Romantic depiction of Chatterton epitomises the quintessential concept of the tortured artist. Described as 'the poor boy who aspired to fame and was compelled to write for his living' (*Morning Chronicle*, n.p.) but with little to no success, the financial, personal, and professional failures that precipitated Chatterton's suicide find a conspicuous parallel in Wainwright's imagery of Branwell. But where Chatterton was retrospectively hailed a romantic hero by Wallis in 1856, *To Walk Invisible* asserts Branwell is merely a 'flaked out' waster (Wainwright, 2016: 28) (see Figure 13.1).

'Stop looking at me!': masculinity and failure

While Wainwright's evocation of Wallis's painting warns of Branwell's future demise, this scene is also one of many whereby the drama connects Branwell's alcoholism to notions of failure. Here that failure is both personal *and* professional; on a personal level, he has fallen asleep in his clothes, but on a professional level, the inclusion of Branwell's infamous unfinished manuscript reminds the viewer that, unlike his sisters, the only Brontë son was unable to finish a book. Notably, *To Walk Invisible* also insists upon correlating Branwell's 'failures' with what it perceives as his masculine inadequacies. Crucially, one of the ways the series re-mythologises Branwell's alleged incompetence is to pathologise his failures, which are habitually intertwined with his body and (ill) health. Throughout, he is rendered weak, frail, vulnerable, unmasculine, and undignified. Indeed, like the evocation of Wallis's *Chatterton*, across many scenes we see Branwell in various states of physical helplessness, often lying on the ground after collapsing, unable to walk due to drunkenness or prostrate unconscious. He is often depicted through high-angle shots that work purposefully to underscore his diminutive status both on a physical and moral level.

Branwell's masculinity is also pathologised by being presented in terms of frailty, infirmity, and emotionality. Bodily fluids become a visual motif registering his lack of self-control and personal degradation. In the opening scene, spit runs down Branwell's beard after the frenzied argument with his father and aunt. This scene is followed by various moments where he cries, vomits on himself, sits on a chamber pot, or spews blood. Branwell's humiliation reaches a climax when he returns from The Black Bull drunk and emotionally distraught after hearing news that Lydia, despite her husband's death, refuses to see him. As he looks directly at his family, pleading with them to 'stop looking at me', we are reminded in this moment of 'anguished crying' (Wainwright, 2016: 59) that he feels perpetually judged by them. The scene evokes the notion of 'the gaze', a 'being-looked-at-ness' (Mulvey, 1975: 11), to use Laura Mulvey's term, but in such a way that is re-coded from an erotic gaze to a judgmental one. The scene is constructed so as to align our sympathies with both the sisters and Patrick who are rendered victims of yet another outburst, and specifically with Charlotte who looks on with impatience and disgust. Wainwright pairs shots of a teary Patrick and repulsed Charlotte with shots of a crazed Branwell whose face is soaked with tears and mucus. It is a composition that simultaneously evokes compassion for the family and pitiful repugnance for him.

Tellingly, Wainwright's script also suggests that the only bodily fluid Branwell cannot successfully produce is the most masculine of all: semen. The nightmare scene, described earlier, strongly suggests Branwell's sexual impotence. Nagaitis contends that the scene symbolises Branwell's 'complete inability to connect to his masculinity' and communicates how he is 'terrified of manhood and is trapped as a boy', a view that is supported by Wainwright's script direction: 'MRS. ROBINSON wants sex with anyone and everyone. All except BRANWELL. Pathetic little BRANWELL' (Wainwright, 2016: 74). Here, Wainwright adds insult to injury. Not only is Branwell framed as a miserable ne'er-do-well but the implication of his sexual debility insinuates his fundamental failure as a man.

The culmination of these scenes demonstrates that Wainwright moves away from a medical narrative into a judgmental, stigmatising, and, seemingly, anti-Branwell one. The view that Branwell's alcoholism is a choice and, therefore, a personal failure rather than a symptom of a wider mental health disorder is underscored by a pivotal scene where, as mentioned earlier, Lydia's coachman delivers news of Mr Robinson's death and warns

Branwell 'to stay away' (Wainwright, 2016: 54). In the next scene, after Allison's departure, we see John being summoned to The Black Bull where Branwell is collapsed on the floor, crying and paralytically drunk. Again, Wainwright maintains that Branwell's longing for Lydia is *the* reason he drinks. If there was any doubt of this angle, Patrick articulates this point to his daughters after Dr Wheelhouse's visit:

> PATRICK
> There is hope ... His body has suffered the ravages of gross neglect.
> And ...
> (he hates saying it)
> abuse. Self-inflicted. And yet I cannot – in my conscience – do other than blame that woman. That sinful, hateful woman ... Who with her more mature years and her social advantages should surely have known better responsibility. (Wainwright, 2016: 72)

Although Wainwright here redirects the blame onto Lydia, there is a symptom of denial that refuses to acknowledge there may have been an underlying medical reason for Branwell's symptoms and therefore a resistance to medicalise alcohol dependency.

Conclusion

Daphne Du Maurier once wrote that

> it would be heartening to think that after two biographies to himself within eight months, Branwell Brontë will be remembered in future for his early brilliance, not for his later failings, and that the thousands of visitors who walk through the Parsonage during the years to come will remember the youthful, happier days of all four Brontës and not dwell upon the last, sad scenes. (Du Maurier, 1998: 155)

Sadly, this is not the case in *To Walk Invisible*. As we have shown, the drama not only dwells on Branwell's 'later failings' but also emphasises his complicity in his own demise, something at odds with medical perspectives of the past and present. The possible medical explanations that challenge myth-based notions of Branwell's habitual dependency are overlooked and what little acknowledgement of medical science there is is problematic. In this respect, it is worth noting that the drama also entirely overlooks speculation that Branwell might have suffered from seizures since his childhood that may suggest a long-standing physiological condition, or that he also self-medicated through the use of opium. Instead, through select letters and ghostly voices we are reminded that Branwell's health and personal challenges were the social and psychological adversity that his sisters overcame to achieve literary success. Undoubtedly, there is something of a sad truth to this narrative, but it is a dominant and one-sided perspective on the Brontë family story, and one that elides Branwell's view entirely.

To Walk Invisible closes with a present-day view of the Parsonage. We follow a young boy running into the museum's 'happy' book shop and see first-hand the powerful tourist legacy that the sisters' literary success enabled (Wainwright, 2016: 117). The camera pans from inside into the museum's courtyard and rests on a bronze sculpture of the sisters. Wainwright's script indicates that, originally, this closing image in *To Walk Invisible* was meant to be followed by another scene on the Rochdale Canal in Sowerby Bridge. There the viewer was meant to see a final image of a different Brontë statue:

> A badly decayed 15' tall wooden statue labelled 'Branwell Brontë' 1817–1848' [...] One of the eyes is hollow, both his hands have rotted away, and down by his crotch the Sowerby Bridge piss-heads have put an empty Budweiser bottle, among other modern-day debris around the dank little picnic site. (Wainwright, 2016: 117)

This scene was never filmed because by the time drama went into production, the statue of Branwell had been destroyed, 'burnt down', we were told by one local when we went looking for it ourselves in August 2019. That this scene was never produced is, perhaps, positive, for the juxtaposition would only have served to reinforce Branwell's tragic history and the unfair comparison of him to his celebrated sisters. While the series empowers the sisters' narrative in innovative and very modern ways through a feminocentric focus on their plights and achievements in a world hostile to women's intellectual pursuits, the misfortune is that *To Walk Invisible* not only persists but is complicit in presenting Branwell, as Leyland lamented 130 years ago, in a 'spirit' decidedly 'unfriendly to him'.

Acknowledgements

We would like to thank Mary Mifflen, MA, L Psych, and Dr John J. Ross, Assistant Professor of Medicine at Harvard Medical School, for taking the time to share their professional medical perspectives on Branwell's health with us. Their views have been invaluable to us in formulating our thoughts on Branwell. We would also like to acknowledge Chris Sutherns at Tate Images for his support in granting us permission to reproduce Henry Wallis's *Chatteron* (1856). Finally, we would like to thank Adam Nagaitis – Branwell himself in *To Walk Invisible* – for taking the time to share his thoughts on Branwell's challenges and his approach to presenting him onscreen.

Notes

1 While we recognise that the terms 'alcoholism' and 'alcoholic' are anachronistic because they only came into being in 1849 via Magnus Huss's influential work 'Alcoholismus Chronicus', we use them throughout this chapter in recognition of their use in contemporary culture.

2 Alcohol dependency was first recognised as a medical disease in the United States in 1935 with the creation of Alcoholics Anonymous (AA). The American Psychiatric Association (APA) officially medicalised alcohol abuse in 1952 with the publication of the DSM-2. See www.sciencedirect.com/topics/medicine-and-dentistry/dsm-ii (accessed 5 October 2020).

3 As the organisation's website indicates, 'The only requirement for membership is a desire to stop drinking', something they achieve through their infamous Twelve Step recovery programme. The AA are also clear that they do 'not engage in the fields of alcoholism research, medical or psychiatric treatment, education, or advocacy in any form' (Alcoholics Anonymous UK, 2019: n.p.). In other words, it is a 'self-help' organisation, rather than one that practises medicine or psychiatry.

4 Both Branwell and Patrick were also involved with Haworth's temperance society across the 1830s.

5 Patrick's implied belief in the hereditary nature of insanity underscores nineteenth-century writing on the topic.

6 The BBC received numerous complaints about the show's audio quality. For more on this, see Helen Kelley's article in *The Express*, '"So disappointed!" Viewers slam *To Walk Invisible* over "inaudible mumbling"': www.express.co.uk/showbiz/tv-radio/748364/To-Walk-Invisible-slammed-inaudible-mumbling-Bronte-sisters-BBC-Sally-Wainwright (accessed 5 October 2020).

7 Interestingly, Dr Wheelhouse is described in the script as 'a rather charmless, awkward man, who is in fact an alcoholic himself' (Wainwright, 2016: 75).

8 Nagaitis argues that while there is no direct evidence to indicate Branwell suffered from a particular mental health disorder, there is circumstantial 'proof' there was 'something there', evidenced by an inability to complete tasks or finish projects, a propensity to self-medicate, and an overwhelming sense of personal failure.

9 See Sally Wainwright, 'I didn't want *To Walk Invisible* to be just another period drama', *Radio Times*, 29 December 2016, www.radiotimes.com/news/2016-12-29/sally-wainwright-i-didnt-want-to-walk-invisible-to-be-just-another-period-drama/ (accessed 5 October 2020).

References

'A Parthian Glance at the Royal Academy Exhibition' (1856). *The Morning Chronicle*, 8 August 1856 (27963).

American Psychiatric (2013). *Diagnostic and Statistical Manual of Mental Disorders* (DSM-5). 5th edn. Washington, DC: American Psychiatric Association.

Anon, 'What is AA? An Introduction', Alcoholics Anonymous UK. www.alcoholics-anonymous.org.uk/# (accessed 10 September 2019).

Carpenter, W. B. (1876). *Principles of Mental Physiology: With Their Applications to the Training and Discipline of the Mind, and the Study of Its Morbid Conditions.* London: Paternoster Row.

Cocozza, P. (2016). '"They Had Issues": Sally Wainwright and Tracy Chevalier Discuss the Brontës', *The Guardian*, 16 December 2016. www.theguardian.com/tv-and-radio/2016/dec/16/they-had-issues-sally-wainwright-and-tracy-chevalier-in-conversation-about-the-brontes (accessed 7 September 2019).

Du Maurier, D. (1998). 'Second Thoughts on Branwell', *Brontë Society Transactions*, 23 (2) (October 1998), pp. 155–158.

Fan, J. (2018). '*To Walk Invisible* Review', *The New Yorker*, 20 February 2018. www.newyorker.com/recommends/watch/to-walk-invisible (accessed 23 May 2019).

Gaskell, E. ([1857] 2009). *The Life of Charlotte Brontë*. Oxford: Oxford University Press.

Gilbert, S. (2017). 'PBS's *To Walk Invisible* Finds Fire in the Lives of the Brontë Sisters', *The Atlantic*, 26 March 2017. www.theatlantic.com/entertainment/archive/2017/03/to-walk-invisible-bronte-sisters-pbs/520749/ (accessed 23 May 2019).

Grindrod, R. B. (1839). *Bacchus: An Essay on the Nature, Causes, Effects, and Cure of Intemperance*. London: Johnston and Barrett.

Lewis Shiman, L. (1988). *Crusade against Drink in Victorian England*. Basingstoke: MacMillan Press Ltd.

Leyland, F. A. ([1886] 2005). *The Brontë Family: With Special Reference to Patrick Branwell Brontë*, Volume One and Two. Honolulu: University of the Pacific Press.

Macnish, R. (1828). 'Anatomy of Drunkenness', *Blackwood's Edinburgh Magazine*, 23, pp. 481–499.

Mangan, L. (2016). '*To Walk Invisible* Review – A Bleak and Brilliant Portrayal of the Brontë Family', *The Guardian*, 30 December 2016. www.theguardian.com/tv-and-radio/2016/dec/30/to-walk-invisible-review-a-bleak-and-brilliant-portrayal-of-the-Brontë -family (accessed 23 May 2019).

Mulvey, L. (1975). 'Visual Pleasure and Narrative Cinema', *Screen*, 16 (3) (October 1975), pp. 6–18.

Nagaitis, A. (September 2019). Email and phone interviews.

Trotter, T. (1804). *An Essay, Medical, Philosophical, and Chemical, on Drunkenness, and Its Effects on the Human Body*. London: Paternoster Row.

Wainwright, S. (Dir.) (2016). *To Walk Invisible*. Shooting Script, 26 April 2016.

14

'After I left England, they thought I was mad. But they taught me to use it – now it's a gift': representations of mental illness in the period dramas of Steven Knight

Dan Ward

One of the most striking developments in recent period drama has been the emergence of Steven Knight as a prominent voice within the genre. Through shows like *Peaky Blinders* (BBC, 2013–) and *Taboo* (BBC, 2017–), Knight has brought a distinctive authorial style to the format which grounds itself in what he calls 'the mud on your boots, the blood, the violence' (Singh, 2013), the visceral underbelly of Britain's history so often obfuscated by the heritage tendency in British period drama. While Knight's stories are conspicuously concerned with addressing the issues of social class, economics, and political intrigue he sees as underrepresented within period drama more broadly, another key theme underpinning several of his most intriguing characterisations is that of mental illness. This features prominently even within his work outside of the period genre: both *Hummingbird* (Knight, 2013) and *Locke* (Knight, 2013), films which Knight wrote and directed, feature protagonists undergoing mental breakdowns, so the issue is clearly one which holds personal interest to him as an author. Probably the most prominent example within Knight's period dramas comes in *Peaky Blinders*' consideration of 'the trauma of WW1 and what it visited upon the industrial working class' (Ellis, 2013). Returning to Birmingham in the immediate aftermath of the Great War, the leaders of the Shelby crime family act as avatars of the enduring impact of the war on the men who survived it, its nihilistic chaos pervading the shattered psyches of these men, and projected through them into the urban warfare they unleash on the streets of Small Heath and beyond. While the centrality of war trauma in *Peaky Blinders* has been discussed at length in critical studies of the series (Taddeo, 2018), this is by no means the only representation of mental illness in Knight's work. It is also visible within the same series in Polly Gray's (Helen McCrory) mental breakdown following her late reprieve from the gallows, and madness functions as a central motif in Knight's other BBC period text, *Taboo*. The ways in which madness and mental illness are represented in *Peaky Blinders* and *Taboo* raise stark questions around contemporary attitudes to gender, lineage, superstition, and the ability of the developing field of medicine to effectively treat maladies of the mind.

'You know, gentlemen, there is hell, and there is another place below hell'

Peaky Blinders draws heavily on the iconography of the gangster genre, steeped as it is in machismo and heavily stylised portraits of violent, uncompromising alpha males. The series was originally conceived from Steven Knight's childhood memories of stories his parents and grandparents would tell about the feared and respected gangs who inhabited his native Birmingham years before his birth, in particular the infamous 'Peaky Blinders' group. In conveying the young Knight's sense of cautious wonder and imagined nostalgia at these tales, the series employs a visual aesthetic that echoes what Knight calls the 'mythological' aura such stories evoke (Wright, 2016). This is apparent in everything from the striking vintage fashions the characters are clothed in (which have inspired notable copycat trends at the bars and racecourses of twenty-first-century Britain), to the series' memorable opening sequence, in which Thomas Shelby (Cillian Murphy) rides a horse down a narrow street in a scene deliberately contrived in such a manner as to reference western films (Wright, 2016). While such portrayals might be understandably read as romanticising the brutal men and illicit lifestyles the series documents, this is only part of the story which *Peaky Blinders* tells of crime and its consequences.

Just as the series lays down a marker in one respect through its iconic opening horse-riding sequence, it also signals its intentions in a very different sense from its outset through the heavy focus on war trauma. Long (2017: 174) observes that 'while some (in the series) wear the physical scars of war, all appear to bear at least some mental scars that have conditioned them, and distinguish them from those they left behind'. Although the psychological scarring which the war has left on Tommy and Arthur Shelby (Paul Anderson) is evident in the opening episode (and will continue to be as the series progresses) through nightmarish flashbacks to the cold brutality of the trenches and tunnels, the most jarring example of post-traumatic stress disorder (PTSD) featured appears in the character of the Shelby brothers' friend and wartime comrade Danny Whizz-bang (Samuel Edward-Cook), who 'cannot stop his headaches and rage' (Taddeo, 2018: 179). Danny has been irreparably damaged by the war, to the extent that he imagines himself 'as an exploding shell, so creating havoc wherever he goes' (Long, 2017: 174). These sporadic outbursts of panic and misdirected violence ultimately culminate in a fatal scuffle with a local Italian, which embroils the Shelbys in the first of many conflicts in the series with rival criminal factions. While Tommy is apparently able to keep his night terrors hidden from his peers (with the help of opium) for the most part, in Danny's case the trauma has so consumed him that it has become the defining aspect of his persona, his previous personality stripped away and his identity reduced to the 'whizz-bang' of the artillery shells.

These themes are once again revisited in the fifth season of *Peaky Blinders* when Tommy goes to visit his old army comrade Barney Thompson (Cosmo Jarvis), who has been committed to a mental institution (S5E5). The parallels between Barney and Danny are clear: both men are irreparably broken mentally as a result of their experiences in the war, and both maintain an unswerving loyalty to Tommy. In this latter sense as much as the former, the underlying theme of the Great War as one which never really ended for the Shelby gang and their peers is reaffirmed. In drawing these obvious parallels in characterisation, Knight uses Barney as an opportunity to continue to explore some of the issues only touched on before Danny met his fate, an early casualty of the Peaky Blinders' ascendancy of the criminal hierarchy. The key development in this later characterisation is Knight's attempt to represent not only the symptoms of war trauma, but the clinical treatment of its after-effects. Asylums were an integral part of the medical treatment of afflicted soldiers during the war and in its aftermath, with a number of asylums emptied and repurposed as 'war hospitals' from 1915 onwards. The issue of mental illness for soldiers was widespread enough that, by 1920, around 9 per cent of the 440,000 men who had been treated at these 'war hospitals' were 'psychiatric cases; those suffering from shell-shock, nervous breakdowns, delusions, and sheer terror' (Nielson, 2014).

When Tommy comes to the asylum in which Barney is housed, he first enters a dark, drab hallway, to be met coldly by a man wearing an outfit that resembles a butcher's smock. He searches Shelby roughly 'for his own safety', addressing him in coarse, impolite speech. It is unclear if the guard is aware of who Tommy is, and if this motivates his apparent scorn, but the implication is clear: in the asylum, every part of a man's identity in the outside world is stripped from him. Even Tommy Shelby, famous member of parliament, OBE, and feared gang leader, is manhandled and treated disdainfully when he enters, and although Tommy is only a visitor in this scenario, he is nevertheless treated with similar contempt to the inmates. The overriding tone is of dehumanisation, made explicit when the guard tells Tommy that the man he has come to see is nothing but 'a fucking animal'. This attitude is not confined to the inner sanctum of the institution, as Barney is tied to a lamppost by the Shelby gang in the following episode to temporarily restrain him, and at one point we learn that he has 'bit through the fucking rope'. Again, the echoes of Danny's wretched fate are evident. After Danny's manic outburst in The Garrison, Tommy tries to calm him by telling him 'You're not an artillery shell, Danny, you're a man ... You're not a whizz-bang. You're a human being' (S1E1). Such reminders are to little avail, though. Madness takes away the humanity of Tommy's comrades, both in their own eyes and in the eyes of society at large: they become 'whizz-bangs' or 'fucking animals'. Nowhere is this clearer than in the callous, unforgiving environment of the asylum, with the 'huge social stigma' (Nielson, 2014) which institutionalisation carried in the period adding to the isolation of sufferers.

The asylum scene also underscores the theme of confinement in Knight's representation of mental illness. This is physically apparent in the cavernous setting of the asylum itself, and in the intrusive checks which Tommy must undergo in order to be allowed access to the secluded cell now housing his old comrade. When Barney eventually appears, he himself is bound in a restrictive straitjacket, emphasising that he is more prisoner than patient in the institution. As much as the extreme physical confinement is highlighted here, it is also made clear that the prisons the traumatised veterans of *Peaky Blinders* inhabit are mental as well as physical. The purpose of Tommy's visit is to offer Barney two 'escape routes': the first is literal, a proposition for the Shelby gang to break him out of the asylum in order to assist in Tommy's plot to assassinate Oswald Moseley. The other, more permanent form of escape is offered by means of a cyanide capsule laced with opium. Shelby seems surprised when Barney refuses the capsule, and the expectation that his wartime ally might naturally prefer oblivion and the unknown is clearly influenced by the mental turmoil Tommy himself has been increasingly experiencing in the lead-up to the visit. Haunted by visions of his dead wife, Grace, he apparently attempts suicide first by firing a machine gun indiscriminately at a field mined by the Billy Boys, and later by starting the ignition in a car he imagines has been booby-trapped by the intelligence services. Barney and Tommy act as mirrors of each other throughout the scene: the sneering disdain with which Tommy is regarded by the guard makes the dehumanisation of anonymous patients like Barney more resonant to an audience unused to seeing the series' charismatic anti-hero treated in this manner. Barney, meanwhile, acts as a cautionary tale embodying what Tommy might have become after the war, or even what he might yet become as his mental state increasingly unravels.

There is an undeniably exploitative element in Tommy's treatment of Barney, seen in his reassurance, upon seeing his damaged comrade slip naturally back into the role of crack sniper after being freed from the asylum, that all Barney needed to relieve his torment was 'another war'. Particularly given the suicide mission Barney is ultimately sent on, it is hard to ignore the parallels between Shelby – now an influential MP as well as a gang leader – and the wartime British state, having effectively conscripted Barney into his destructive scheme. Even here, though, there are commonalities between exploiter and exploited. Tommy's insistence that 'another war' is the only respite Barney can attain is just as applicable to his own situation, the murderous conflicts the Blinders incessantly engage in being the only focal point apparently powerful enough to sway Tommy's mind from thoughts of self-destruction (yet all the while adding to his burdens). The perverse implication that extreme violence is the only means by which these men can find some grotesque element of 'peace' speaks further to the enduring brutalisation of the living casualties of war in Knight's work, violence constituted as both their mental prison and their release. In these allusions to the shared brutalisation of Tommy and Barney (not to mention Danny and Arthur), this aspect of *Peaky Blinders*' plot reminds its audience that the enduring trauma suffered by such characters was a far more commonplace scenario for returning soldiers than the mythologised tale of social ascendance and conquest that is the series' central thread.

This is not, however, to deny the existence of a certain mythologised element to Knight's treatment of war trauma, in particular shell shock. Historian Jessica Meyer has argued that shell shock has retrospectively been positioned as 'the dominant symbolic wound of the war in British culture' (Meyer, 2014), to the extent of its conflation with other variations of war trauma and 'trench neuroses' within cultural forms such as period drama. Particularly in the case of Danny, Knight seems to draw on the assumed resonance of this trope to signpost the broader theme of brutalisation and ceaseless warfare: the visceral sights and sounds of war continue to play out in Danny's head, just as the violence of the war continues to play out in the lives of the Shelby gang. Again, Knight's representation of these themes is inextricable from personal recollections and family history: discussing his uncle's experiences after returning to civilian life after the war, he references a horrific fight involving two other returned servicemen. The extreme violence employed by the two men apparently illustrated to Knight's uncle that, because of their wartime experiences, 'their boundaries had gone. Everybody who returned from that conflict did so with a fury inside him' (Allen, 2018). Meyer observes that, of the soldiers who returned from the war, there were 'three million men who somehow went through this experience and managed to reintegrate into society' (Meyer, 2014), which suggests a degree of embellishment in Knight's universalisation of the 'fury' inside returning servicemen. Nevertheless, the prominence he affords such discourses in his work suggests his determination to memorialise the scars of war, visible or otherwise, with the same resonance that his uncle's stories had for him.

'I witnessed and participated in darkness that you cannot conceive'

The setting of *Taboo* (a joint creation of Steven Knight, Ridley Scott, and lead actor Tom Hardy) takes place in 1814, at the outset of the nineteenth century. Chronologically, this places it in a quite different space to *Peaky Blinders* as far as attitudes to mental illness are concerned. While the latter's representation of asylums depicts a somewhat primitive and underdeveloped approach to the treatment of psychiatric disorders, this was even more so the case more than a century earlier. The modern medicalisation of mental health was in its infancy in the early nineteenth century; Tom Hardy, who plays protagonist James Delaney and also co-produces the series, summarises prevailing attitudes in the years surrounding *Taboo*'s setting: 'if you had something wrong with you, you were sent to Bedlam and were mad, there was no mental health. You were just fucking mad' (Travers, 2017). 'Bedlam' is the familiar name for Bethlem Royal Hospital, a London hospital for the insane. In tracing the history of Bethlem, Ruggeri (2016) describes how 'Bedlam' became so iconic in the field that it developed as a synonym not only for asylums in general, but also as a kind of idea in a broader sense, 'coming to mean not just "insanity" but chaos in general'. Incarceration in Bedlam was the fate of Delaney's late mother, Salish (Noomi Rapace). According to Michel Foucault in his seminal work *Madness and Civilisation* (1965), the period in which Salish would have been institutionalised was one in which the central purpose of confinement was to physically separate the afflicted from the rest of society, and this physical separation helped to establish the conceptual barrier between madness and rationality. For Foucault, it was only around the turn of the nineteenth century when the confinement of the mentally ill in asylums began to merge with the additional goal of curing madness (as discussed elsewhere in this collection). Thus, for the tentative strides beginning to take place in this period, what we are presented with in *Taboo* is an impoverished and somewhat mystified conception of mental affliction and its treatment.

James Keziah Delaney, the central protagonist of *Taboo*, shares many similarities with Tommy Shelby. Both men are effective strategic planners, and as adept in the use of violence as they are in their plotting. Both have a military background: while Shelby and his brothers were among the many working-class conscripts in the Great War, Delaney was given over into the service of the East India Company as a cadet by his father at a young age. The most significant similarity Delaney shares with Tommy, as far as the concerns of this chapter extend, is that he has undergone traumatic experiences which leave him haunted, with Tom Hardy suggesting that he may be 'so damaged from trauma that his processing is literally the affectation and a symptom of traumatic experience' (Travers, 2017). Like Tommy, Delaney suffers from recurring, nightmarish visions, often involving his dead mother, but also featuring the men who perished in the sinking of a Company ship manned by Delaney, on route to being trafficked into slavery. In one such vision of the latter type, Delaney imagines himself alternately on board a ship taking in water, and in a room surrounded by bodies on mortuary slabs (S1E1). His internal conflicts are made explicit as he attempts to argue against the hallucinations in his own mind, telling them 'I have no fear to feed you with', and speaking in foreign tongues to the figures he sees. As he grows more defiant, Delaney begins walking around the room, pulling sheets from the bodies as he addresses them. The last body he uncovers, that of a large, black male, appears not to be dead at all, as it thrashes and convulses on the slab. Perceiving this unrest, Delaney grows all the more adamant, bringing his face up close to that of the convulsing corpse as he tells it 'you are not here. I have no fear for you and I have no guilt for you.' At this, the corpse opens its eyes and rises, walking slowly and mechanically towards Delaney until it finally faces him, towering over him with manacles and chains clanking. Delaney continues: 'I did as others did and as others had me do, and we are all owned and we have all owned others – so don't you dare judge me.' The imagery interspersed with the confrontation shows water engulfing the men in the ship's hold, as a hand – presumably Delaney's – nails it shut. The hulking apparition only retreats and fades from focus when Delaney points a bloody finger at it, telling it 'today I have work to do'. The bloody hand gives the lie to his claims not to feel guilt, and the 'work' he is setting out to do likely involves the revenge he is plotting against the Company for this and other crimes. Like Tommy Shelby's stark wartime flashbacks of the enemy bursting through the tunnel walls, Delaney's nightmare is clearly framed as a remembered horror, one that has left indelible scarring on his psyche (Figure 14.1).

Notwithstanding the parallels between the two characters, where Shelby and Delaney diverge most sharply is in the latter's position as an outsider in society. Although Shelby is an outlier in some respects, existing as he does outside the law, he still possesses sufficient social acuity to blend in in a variety of environments – including those settings where fear and menace alone are not enough to sustain his position, as seen by his rise in the political sphere. Delaney, while an intelligent and crafty operator, shows little regard for the kind of acceptance in respectable society that Shelby strives toward. Rather, he is regarded as something of an oddball, and a deviant. In his historical account of the development of madness as a concept, Petteri Pietikainen observes that, consistently throughout human history, 'people who have been perceived and treated as mad have behaved in ways that deviate from the so-called average behaviour more than the strictures of normality allow' (Pietikainen, 2015: 3). This is certainly true in the case of

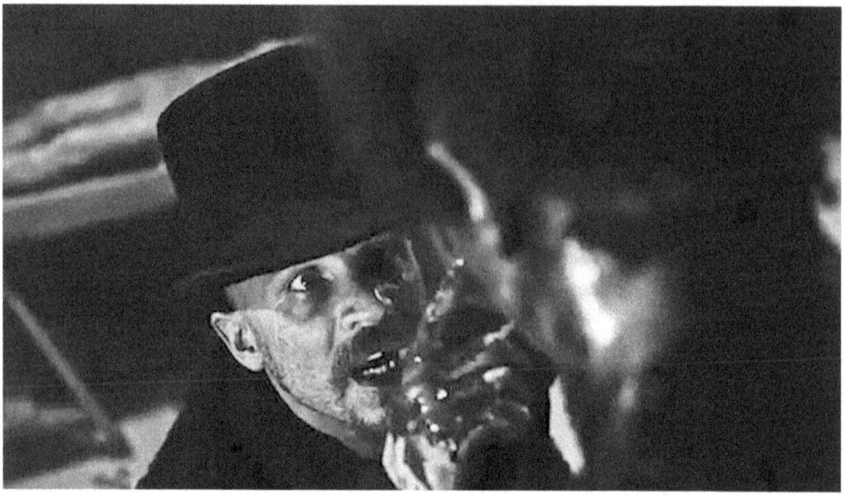

Figure 14.1 James Delaney confronts his visions (*Taboo*)

James Delaney: the title of the series alludes to the proscribed behaviours he is implied to have partaken in, such as incest and cannibalism, and he seems to have little concern for refuting or dispelling the rumours which circulate around such predilections. Delaney is associated strongly with the exotic and mythologised Other, particularly in light of his return from Africa: James's contemptuous and envious brother-in-law, Thorne, refers to Delaney pejoratively as 'that animal from Africa' and 'that nigger', while an East India Company board member speculates about his 'true savage nature' in the course of tracing Delaney's history with the Company (S1E1). These slurs harken back to the theme of dehumanisation in Knight's work, in this case drawing parallels between the shunning and isolation of the 'mad' and the apparent disdain with which ruling classes and members of 'respectable' society perceive the colonies in the text.

Though he appears unremarkably Caucasian, Delaney's mother is Native American, purchased by his father as part of the trade which also saw him take ownership of the contentious territory of Nootka Sound. Like Nootka Sound itself, Salish Delaney is spoken about in the series but never seen (except in the feverish hallucinations of her son), and is similarly perceived as something mysterious and dangerous. The racialised discourses pervading around Delaney associate him with foreign behaviours and practices – his torso is etched with tribal tattoos, and he appears to engage in ritualistic murmurings around the dead – and position him as heathen to the religious hegemony of contemporary society. As such, Delaney is often referred to as 'the devil'. Deviancy and otherness is a threat that must be cast out; while confinement such as befell Salish Delaney is one means by which this might have been achieved in the period, we are also presented with a more aggressively theistic model of 'treatment' when a vengeful, cuckolded Thorne Geary (Jefferson Hall) attempts to 'cure' his wife Zilpha (Oona Chaplin) of her attraction to her brother, James, by pronouncing her possessed by demons (S1E5). When an increasingly jealous and humiliated Thorne grows progressively more cruel in his treatment of his recalcitrant wife, including beating and apparently raping her, he finally brings in a supposed exorcist to drive the imagined demons out of Zilpha. The ordeal she undergoes, in which she is roughly restrained by her husband and clumsily groped by the 'exorcist' as he chants Latin mantras atop her, underscores an uncomfortable irony in some of the bizarre and disturbing treatments historically visited upon individuals declared insane by those supposedly of sound mind. The fact it is the increasingly hysterical Thorne who pronounces his wife as 'mad' in this instance also raises troubling questions about the gender politics underlying the ways in which madness has historically been conceptualised, particularly where recourse is taken to institutionalisation: Marland (2013) notes that women in the Georgian period were at risk of being admitted to private asylums on minimal evidence, 'notably those who contravened expectations concerning their modesty, conduct, duties or behaviour or those who would not bend to their husbands' will'. By the nineteenth century, the proportion of female admissions had risen, and along with the aforementioned social and cultural pressures, 'women were deemed likely to fall prey to disorders of the mind related to their biological vulnerability and the female life cycle'. Though other characters speak sympathetically of the late Horace Delaney, it is clear that James blames his father at least in part for his mother's institutionalisation, so the theme of men exercising this punitive diagnostic power over their spouses in *Taboo* seems to be one that crosses generations.

'They blew God right out of my head'

Religious belief, or absence thereof, is a recurrent theme in Knight's work, one which is often entangled with the way crises of the mind are represented. This entanglement is perhaps most starkly vocalised in *Peaky Blinders* when Danny Whizz-bang laments his inability to pray, because of 'those fucking guns – they blew God right out of my head' (S1E1). Just as the war left its indelible imprint on the psyches of those consumed by its devastation, it also severely impacted religious faith in the people and places it touched. While some found refuge in their faith, others turned to fatalism. For many, 'the futility and brutality of the lethal conflict destroyed any vestige of faith' (Shaw, 2014). This disparity of personal responses and subject positions is encapsulated in the Shelby family and again is acutely bound up with issues of internal strife.

At numerous points of the series, Tommy Shelby reaffirms his personal tendency toward fatalistic rationalism, which stands in contrast to the religious faith of other family members (most notably Arthur and Polly). However, one senses his insistence that religion is 'a foolish answer to a foolish question' (S3E3) is as much an attempt to erect a bulwark against the sporadically irrational workings of his mind as it is a sincere profession of faithlessness; after all, there are other aspects of his belief system which contradict his apparent adherence to logic above all, such as his insistence that 'a black cat dream is never wrong' after he has a supposedly symbolic premonition of coming betrayal by a family member (S5E2). Shelby seeks in rationalism a reliable barrier against the visions, paranoia, and superstitious mysticism that increasingly intrude upon his thoughts, particularly as his criminal career progresses and the casualties mount up. This stands in stark contrast to his brother Arthur, whose periodic turns toward devout Christianity are explicitly positioned as increasingly doomed efforts to resist his pathological violent tendencies. The ineffectuality of this strategy for Arthur is made clear when, with his marriage in crisis, he confronts a Quaker he suspects of sleeping with his exasperated wife Linda (S5E3). After brutally beating and ultimately maiming the man, Arthur begins to wail despairingly over his prostrate victim: 'I'm a good man … a God-fearing man. There is good in my heart! But these hands … these hands belong to the Devil!' Arthur's vocalisation here of a struggle between body and soul, in biblical terms a clash between God and the Devil, represents his attempts to make sense of the mental anguish that manifests in his own brutality. Whether his search for God is an attempt to find a stable focus for his troubled mind or a desperate hope for divine intervention against his many vices, each relapse he undergoes seems to take Arthur more violently and decisively towards an unhappy fate. The notion of being fated to madness, and in particular the role of religious symbolism in this, seems to be an underlying belief in the Shelby family; Arthur and Tommy's mother is said to have believed that it was their gypsy ancestors who made the nails for Jesus's crucifix, and thus they are cursed never to be still or settled 'or the guilt catches up with you' (S5E6). Periodic returns to superstitious explanations for mental disturbance underscore the uncertainty belying the Shelby family's brash exterior, but also speak to an enduring ambiguity in Knight's representation of the issue. The mythic, poetic aspects of the text occasionally invest superstition and folk tradition with some ambivalent semblance of credence and stand as a persistent counter-narrative to the rationalist medical discourse also apparent in the work.

'All of those that I gather are damned'

The implication that madness is fated lends itself naturally to the more ethereal and enigmatic aspects of Steven Knight's narratives, along with phenomena like Polly's supposed 'second sight' or the allusions to James Delaney's apparent ability to communicate telepathically with his sister and father. The notion of people as 'damned' from birth would certainly seem to provide justification for the fatalistic worldview of characters like Tommy Shelby. However, such speculations are underpinned by more sober diagnoses about the nature of cross-generational affliction. Recent medical research by the Cross-Disorder Group of the Psychiatric Genomes Consortium has found that significant psychiatric disorders such as bipolar disorder, schizophrenia, and major depressive disorder may be genetically linked (*The Lancet*, 2013), with the coda that these genetic risk factors are not in isolation enough to predict such conditions, but may increase susceptibility in combination with particular environmental factors. The idea that mental illness may indeed be hereditary is implied very strongly in the characterisation of Knight's protagonists. In *Peaky Blinders*' fifth season, Tommy, who has been spiralling into depression and despair as the series progresses, finally learns from Charlie that his mother ended her own life when Tommy was a child. 'She just stepped into the canal', he tells him. More pointedly, he informs him that 'your grandfather, he went the same way – suicide. Sometimes these things run in the family' (S5E6). As previously discussed, we are made aware throughout the series that Tommy has been contemplating suicide, tempting death more recklessly than usual on several occasions, and in earlier years Arthur has attempted suicide at least twice.

In James Delaney's case, it is suggested that both parents suffered from mental disturbances to varying degrees. As early as *Taboo*'s first episode, we learn that his mother was previously committed to Bedlam, with an East India Company official emphasising the implication of hereditary madness in telling the board that 'in temperament, he takes after his mad mother', and surmising that Delaney's growing confidence as a youth 'allowed his mother's madness to emerge' (S1E1). As well as Salish 'Anna' Delaney's instability (which had apparently made her a danger to the young James as well as to herself), it is also strongly implied that his father increasingly lost his mind to paranoia and grief in his later years. Brace, the Delaney family's loyal steward, describes the late Horace as 'a madman' who 'was half human in the end', and would 'make deals with ghosts in the flames'. Although inheritance came to prominence in psychiatry gradually over the course of the nineteenth century, historian Theodore Porter insists that heredity in mental ailments was already an established 'folk category' by

1800 (Porter, 2018), with family members of asylum patients often reporting other afflictions in the family (perceived or otherwise) to doctors as potential contributing factors; so this theory would likely have had at least some traction in popular discourse at the time of *Taboo*'s setting. More recently, studies have found that the risk for psychiatric disorders such as bipolar disorder or schizophrenia, which is typically around 1 per cent for the general population, increases to around 15 per cent when one parent is afflicted, and up to 50 per cent in cases where both parents are sufferers (Barlow-Stewart, 2012). In James Delaney's case, the risk would seem to be at the high end of this scale, depending on the specific nature of his parents' disorders. Both Horace and James appear to experience hallucinatory visions and communicate with apparitions, suggesting some degree of crossover between their maladies. Viewed from this more rationalistic perspective, then, the tormented protagonists of *Taboo* and *Peaky Blinders* are not so much 'damned' as they are placed at a heightened risk of sustained mental illness due to a troubled family history. Most likely, it is the extreme violence and brutality that these characters are steeped in from an early age that provide the trigger to realise that risk.

'In all the world, violent men are the easiest to deal with'

The connection between violence and mental illness is a consistent theme within Knight's work, and much of the trauma we encounter therein is framed as a consequence of the suffering or infliction of violence. Helen McCrory, who played Polly (she sadly died recently) has suggested that the mental disturbances experienced by characters like Tommy and Arthur function within the narrative as a punishment of sorts; considering the rationale behind what she calls the 'disgusting' violence depicted in the series, McCrory argued that 'you should have the people who are responsible for the violence unable to self-medicate or having mental health problems, or all the things that do happen if you kill other people' (Harp et al., 2018). Violence, particularly in its most extreme form, is presented as both a cause and a symptom of mental disturbance. As previously discussed, Arthur's unprovoked mauling of Linda's Quaker friend provokes his hysterical outburst about having the Devil's hands. In the case of Tommy, while we regularly see him kill dispassionately in the name of personal gain or self-preservation, the first time we see him personally driven to an act of savage, sadistic violence has particular resonance for this issue. The event occurs when he attempts to blind a bound and defenceless Vincente Changretta (S3E3) after a hitman working for Vincente (Kenneth Colley) botches an attempt on Tommy's life, the misfire resulting in the death of Tommy's wife,

Grace (Annabel Wallis). Although blinding is an established tactic that gives the Shelby gang their name, this is the first time in the series we see Tommy attempt it, and it is made clear that the brutality is motivated more by a grief-crazed lust for revenge than as a stark message to deter the Changrettas or other gangs from trying similar attacks in future. The series' anachronistic soundtrack plays no small part in adding resonance to the depiction of Tommy's mental turmoil here, particularly through the use in the scene of Nick Cave's stirring song 'Tupelo'; the lyrics of the song ominously reference 'a big black cloud come', and 'distant thunder', which rumbles 'hungry like the beast'. The volatility and sense of brooding dread evoked by the lyrics echo the storm raging in Tommy's head. As the scene progresses and Tommy's bloodlust boils, we see him increasingly experiencing a kind of mania, self-reproach, and uncharacteristic rage as he finally storms toward Changretta with his blade at the ready, before the act is ultimately prevented by a merciful bullet from Arthur's gun, killing the Italian before Tommy can torture him. The scene underscores the cyclical nature of violence as the death of reason: the usually calculating Tommy is driven mad with grief as a result of the chaos unleashed by his cold, dispassionate acts in the past.

Knight himself echoes McCrory's framing of trauma as the 'consequences' of inflicting violence 'rather than the characters dusting themselves off and they're fine again' (Jenkins, 2019). In this reading, then, the parallels between warfare and urban gang culture are made explicit not only in the extreme violence of both, but also in the depiction of their after-effects. Smith (2017) argues that this was a familiar concern within contemporary society in regard to the 'damaged man' returning to society in the aftermath of war: 'the attraction of the alienated demobilised soldier to the criminal underworld or to political violence was something feared by many across the Western world and has continued to shape how we see the returned soldier in the socio-economic and political chaos that plagued the inter-war period' (Smith, 2017: 279).

James Delaney is also shown to be capable of acts of extreme brutality which reinforce the perceptions his peers hold of him as animalistic, primarily revealed in the savage fashion in which he deals with would-be assassins. A Malay working for the East India Company is ultimately dispatched when a wounded Delaney tears his throat out with his teeth, while a larger thug who temporarily incapacitates Delaney with a club ends up mutilated with knives and disembowelled against a post. In contrast to the previous discussion of *Peaky Blinders*, there is no explicit suggestion that these acts of savagery have any identifiable consequences for Delaney's state of mind, although it should be noted that he is more consistently depicted as 'mad' throughout the series than Shelby is: perhaps Delaney's ability to engage in extreme violence without easily identifiable mental consequences is testament to the degree of damage to his psyche already done by the time we are first introduced to the character. It is arguable that this, along with his apparent 'shamanistic' qualities and recklessness, is the 'gift' that Delaney has been darkly blessed with through madness. Just as the post-war society feared the damaged man irreversibly altered by exposure to the netherworld of war, so 'the devil Delaney' is feared for his prolonged exposure to the dark continent, ostensibly for Orientalist fears that he has 'gone native'. In reality, the damage in this latter case has been done in no small part, not dissimilarly to the Shelbys, by the brutalisation inherent in exposure to the crimes and culture of colonial militarism in service of the East India Company.

In Delaney's case, then, trauma provides a kind of inoculation, and we can see a similar development in Polly Gray in the wake of her late reprieve from the gallows (S4E1). In Polly's case, the trauma is caused not by lethal violence committed by her, but by that threatened and almost inflicted upon her. In the gallows scene, Polly's immediate horror turns to a kind of euphoria as she begins communicating with visions, imploring that they use the hanging rope to pull her up to heaven. After she is saved at the last minute by Tommy's manoeuvring, she initially struggles to cope with the banalities of everyday life, retreating into substance abuse and a flirtation with the supernatural, holding séances and talking to apparitions. Interestingly, Tommy's prospective solution to this is for Michael to 'believe the spirits are real – believe it with her'. In contrast to his own adherence to cold rationalism in his efforts to keep his torment at bay, he proposes indulgence of Polly's otherworldly dabbling as a means of distraction from the horrific memory of her brush with death, and this is indicative of his paternalistic, arguably patronising tendencies toward Polly as separate from the Shelby men. However, Polly's ultimate means of dealing with the trauma is to develop the kind of fatalistic attitude which Tommy himself brought back from the war: 'I was dead in that noose, and then I was saved. So everything from now on is extra. What I didn't understand until today is when you're dead already, you're free' (S4E2). Throughout the series, Polly has been positioned as a mirror to Tommy in her stabilising, authoritative influence on the family, assuming control of the Shelby business while the men were away at war, though it is clear that this has not always been acknowledged or appreciated because of the gender politics of the period. The final tragedy for Polly is for this closeness to be revealed most emphatically in shared trauma.

Conclusion

Madness is a persistent theme in Knight's work, with the repeated presence of Tom Hardy acting as an intertextual reminder of this: Hardy's characters from *Locke* to *Taboo* and *Peaky Blinders* display various degrees of mental disturbance, with even the oddball charisma of Alfie Solomons a feint from the pervasive instability and paranoia which becomes ever more evident as the series progresses. Knight invites viewers to draw connections across his texts, and also across epochs: even across the divergent timeframes of *Taboo* and *Peaky Blinders* we see commonalities between the degraded institutionalisation of Salish Delaney and Barney Thompson, and between the brutalisation in service of the state and its organs undergone by James Delaney and the Shelby brothers. But beyond the timeframes ostensibly represented, Knight uses history symbolically as a mirror to the present day: much as *Peaky Blinders*' representation of the rise of Moseley draws parallels with the polarisation of Western politics in recent times, so too does Knight's treatment of issues like war trauma invite comparisons with PTSD suffered by combatants in places like Afghanistan, which he researched while working on *Hummingbird*. According to Knight, the recollections of some of the afflicted Royal Marine commandos he interviewed for the film 'shaped the personalities and demons of Tommy and Arthur Shelby' (Allen, 2018), indicating his desire not only to elucidate contemporary concerns through a period lens, but to draw attention to the aspects of our culture which appear stubbornly resistant to change over time. Knight's tendency towards mythologised and occasionally universalised narratives functions as a means of impressing the resonance of these comparisons on his audience.

References

Allen, M. (2018). 'The dark, emotional forces that haunt Tommy Shelby in Peaky Blinders are still prevalent 100 years on', *BBC Sounds*, www.bbc.co.uk/programmes/articles/14fK3CnYGqryd95SkcVr89B/the-dark-emotional-forces-that-haunt-tommy-shelby-in-peaky-blinders-are-still-prevalent-100-years-on (accessed 17 January 2020).

Barlow-Stewart, K. (2012). 'Mental illness and inherited predisposition – schizophrenia and bipolar disorder', Centre for Genetics Education, www.genetics.edu.au/genetics/Genetic-conditions-support-groups/FS58KBS.pdf (accessed 2 September 2019).

Cross-Disorder Group of the Psychiatric Genomics Consortium (2013). 'Identification of risk loci with shared effects on five major psychiatric disorders: a genome-wide analysis', *The Lancet*, 28 February, DOI: https://doi.org/10.1016/S0140-6736(12)62129-1 (accessed 20 September 2019).

Ellis, J. (2013). 'BBC goes steampunk: Ripper Street, Peaky Blinders and the memorialisation of history', *CST* Online, https://cstonline.net/bbc-goes-steampunk-ripper-street-peaky-blinders-and-the-memorialisation-of-history-by-john-ellis/ (accessed 2 March 2019).

Foucault, M. (1965). *Madness and Civilisation: A History of Insanity in the Age of Reason* (New York: Vintage).

Harp, J., et al. (2019). 'Peaky Blinders season 5 star says show is "disgustingly violent" and that's just how it should be', *Digital Spy*, www.digitalspy.com/tv/a28651996/peaky-blinders-season-5-star-show-disgustingly-violent/ (accessed 15 January 2020).

Jenkins, K. (2019). 'Peaky Blinders creator defends violence after cast member labels it "disgusting"', *Mirror*, www.mirror.co.uk/tv/peaky-blinders-creator-defends-violence-18954217 (accessed 3 September 2019).

Long, P. (2017). 'Class, place and history in the imaginative landscapes of Peaky Blinders', in D. Forrest and B. Johnson (eds), *Social Class and Television Drama in Contemporary Britain* (London: Palgrave Macmillan).

Marland, H. (2013). 'Women and madness', Warwick University Centre for the History of Medicine, https://warwick.ac.uk/fac/arts/history/chm/outreach/trade_in_lunacy/research/womenandmadness/ (accessed 20 August 2019).

Meyer, J. (2014). 'Shell shock, emotional resilience and the cultural memory of the First World War: A literary perspective', Freud Museum London: *Psychoanalysis Podcasts*, www.freud.org.uk/2014/10/02/shell-shock-emotional-resilience-cultural-memory-first-world-war-literary-perspective/ (accessed 14 January 2020).

Nielson, C. (2014). 'The other war dead: Asylum patients during the First World War', *Beyond The Trenches*, http://beyondthetrenches.co.uk/the-other-war-dead-asylum-patients-during-the-first-world-war/ (accessed 9 September 2019).

Peaky Blinders (2013–2019). BBC.

Pietikainen, P. (2015). *Madness: A History* (Abingdon: Routledge).

Porter, T. (2018). 'Theodore Porter on genetics in the madhouse', Princeton University Press, https://press.princeton.edu/ideas/theodore-porter-on-genetics-in-the-madhouse (accessed 17 January 2020).

Ruggeri, A. (2016). 'How Bedlam became "a palace for lunatics"', BBC, www.bbc.com/culture/story/20161213-how-bedlam-became-a-palace-for-lunatics (accessed 3 July 2019).

Shaw, M. (2014). 'Faith, belief and superstition', British Library, www.bl.uk/world-war-one/articles/faith-belief-and-superstition (accessed 14 March 2019).

Singh, A. (2017). 'Taboo writer Steven Knight: Blood and guts is the modern way to do costume drama', *Telegraph*, https://telegraph.co.uk/tv/2017/01/06/taboo-writer-blood-guts-modern-way-do-costume-drama/ (accessed 14 March 2019).

Smith, E. (2017). '"Brutalised" veterans and tragic anti-heroes: Masculinity, crime and post-war trauma in Boardwalk Empire and Peaky Blinders', in M. Walsh and A. Varnava (eds), *The Great War and the British Empire: Culture and Society* (Abingdon: Routledge).

Taboo (2017). BBC.

Taddeo, J. (2018). '"The war is done. Shut the door on it!": The Great War, masculinity and trauma in British period television', in K. Byrne, J. Leggott, and J. Taddeo (eds), *Conflicting Masculinities: Men in British Television Period Drama* (London and New York: I.B. Tauris).

Travers, B. (2017). 'A chat With Tom Hardy: Is his "Taboo" killer a true shaman or "just f***ing mad"?' *IndieWire*, www.indiewire.com/2017/02/tom-hardy-interview-taboo-shaman-madman-1201783839/ (accessed 6 September 2019).

Wright, J. (2016). 'Peaky Blinders: Behind the scenes with creator Steven Knight', *HistoryExtra*, www.historyextra.com/period/20th-century/peaky-blinders-behind-the-scenes-with-creator-steven-knight/ (accessed 6 September 2019).

15

Bitter living through science: melodramatic and moral readings of gay conversion therapy in *A Place to Call Home*

Gordon R. Alley-Young

On 28 April 2013, *A Place to Call Home* (*APTCH*) (2013–2018) premiered at 8:30 PM in *Downton Abbey*'s (*DA*) timeslot on Australian TV. *APTCH* revolves around Sarah Adams (Marta Dusseldorp) who meets the Bligh family of Ash Park, Inverness, members of Australia's squattocracy, while nursing on a ship sailing from England to Australia in 1953 (S1E1). Sarah bonds with widower George (Brett Climo) while treating his formidable mother Elizabeth (Noni Hazlehurst). One evening, Sarah stops George's son James (David Berry), a closeted homosexual travelling with English bride Oliva (Arianwen Parkes-Lockwood), from death by suicide. Post-voyage, Sarah's Catholic mother rejects her for converting to Judaism so Sarah takes a district nursing job near the Blighs. Elizabeth blocks Sarah's access to the family fearing she will expose James's secret. While George and Sarah's difficult road to happiness is *APTCH*'s main storyline, this chapter focuses on James's struggle to change, and later accept, his homosexuality. Specifically, how James's homosexuality is medically pathologised will be analysed using media, moral, medical/scientific, and socio-cultural discourses of the era. This includes considering the verisimilitude of James's experience and the efficacy of representing it within a historical/period drama that critics have labelled a soap opera or melodrama. Understanding James's storyline, and those he represents, requires understanding how post-war Australian society was defined by one's place in the white heteronormative family.

The white heteronormative family in post-war Australia

Post-war Australian society was built around the white, middle-class, heteronormative, nuclear, patriarchal family (Arrow, 2018). The working poor, people of colour, and gender/sexual non-conformers were marginalised as social ills (Arrow, 2018). Victorian sexual attitudes (i.e., the female body as morally/physically vulnerable; homosexuality as illness) persisted into the twentieth century (Brown, 2015; Featherstone, 2010). The Victorian social order opposed suffrage and declining birth rates as threats to this heteronormative family (Featherstone, 2010). Yet upholding the mantle of the heteronormative family was difficult, as a 1944 Australian government medical inquiry learned when it received 1,400 letters from women seeking family planning (Arrow, 2018). Concurrently, doctors (1940–1970) started to problematise women as sexually frigid (Margolin, 2017). Post-war society expected large families, women's domesticity, and male dominance.

Australia lacked family support programmes from the 1930s to the 1970s and women became solely responsible for childcare while the children of widowed/abandoned/unwed mothers and single fathers (i.e., deemed ineffective as caretakers) were often put into state care (SSCCA, 2005). This relegated women to domestic roles, many after having left wartime workplaces (e.g., Australian Women's Land Army). As Friedan (1963) argued, foisting such domestic role expectations on women, post-WWII, created a disillusioned and unhappy generation of women. Alternately, Haggett (2009), in her study of post-war British wives/mothers, found that women cited partner infidelity, marriage breakdown, partner's mental health, marriage migration (i.e., to the US/Australia), and consecutive pregnancies more often than domesticity as aggravating factors for their anxiety and depression.

Post-war men and women faced increased scrutinisation of their socially prescribed gender roles. Heteronormative society, in facing some of these challenges, turned to medical science for answers. For instance, Australian courts and society struggled to understand male homosexuality with the courts alternating between behavioural (i.e., penetration) and mental health (i.e., illness) definitions of homosexuality (Smaal, 2013). US and Australian psychoanalysts and psychiatrists, influenced by Freud's attempts to cure some forms of homosexuality in the 1920s, attempted to *cure* homosexuals, rather than imprison them, in the 1950s onward and thus return them to the heterosexual social order (Rubinstein, 2010; Smaal, 2013).

Today medical science largely rejects sexual orientation change efforts (SOCE) as brutal interventions justified by pseudo-science/medicine and religious organisations (McDermott, 2018). SOCE included insulin comas, lobotomies, electroconvulsive therapy, shocks, anti-psychotic drugs, induced vomiting, and chemical castration that were used in the name of medical treatment from the 1950s to the 1970s, when they fell into disuse medically when the pathologising of homosexuality was challenged (Dean, 2016; McDermott, 2018; Scot, 2017). Wartime codebreaker Alan Turing died by suicide two years after being chemically castrated in 1952, and many previously healthy lobotomy patients required lifelong care (Dean, 2016; Scot, 2017). Esterberg (1990) finds in her study of the first nine years (1956–1965) of the first US publication for lesbians, *The Ladder*, that the early issues of the magazine reflected, unquestioned, the medical profession's diagnosis of homosexuality as a mental illness, a fact that she argues likely caused enormous damage to readers (i.e., who were being told they were mentally ill). Jennings (2015) notes that from 1956 onward *The Ladder* had an Australian readership as evidenced by reader letters, and subsequently some Australian readers reported having their copies of this and other LGBTQ+ magazines seized by customs in the 1960s.

SOCE endured even though Freud had said that homosexuality was not an illness in 1935 and after medical/social activists had homosexuality declassified as a mental illness in 1973 (Chiang, 2008; Vider and Byers, 2015). From the 1970s onward, religious organisations adopted SOCE practices, using SOCE's previous associations with medical science as a claim to its legitimacy (McDermott, 2018). In 2018 members of Victoria, Australia's Liberal Party, tried (unsuccessfully) to legislate to allow legal access to SOCE for children (Hegarty, 2018). SOCE is not relegated to medical history, for as recently as 2008 a doctor in Sydney, Australia, Dr Mark Christopher James Craddock, was banned from medical practice after prescribing chemical castration to treat an eighteen-year-old patient's homosexuality (i.e., Cyprostat, a drug that lowers libido by reducing testosterone) (Petersen, 2012). Many Australians have recently come forward with accounts of enduring electroconvulsive therapy (also called electroshock therapy) and/or chemically induced nausea in response to homosexual stimuli to cure homosexuality from the 1950s to the 1970s at the hands of Australian doctors, care homes, and religious institutions (Daley, 2018; Donovan, 2015; Hegarty, 2018).

A Place to Call Home depicts how LGBTQ+ people (and progressive women) were perceived as threats to the dominant heteronormative social order and thus subject to interventions or eradication by intersecting and interdependent moral and medical discourses. James, as a closeted homosexual, is forced to live an inauthentic heterosexual public life all the while fearing exposure and social death. James seeks SOCE doctors who would cripple him mentally, emotionally, and physically to make him fit into his heteronormative family using barbaric methods. Ultimately *APTCH* criticises the 1950s post-war Australian family and champions its evolution. By series' end, *APTCH* presents a reconfigured Bligh family based on fellowship, cultural diversity, inclusion, and community support as the basis for family and community health.

Melodrama, medicine, and the marriage survey

APTCH's emotional intensity and relational focus (i.e., melodrama) have led television critics in the US and Australia to define the series as soap opera/melodrama (Blundell, 2016; Hale, 2017). Soap operas originally were daytime radio/TV serials sponsored by soap companies but today this label has been expanded to include serial TV dramas, dealing with home/family/intimacy issues in melodramatic fashion (Soukup, 2016). Critics, however, question the usefulness of melodrama for mediating LGBTQ+ lives. Johnson (2013) argues that TV critics stereotype gay audiences with graphic sexuality and melodrama, and thus dismiss programmes like *Queer as Folk* (*QAF*, 1999–2000) despite the fact that they tackle important social issues. Cherniavaky (1998) argues that HIV/AIDS melodrama fails in trying to domesticate HIV+ gay masculinity as heteronormative reproductive femininity. Similarly, Skvirsky (2008) argues that while melodrama provides satisfying moral clarity with its virtuous victims, it is not suited to contemporary injustice. Ultimately, LGBTQ+ lives are more complex than victim archetypes and discrimination is more complex than social ostracism. While *APTCH* participates in domesticated heteronormative constructions of LGBTQ+ relationships (e.g., Henry Polson [Dominic Allburn] and Dr Harry Fox [Tim Draxl]), characters also break from these archetypal models to define their own relational happiness and success (e.g., James).

James's public–private life divide fits the classic melodrama protagonist, initially and stoically choosing conformity over happiness (i.e., suffering in silence) (Simmons, 2005; Skvirsky, 2008). James asks his aunt for a doctor for Olivia's 'anxiety' but he's actually seeking out SOCE for himself (S1E12). The first day in the clinic, James receives electroconvulsive therapy (S1E13). The Blighs are dissuaded from visiting and when they do James is sedated in an insulin coma (S2E2). Subsequently, James vomits as he views gay images (S2E3), and his doctor is shown planning a trans-orbital lobotomy (S2E3) before George intervenes (S2E4). After SOCE James is weak, has flashbacks, and electroconvulsive therapy has erased memories of his ex-lover, farmhand Harry Polson (S4E5).

James's SOCE storyline fits melodramatic conventions of private suffering and emotional storytelling, but not of exaggeration. Actual SOCE survivor accounts are more extreme. SOCE survivors report receiving shocks directly to their genitals while seeing homoerotic images, some being forced to marry, and others feeling suicidal afterwards (Hegarty, 2018; Jones et al., 2018). LGBTQ+ US federal employees (1950–1960) could be fired and committed to St Elizabeth's, Washington DC's federally funded psychiatric hospital, like Thomas H. Tattersall who spent weeks in insulin comas (McDermott, 2018). Dr Walter Freeman, who created and popularised the trans-orbital lobotomy with Dr James Watts, began his career at St Elizabeth's; 30 to 40 per cent of Freeman's lobotomies were on LGBTQ+ people, many of whom required extensive aftercare (McDermott, 2018; Scot, 2017).

Johnson (2013) argues, though critics disagree, that melodramas can realistically depict LGBTQ+ health issues. The scholarship supports *APTCH*'s depiction of SOCE medicine as accurate and even *APTCH*'s frivolous plotlines symbolise real post-war anxieties. For example, drug-addicted, hypersexual villain Regina (Jenni Baird) reifies societal fears about post-war female promiscuity (i.e., the unscrupulous temptress) and addiction (Romm, 2015; Trickey, 2018). Regina's madness and institutionalisation symbolise the perception of unattached women in the 1950s as social outliers. British expat Olivia's fears about her son Georgie's illegitimacy and James's homosexuality symbolise fears of surviving in 1950s society without blood, marital, or shared cultural bonds to a heteronormative family. When Anna becomes pregnant before marriage with her future husband Gino's (Aldo Mignone) baby (S1E10) she considers abortion before she accidentally miscarries (S1E12). After their marriage, Gino learns the miscarriage left Anna unable to bear children, so he annuls their marriage. Later Anna is happily surprised to find herself single and pregnant and initially, she faces her family's and society's disapproval. James's amnesia (a plot device typical of soap operas) symbolises the erasure of LGBTQ+ people from the family/society. Medicine and religion both promoted large families and suppressed homosexuality via SOCE from the 1950s onward (Jones et al., 2018). *Call the Midwife* (2012–) also explores amnesia within LGBTQ+ relationships when Delia Busby (Kate Lamb) temporarily forgets her lover Patience 'Patsy' Mount (Emerald Fennell) after a car accident (S4 and S5). Johnson (2013) argues that melodrama's capacity to engage viewers emotionally (e.g., love lost through amnesia or other narrative devices), creates an outlet for long-silenced voices via connections to LGBTQ+ characters.

APTCH aired James's SOCE plot around the same year, 2014, as *Downton Abbey*'s butler Thomas Barrow (Rob James-Collier) discovers a newspaper advert urging him to Choose Your Own Path (S5E3). Brown (2015) argues that period dramas *Downton Abbey* and *Upstairs, Downstairs* (*UD*, 1971–1975) write homosexual and hidden lives back while negotiating both historical and modern morals. For example, in *UD* when head maid Rose equates footman Alfred's homosexuality with mental illness (i.e., she says he's 'not right in the head' [S3E5]), she echoes 1970s audiences' attitudes (i.e., homosexuality was only declassified as a mental illness in 1973). Similarly, when Thomas in *DA* develops an abscess from injecting a useless cure, Miss Baxter's (Raquel Cassidy) empathy and respect for Thomas reflects modern acceptance of LGBTQ+ people. Tempering this twenty-first-century attitude with some twentieth-century realism, Dr Clarkson, however (David Robb), is pessimistically tolerant in advising Thomas to accept his unchangeable lot and make the best life possible (S5E6). Alternately, just as Thomas is attempting to 'cure' himself, Lady Mary (Michelle Dockery) is compelled by Dr Marie Stopes's book *Married Love or Love in Marriage* (Stopes, 1918) to purchase a diaphragm so she can have sex with prospective fiancée Anthony Gillingham (Tom Cullen) (S5E2). Stopes's (1918) work was progressive for encouraging women to take charge of family planning and for advocating that women and men have a right to enjoy sexual pleasure as these things, Stopes (1918) argued, would strengthen the heterosexual couple bond. However, unfortunately, Stopes was also known for advocating eugenics, including the elimination of homosexuals whom she grouped together with perverts (Williams, 2011). Stopes likely would have supported Lady Mary's sexual freedom but not Thomas's or James's.

Meanwhile, as the conservative voice at Downton, head butler Mr Carson (Jim Carter), who previously called Thomas 'foul' (S3E8), grew up (b. 1856) with the miasma theory of disease (i.e., foul-looking air transmitted diseases like cholera) (Halliday, 2001). The word 'foul' connotes Thomas with decay/disease/contagion, blends medical and moral discourses, and reflects Carson's Edwardian morals/beliefs. After germ theory overtook miasma theory in the late nineteenth century, urban exploration writers still conflated visible dirt, poverty, disease, and moral decay, thus linking physical and spiritual uncleanliness (Kvistad, 2018). Miasma beliefs surface in *APTCH* when James's lover Harry is evicted by his sister Evie and her fiancé Burt (i.e., 'cleaning house') (S1E12). Burt calls Harry filth and Evie states that Harry cannot be around her son Collin (i.e., risk of infection). Later in the series when Harry is gay-bashed and Sarah goes to him, she is told by a nurse that Harry was beaten in a laneway (i.e., an alley), the nurse adding, 'the sort of place his type do their filth' (S4E3). The nurse's comment conflates a dirty urban space with a homosexual act she perceives to be morally perverse. The connection of dirt and morality is made visually with James in various scenes in the SOCE clinic when he looks dirty and dishevelled in vomit-stained pyjamas (Figure 15.1).

Twentieth-century medicine theorised homosexuality in three main ways: as stunted development (i.e., sexual immaturity), as natural variation (i.e., people are born this way), or as pathology (i.e., a disease requiring mental health attention) (Drescher, 2015). Theorists, some morally opposing homosexuality, labelled potential internal defects (e.g., intrauterine hormonal exposure) or external pathogenic agents (e.g., excessive/hostile parenting) as causes of homosexuality (Drescher, 2015). When homosexuality was declassified as a mental illness in 1973 the discourse of pathology persisted. For example, Ehrlich's (1980) pro-LGBTQ+ research framed closeted homosexuality as a pathogenic secret that causes physical and psychological dysfunction. Also, biologist, Paul W. Ewald, and physicist, Gregory Cochran, controversially hypothesised, without proof, that a germ/pathogen may cause homosexuality (Crain, 1999).

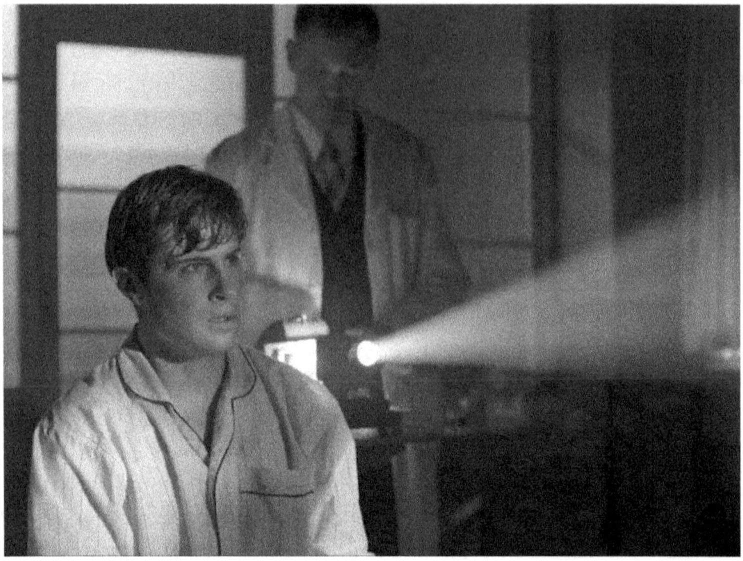

Figure 15.1 James is bombarded with homosexual images while being dosed with vomit-inducing drugs (*A Place to Call Home*)

APTCH's Dr Milson (Andrew McFarlane) blends pathology and moral discourse when justifying SOCE, saying, 'Your kind lacks moral fibre, James, and I'm here to provide it for you' and 'You are not the deviant within. We will defeat him, together' (S2E2). The latter comment equates homosexuality with psychological/spiritual possession and frames SOCE as medical exorcism. SOCE leaves James rigidly heteronormatively moral so when Dr Henry Fox's gay male friends wrestle at the beach James gives a disapproving look. Henry's friend, a minister, notices James's look and reframes the scene ('it's just playfulness. It's not sexuality' and 'We come in all shapes and sizes, James' [S4E2]). Here James's SOCE storyline shifts from pathologising homosexuality to a discourse of natural variation. James's reaction (i.e., when Henry's friend says, 'Even our own sometimes fear us', he is addressing James's reaction) is framed as a pathogenic secret.

Not all period dramas, however, reinforce dominant discourses of homosexuality as illness. *Father Brown* (2013–), set in the 1950s Cotswolds, blends moral and medical discourse when Father Brown (Mark Williams) offers to listen non-judgementally to a gay atheist widower in the series pilot, saying, 'I won't try to convert you' (S1E1). Brown also enthusiastically delves into a book with a lesbian plotline to solve a murder (S5E5), gives his blessing to a postulant who chooses her female partner over a life of religious service (S6E4), and persuades Mrs McCarthy (Sorcha Cusack) that two bell ringers at St Mary's in a lesbian relationship deserve to be happy (S7E2). In 1950s-set crime drama *Grantchester* (2014–), Detective Inspector Geordie (Robson Green), Reverend Sidney (James Norton), and Reverend Will (Tom Brittney) accept Reverend Leonard (Al Weaver) as gay while housekeeper Mrs Chapman (Tessa Peake-Jones) makes Leonard bar his partner Daniel (Oliver Dimsdale) from the vicarage (S4E6). An ardent Anglican, Mrs Chapman promotes celibacy but not SOCE, jail, or exposure. Britain's 1950s SOCE doctors, in hindsight, report shame, ignorance of SOCE's impact, efficacy doubts, and ethical conflicts (i.e., administering SOCE so that patients could avoid prison) (King et al., 2004). Unfortunately, in *APTCH*, Dr Milson lacks this hindsight while Dr Jack Duncan (Craig Hall) is morally conflicted (i.e., he calls gays 'shirt lifters') but still opposes SOCE (S6E4).

In *APTCH* James does not face prison or chemical castration (i.e., oestrogen pills), a practice with roots in Austrian endocrinologist Eugen Steinach's experiments of transplanting heterosexual donors' testicles into castrated homosexuals in the 1920s (Blakemore, 2018). James references British Lord Edward Montague's twelve-month imprisonment in 1954 for consensual homosexual offences (S4E11). Montague's and others' cases led to 1957's Wolfenden Report that argued for decriminalising private consensual homosexuality, as did happen in 1967, while Australian states decriminalised homosexuality between 1975 (i.e., South Australia) and 1997 (i.e., Tasmania) (Arrow, 2018). Post-SOCE, James's power and connections allow him a secret relationship with Henry. James first visits and then moves to the south of France with his first love William, Olivia's brother, where homosexuality is legal (S5E7). Starting in the 1970s Australian LGBTQ+ advocates would fight for the right to be LGBTQ+ publicly (Arrow, 2018).

While James's wealth and social privilege allow him to escape SOCE and find happiness, other gay characters in period dramas face bleaker futures. In *Call the Midwife*, Tony (Richard Fleeshman), husband of new mother Marie (Cara Theobold), is arrested for homosexual solicitation in 1960s London and he opts for chemical castration (i.e., oestrogen treatment) over jail (S4E3). Dr Turner (Stephen McGann) sympathetically warns that chemical castration can cause impotence, breast growth, and hair/muscle/libido loss. While the episode ends on an upbeat note when Tony goes to support Marie at her beauty pageant, in reality, long-term chemical castration causes depression (Han et al., 2018) and as previously noted, is believed to have contributed to WWII codebreaker Alan Turing's death by suicide. In *APTCH*, Dr Duncan, who battles depression and alcohol, injects testosterone after a forced orchiectomy as a Japanese POW and through him, we get a glimpse of the psychological pain that results from castration (S2E1). Jack's struggle with castration mirrors SOCE's attempts to castrate homosexual characters like James and Tony and their real-life counterparts.

Melodrama has historically been dismissed as women's films for their emotional/relational focus as well as exaggerated situations (Malone, 2017). Yet TV soap operas have affected great social changes, thus the United Nations Population Fund (UNPF) uses them for education (Jensen, 2006). American soaps like *Days of Our Lives* (1965–) depicted the acceptance of gay characters and one of the first gay kisses on American daytime TV in 2007; likewise, Australian soap *Number 96* presented a transgender actor playing a transgender character in 1973 and UK soap *EastEnders* depicted Britain's first televised mouth to mouth male–male kiss in 1989 (Baden, 2018; Brown, 2015). The UNPF was able to increase condom use with a Tanzanian radio soap due to audience/character identification, and Mexican sociologists argue that having a popular telenovela depict a gay man finding social/family acceptance helped to legalise same-sex marriage (Tate, 2014; Jensen, 2006). The UNPF's soap formula introduces sensitive content slowly, allowing audiences to bond with characters emotionally while giving them a vocabulary to be able to speak freely about challenging social issues (Jensen, 2006). Television critics have criticised *DA* and *CTM*, along with other period dramas, for altering history by transplanting modern attitudes and social politics regarding feminism, sexuality, and sexual violence into historical contexts where they would not have existed (Byrne, 2014; Fitzgerald, 2015; Lawson, 2017). *APTCH*, being a 1950s period drama, has managed to balance representing previously hidden LGBTQ+ lives and opening up the discussion on the destructive legacy of SOCE in Western medicine with achieving a realistic depiction of anti-LGBTQ+ attitudes and pseudo-treatments that characterised this period.

APTCH modifies UNPF's formula of introducing socially sensitive content slowly, because James's homosexuality is revealed early in series one, as a secret, and his family seeks a cure, but it is acceptance of James and other LGBTQ+ characters in the series (e.g., Harry, Henry) by the family and community that happens slowly, throughout the entire series. Elders Roy Briggs (Frankie J. Holden) and Doris Collins (Deborah Kennedy) become gatekeepers for community standards. Roy, a widowed farmer, is an archetypal Aussie working-class bloke. Whitman (2013) describes this archetype as having a normative sexuality, gender, and ethnicity that position him as unquestioningly Australian in opposition to culturally elite outsiders. Yet Roy extends his cultural privilege to gay, Jewish, and Aboriginal community outsiders in *APTCH*. Roy is surprised by James and Harry's sexuality but accepts them (S4E4). Roy's identity also fits the lone frontier man archetype, originally an identity that historically prioritised male bonds as there were few women in Australia's early period but 'frontier mythologies silenced alternative views of masculinity, including homosexuality' (Featherstone, 2010: 347). One could argue that *APTCH* engages the heteronormative by emphasising the hypermasculinity of LGBTQ+ characters like Henry and James (e.g., Roy initially refuses to believe Harry, a ruggedly athletic farm-worker, is gay for this reason [S4E4]) and by using heterosexual-identified actors like David Berry to portray James (who plays another homosexual character, Lord John Grey in *Outlander* [2014–]). Another possible reading is that the series is interrogating the social phenomenon of straight-acting, whereby gay men use hegemonic masculinity to overcome their culture's feminised stereotype, and punishment, of male homosexuals (Eguchi, 2009). Roy encourages Doris to accept Harry and Henry after she finds them kissing (S6E6). Doris is representative of the anglicised colonial identity that Mohanram (1999, p. 165) argues of women who reconstructed 'British homes in foreign spaces, functioning as metonyms of home and of Brittania [*sic*]' and civilised bachelors. Doris initially attempts to find Harry a wife (S6E4) and continues to bake for him upon learning he is homosexual. Elizabeth, represented by her English rose garden and Victorian morals, is similarly a British colonial metonym, who comes to accept her grandson's homosexuality by the series' end.

APTCH's cast, in real life, assumed the roles of social gatekeepers in their efforts to persuade Australians to vote yes on the 2017 marriage equality survey. Actors Sara Wiseman (Carolyn) and Craig Hall's (Jack) social media video mocked the government, the plebiscite expense, and urged Australians to vote 'yes' (FOD, 2017). Actor Marta Dusseldorp (Sarah) staged a human rainbow with Sydney's fashion/creative professionals in Hyde Park (Clarke, 2017). Noni Hazelhurst (Elizabeth) signed a petition against the marriage plebiscite and for a free parliamentary vote (Kirk, 2016). The impact of James's SOCE storyline and cast member advocacy has not been studied but the programme's main demographic, aged fifty-five and older (Anderson, 2014), also submitted the most surveys (i.e., ages fifty-five to eighty-four) (Beaumont, 2017). Fixed address respondents had higher survey submission rates, but the age eighteen to twenty-four demographic most likely to vote for equality were less likely to use postal mail or have fixed addresses (Faruqi, 2017). Thus, outreach to *APTCH*'s main demographic aged fifty-five and over, the most active survey respondents, is significant and speaks to the power of period dramas like *APTCH* to enact change.

Conclusion

APTCH has been labelled a historical drama but also a soap opera/melodrama and both categories seek to achieve realism to attract viewers but they face challenges in reaching this goal. Soap opera melodrama must balance the desire to attract viewers with emotionally gripping stories while maintaining the integrity of their storylines that are meant to educate viewers about social issues. Johnson (2013) argues that melodrama, by expressing emotion, can create an outlet for long-suppressed LGBTQ+ voices. *APTCH* does seem to realistically channel the pain and oppression that is embedded in the real-life accounts of SOCE survivors used in the construction of this chapter. At the same time, the fear is that viewers will discount such representations because of the cultural devaluation of programmes labelled as soap operas or melodramas. As previously noted, historical dramas must balance accurately representing the period with the audience's desire to see their attitudes, beliefs, and values reflected on the screen. *APTCH*'s representation of James's life does reflect the reality of generations of LGBTQ+ who underwent SOCE treatment. At the same time, James's story is one of a socially privileged character, who has agency and a somewhat supportive family. Perhaps as a result James is able to break from SOCE easier and with less damage (i.e., he escapes a lobotomy, and stops electroconvulsive sessions before experiencing long-term memory loss) as opposed to other real-life survivors who lacked these social supports and resources and as a result, faced significantly greater challenges. Historical drama has been critiqued for its privileged perspective. Ridderstrøm's (2018) study of *DA* found that the focus on socially privileged characters and worldviews had the effect of obscuring or hiding the exploitation of less privileged classes. Likewise, James's story in *APTCH* cannot speak to the social diversity of SOCE survivors' experiences, though he provides a window into an underexplored time in LGBTQ+ medical history.

APTCH also connects LGBTQ+ characters' 1950s civil rights struggles to the modern fight for marriage equality. At series end, we learn that nonagenarians Henry and Harry marry legally in January 2018 (S6E10). However, closing the couple's storyline with same-sex marriage suggests that the socio-political struggles of LGBTQ+ people have ended when Australia in 2018 had not yet federally banned SOCE, LGBTQ+ people still faced violence/death, and health care challenges faced by LGBTQ+ Indigenous/Australians of colour remain unaddressed (Power, 2017). Similarly, ending James's storyline with his death in 1986 from AIDS memorialises a lost LGBTQ+ generation but also places series finale viewers in a post-AIDS moment despite an HIV+ population of thirty-seven million people globally.

Given what we know about James's experiences with the medical profession via SOCE, this begs the questions, how did surviving SOCE figure into James's HIV/AIDS health? Did SOCE leave James wary of health care, make him withhold information from his doctor, and be less likely to receive health-saving information/tests/treatment? Did James's social privilege and wealth allow him greater access to expensive experimental treatments that the average person could not afford? Furthermore, how prepared was the medical profession, given its discriminatory history, to provide access to quality care and support to patients like James? James, as a fictional SOCE survivor and a person living with HIV/AIDS (PWA), is a placeholder for the diversity of real people whose stories he represents. The fact that we do not know more of his PWA story is representative of the invisibility and marginalisation of LGBTQ+ people in social and medical history.

Before the 2017 marriage equality survey, the Australian Medical Association (AMA) asked the government to end debate and legislate same-sex marriage. In doing so, it acknowledged the damage caused to LGBTQ+ communities by the medical profession and said that not legislating marriage furthered the institutionalised discrimination that was detrimental to LGBTQ+ mental/physical health (AMA, 2017). The AMA cited a 'long history of institutional discrimination' such as the classification of homosexuality as mental illness as contributing to worse health care outcomes for modern LGBTQ+ people (AMA, 2017). While the AMA's move to acknowledge a history of discrimination is an important first step, it should not be done in a way that connotes that discriminatory medicine is a thing of the past.

If James's SOCE doctor lived today he might express regret in retrospect or he might think like Dr Pansy Lai. Dr Lai publicly opposed changing the definition of marriage, actions that brought public threats and petitions to deregister her as a doctor. The AMA defended Dr Lai's right to her opinion, but same-sex marriage became law in Australia in 2018. While Dr Lai's stance has slipped from the headlines, this does not mean that the anti-LGBTQ+ medical discourses represented by her rhetoric, or those who think like her but who decline to speak publicly, have ceased to make an impact. James may have died in 1986 but the medical legacy he represents endures today in how medical care is structured, delivered, and represented, and by the LGBTQ+ people who continue to advocate for inclusive and self-determined medical care.

References

AMA: Australian Medical Association (2017). *Marriage equality –2017*. Available at: https://ama.com.au/position-statement/marriage-equality-2017 (Accessed 6 August 2019).

Anderson, D. (2014). *A Place to Call Home: Not Australia's Downton Abbey – yet*. Available at: www.theguardian.com/culture/2014/nov/05/a-place-to-call-home-not-australias-downton-abbey-yet (Accessed 23 September 2019).

Arrow, M. (2018). '"These are just a few examples of our daily oppressions": Speaking and listening to homosexuality in Australia's Royal Commission on Human Relationships, 1974–1977', *Journal of the History of Sexuality*, 27(2), pp. 234–263, *LGBT Life with Full Text via EBSCO Host* [Online]. Available at: http://web.ebscohost.com (Accessed 12 August 2019).

Baden III, A. G. (2018). 'Soap operas and social change', *Gay & Lesbian Review Worldwide*, 25(6), pp. 27–29, *LGBT Life with Full Text via EBSCO Host* [Online]. Available at: http://web.ebscohost.com (Accessed 14 August 2019).

Beaumont, A. (2017). *Same-sex marriage survey by the stats: A resounding 'yes' but western Sydney leads 'no' vote*. Available at: https://theconversation.com/same-sex-marriage-survey-by-the-stats-a-resounding-yes-but-western-sydney-leads-no-vote-87258, (Accessed 23 September 2019).

Blakemore, E. (2018). *Gay conversion therapy's disturbing 19th-century origins*. Available at: www.history.com/news/gay-conversion-therapy-origins-19th-century (Accessed 22 June 2018).

Blundell, G. (2016). 'Knowing its place,' *The Australian*, 10 September, p. 31. LexisNexis via Nexis Uni [Online]. Available at: www.lexisnexis.com (Accessed 7 February 2020).

Brown, L. (2015). 'Homosexual lives: Representation and reinterpretation in *Upstairs, Downstairs* and *Downton Abbey*', in Leggott, J. and Taddeo, J. (eds), *Upstairs and downstairs: British costume drama television from The Forsyte Saga to Downton Abbey*. Rowman and Littlefield, Lanham, pp. 263–274.

Byrne, K. (2014). 'Adapting heritage: Class and conservatism in *Downton Abbey*', *Rethinking History*, 18(3), pp. 311–327, Academic Search Complete via *EBSCO Host* [Online]. Available at: http://web.ebscohost.com (Accessed 23 September 2019). doi: 10.1080/13642529.2013.811811.

Cherniavsky, E. (1998). 'Real again: Melodrama and the subject of HIV/AIDS', *GLQ: A Journal of Lesbian & Gay Studies*, 4(3), pp. 385–401, Academic Search Complete via *EBSCO Host* [Online]. Available at: http://web.ebscohost.com (Accessed 23 September 2019). doi: 10.1215/10642684-4-3-375.

Chiang, H. H.-H. (2008). 'Effecting science, affecting medicine: Homosexuality, the Kinsey reports, and the contested boundaries of psychopathology in the United States, 1948–1965', *Journal of the History of the Behavioral Sciences*, 44(4), pp. 300–318, Academic Search Complete via *EBSCO Host* [Online]. Available at: http://web.ebscohost.com, (Accessed 23 September 2019). doi: 10.1002/jhbs.20343.

Clarke, J. (2017). *Australia's fashion community strike a pose for the Yes campaign*. Available at: www.smh.com.au/lifestyle/fashion/australias-fashion-community-strike-a-pose-for-the-yes-campaign-20170927-gypqqp.html (Accessed 23 September 2019).

Crain, C. (1999). *Did a germ make you gay*? Available at: www.steamthing.com/gaygerm (Accessed 27 September 2019).

Daley, B. (2018, May 2). *'Treatments' as torture: Gay conversion therapy's deep roots in Australia*. Available at: https://theconversation.com/treatments-as-torture-gay-conversion-therapys-deep-roots-in-australia-95588 (Accessed 1 February 2020).

Dean, E. (2016). 'Shock therapies', *Nursing Standard*, 30(23), p. 25, MEDLINE Complete via *EBSCO Host* [Online]. Available at: http://web.ebscohost.com (Accessed 23 September 2019). doi:10.7748/ns.30.23.25.s24.

Donovan, S. (2015, August 18). *Turana state ward tells of electroshock therapy*. Available at: www.abc.net.au/radio/programs/pm/turana-state-ward-tells-of-electroshock-therapy/6706892 (Accessed 1 February 2020).

Drescher, J. (2015). 'Out of DSM: Depathologizing homosexuality', *Behavioral Sciences (2076-328X)*, 5(4), pp. 565–575, Academic Search Complete via *EBSCO Host* [Online]. Available at: http://web.ebscohost.com (Accessed 27 September 2019). doi: 10.3390/bs5040565.

Eguchi, S. (2009). 'Negotiating hegemonic masculinity: The rhetorical strategy of "straight-acting" among gay men', *Journal of Intercultural Communication Research*, 38(3), pp. 193–209, Communication & Mass Media Complete via EBSCO Host [Online]. Available at: http://web.ebscohost.com (Accessed 7 February 2020). doi:10.1080/17475759.2009.508892.

Ehrlich, L. G. (1980). *The pathogenic secret: A response to discrimination*. Available at: https://eric.ed.gov/ (Accessed 27 September 2019).

Esterberg, K. G. (1990). 'From illness to action: Conceptions of homosexuality in *The Ladder*, 1956–1965', *Journal of Sex Research*, 27(1), pp. 65–81. doi: 10.1080/00224499009551542.

Faruqi, O. (2017). *How the housing crisis could help conservatives win the marriage equality plebiscite*. Available at: https://junkee.com/marriage-equality-housing-plebiscite/117375 (Accessed 23 September 2019).

Featherstone, L. (2010). 'Pathologising white male sexuality in late nineteenth-century Australia through the medical prism of excess and constraint', *Australian Historical Studies*, 41(3), pp. 337–351, Humanities Source via EBSCO *Host* [Online]. Available at: http://web.ebscohost.com (Accessed 12 August 2019). doi: 10.1080/1031461X.2010.493949.

Fitzgerald, L. (2015). 'Taking a pregnant pause: Interrogating the feminist potential of *Call the Midwife*', in Leggott, J. and Taddeo, J. (eds.), *Upstairs and downstairs: British costume drama television from The Forsyte Saga to Downton Abbey*. Rowman and Littlefield, Lanham, pp. 263–274.

FOD: Funny or Die (2017). *Lets get marriage equality in Australia*. Available at: www.youtube.com/watch?v=AGXN7L13X8g (Accessed 5 October 2018).

Friedan, B. (1963). *The feminine mystique*. Norton, New York.

Haggett, A. (2009). '"Desperate Housewives" and the domestic environment in post-war Britain: Individual perspectives', *Oral History: The Journal of the* Oral History Society, 37(1), pp. 53–60, *JSTOR Arts and Sciences VIII via JSTOR* [Online]. Available at: www.jstor.org (Accessed 13 August 2019).

Hale, M. (2017). 'Globe-trotting with a TV remote,' *The Australian*, 2 June, p. 31. LexisNexis via Nexis Uni [Online]. Available at: www.lexisnexis.com (Accessed 7 February 2020).

Halliday, S. (2001). 'Death and miasma in Victorian London: An obstinate belief', *BMJ: British Medical Journal (International Edition)*, 323(7327), pp. 1469–1471. doi: 10.1136/bmj.323.7327.1469.

Hegarty, S. (2018). *Gay conversion therapy survivors share painful legacy of 'ex-gay' treatments*. Available at: www.abc.net.au/news/2018-04-21/gay-conversion-therapy-survivors-on-greg-hunt-comments/9679416 (Accessed 10 August 2019).

Jennings, R. (2015). *Unnamed desires: A Sydney lesbian history*. Monash, Victoria.

Jensen, J. (2006). *Serial melodrama: From selling soap to social change*. Available at: www.unfpa.org/news/serial-melodrama-selling-soap-social-change (Accessed 10 August 2019).

Johnson, M. E. (2013). '"Never the same one twice": Melodrama and repetition in queer as folk', *Genre: Forms of Discourse and Culture*, 46(3), pp. 419–442.

Jones, T., Brown, A., Carnie, L., Fletcher, G., and Leonard, W. (2018). *Preventing harm, promoting justice: Responding to LGBT conversion therapy in Australia*. Available at: www.hrlc.org.au/reports/preventing-harm (Accessed 23 September 2018).

King, M., Smith, G., and Bartlett, A. (2004). 'Treatments of homosexuality in Britain since the 1950s--an oral history: The experience of professionals', *BMJ: British Medical Journal*, 328(7437), pp. 429–432. doi: 10.1136/bmj.328.7437.429.37984.496725.EE.

Kirk, P. (2016). *Public figures call on government to hold free vote on same-sex marriage*. Available at: www.theguardian.com/australia-news/2016/nov/05/public-figures-call-on-government-to-hold-free-vote-on-same-sex-marriage (Accessed 23 September 2019).

Kvistad, E. (2018). 'Bad property: Unclean houses in Victorian City writing', *Victorian Network*, 6(2), pp. 86–108, [Online]. Available at: www.victoriannetwork.org/index.php/vn/issue/view/11 (Accessed 9 September 2019).

Lawson, M. (2017, May 5). *Not in this day and age: When will TV stop horrendously airbrushing history?* Available at: www.theguardian.com/tv-and-radio/2017/may/05/downton-abbey-jamestown-call-the-midwife-when-will-period-dramas-stop-horrendously-airbrushing-history (Accessed 7 February 2020).

Malone, A. (2017). *Backwards and in heels: The past, present and future of women working in film*. Mango, Coral Gables.

Margolin, L. (2017). 'Sexual frigidity: The social construction of masculine privilege and feminine pathology', *Journal of Gender Studies*, 26(5), pp. 583–594. doi: 10.1080/09589236.2016.1152957.

McDermott, W. (2018). *The pernicious myth of conversion therapy: How love in action perpetrated a fraud on America*. Available at: www.nclrights.org/wp-content/uploads/2018/11/Mattachine-Society-Conversion-Therapy-White-Paper-Redacted.pdf (Accessed 27 September 2019).

Petersen, F. (2012, September 5). *Sydney doctor who prescribed chemical castration as 'cure' for gay man banned from practicing*. Available at: www.pri.org/stories/2012-09-05/sydney-doctor-who-prescribed-chemical-castration-cure-gay-man-banned-practicing (Accessed 1 February 2020).

Power, S. (2017). *Indigenous and LGBTI: Who's looking after you?* Available at: www.sbs.com.au/topics/sexuality/agenda/article/2017/03/30/indigenous-and-lgbti-whos-looking-after-you (Accessed 25 June 2019).

Ridderstrøm, H. (2018). 'Class concerns in a heritage setting: Viewers' responses to *Downton Abbey* on IMDb,' *Series: International Journal of TV Serial Narratives*, 4(2), 91–102. Available at: https://series.unibo.it/article/view/7960/8716 (Accessed 7 February 2020). doi: 10.6092/issn.2421-454X/7960.

Romm, C. (2015). *During World War II, sex was a national-security threat*. Available at: www.theatlantic.com/health/archive/2015/10/during-world-war-ii-sexually-active-women-were-a-national-security-threat/409555/ (Accessed 1 September 2019)

Rubinstein, G. (2010). 'Narcissism and self-esteem among homosexual and heterosexual male students', *Journal of Sex & Marital Therapy*, 36(1), pp. 24–34, *SocINDEX with Full Text via EBSCO Host* [Online]. Available at: http://web.ebscohost.com (Accessed 13 August 2019). doi: 10.1080/00926230903375594.

Scot, J. (2017). *Shock the gay away: Secrets of early gay aversion therapy revealed*. Available at: www.huffpost.com/entry/shock-the-gay-away-secrets-of-early-gay-aversion-therapy-revealed_b_3497435?guccounter=1 (Accessed 10 August 2019).

Simmons, G. (2005). 'Paradise lost: *Far From Heaven*', *Screen Education* (40), pp. 103–107, Communication & Mass Media Complete via EBSCO Host [Online]. Available at: http://web.ebscohost.com (Accessed 24 September 2019).

Skvirsky, S. A. (2008). 'The price of heaven: Remaking politics in *All that Heaven Allows*, *Ali: Fear Eats the Soul*, and *Far from Heaven*', *Cinema Journal*, 47(3), pp. 90–121. MLA International Bibliography via EBSCO Host [Online]. Available at: http://web.ebscohost.com (Accessed 14 August 2019).

Smaal, Y. (2013). '"It is one of those things that nobody can explain": Medicine, homosexuality, and the Australian criminal courts during World War II', *Journal of the History of Sexuality*, 22(3), pp. 501–524, Education Source via EBSCO *Host* [Online]. Available at: http://web.ebscohost.com (Accessed 13 August 2019). doi: 10.7560/JHS22306.

Soukup, P. A. (2016). 'Studying soap operas', *Communication Research Trends*, 35(3), pp. 3–55, Communication & Mass Media Complete via EBSCO Host [Online]. Available at: http://web.ebscohost.com (Accessed 7 February 2020).

SSCCA: Senate Standing Committees on Community Affairs (2005). *Inquiry into children in institutional care:* Chapter 3 – *Why children were in homes*. Available at: www.aph.gov.au/Parliamentary_Business/Committees/Senate/Community_Affairs/Completed_inquiries/2004-07/inst_care/report/c03 (Accessed 14 August 2019).

Stopes, M. (1918). *Married love or love in marriage*. Available at: http://digital.library.upenn.edu/women/stopes/married/1918.html (Accessed 26 December 2019).

Tate, J. (2014). 'Laughing all the way to tolerance? Mexican comedic telenovelas as vehicles for lessons against homophobia', *Latin Americanist*, 58(3), pp. 51–65, MLA International Bibliography via EBSCO Host [Online]. Available at: http://web.ebscohost.com (Accessed 14 August 2019). doi: 10.1111/tla.12036.

Trickey, E. (2018). *Inside the story of America's 19th-century opiate addiction*. Available at: www.smithsonianmag.com/history/inside-story-americas-19th-century-opiate-addiction-180967673/ (Accessed 20 August 2019).

Vider, S. and Byers, D. S. (2015). *A half-century of conflict over attempts to 'cure' gay people*. Available at: https://time.com/3705745/history-therapy-hadden/ (Accessed 20 August 2019).

Whitman, K. (2013). *Looking out for the 'Aussie bloke': Gender, class, and contextualizing a hegemony of working-class masculinities in Australia*. PhD. University of Adelaide.

Williams, Z. (2011, September 2). *Marie Stopes: A turbo-Darwinist ranter, but right about birth control*. Available at: www.theguardian.com/theguardian/2011/sep/02/marie-stopes-right-birth-control (Accessed 6 February 2020).

Afterword

Jessica Meyer

As I write this, it is slightly over a year since the World Health Organization declared what has come to be known as COVID-19 a global pandemic. The United Kingdom has just taken the most recent step on its 'roadmap' out of a third national lockdown, which has been in place for over two months; European nations are struggling to contain a third wave of infections currently filling acute wards in Paris, Berlin, and Rome; in Australia and the Americas, vaccine rollouts are embroiled in political debates over mobility and personal freedoms, while China, India, and Russia engage in vaccine diplomacy aimed at extending their global economic influence. For individuals and local communities, forced to isolate, social distance, wash hands regularly, wear masks, and get vaccinated, never have health, illness, and the awareness of the physical body been so great a focus for so many of us for so long.

At the same time, strategies of local and national lockdowns, accompanied by policies of furlough or layoff for workers in shuttered industries, have given many people more time to engage in home-based leisure activities, among which watching television has been one of the most widespread. COVID binge-watching, driven in part by the rise of streaming services, most notably Netflix, has become part of the cultural landscape of our COVID-shaped world.

While the range of programming which has fed this phenomenon has been diverse, including documentaries, contemporary dramas, and nostalgia-driven boxsets of older series such as *The West Wing*, period dramas have made a noticeable contribution to national and international discussions of what everyone is (or, according to the critics, should be) watching. Series four of *The Crown* (Netflix, 2020), set in the 1980s, had viewing figures of twenty-nine million, more than the 28.4 million who watched Charles and Diana's televised wedding in the original 1981 broadcast. *The Queen's Gambit* (Netflix, 2020), set in the 1950s and 1960s, became Netflix's most-watched miniseries within four weeks of its release in October 2020. This has since been overtaken by *Bridgerton* (Netflix, 2020), released, again by

Netflix, in December 2020 which, to date, has had a viewership of eighty-two million households and reached number one in eighty-three countries worldwide.[1]

The international popularity of historical dramas in this time of global health crisis has tended to be viewed by both critics and consumers as a form of escapism. The trials and tribulations of the British royal family, the life of an orphaned American chess prodigy, the froth and frolics of the Regency *ton* all seem at first glance to be as distanced from the quotidian trials of furlough, work-from-home, and homeschooling, or the anxieties of job loss, distance from loved ones, and rising death tolls as one can imagine. And yet health, medicine, and the body are all central to these dramas. Diana's bulimia, Beth's drug addiction, and the perils of sex, pregnancy, and childbirth for a range of characters in *Bridgerton* are all central to the plots of these dramas. Even when medical practitioners and settings are not central, medical encounters serve to drive the plots of television dramas with historic settings.

The centrality of medicine to historical dramas is not, of course, new. As the editors of this collection note, medicine has long been a way of expressing and exploring anxieties about the world, in the past as well as the present. And medicine is itself inherently dramatic. From the operating theatres of the eighteenth century, designed to allow banks of students to act as an audience to medical treatments and vivisection, to the popularity of reality television series such as *One Born Every Minute* (Channel 4, 2010–2018; Lifetime Television, 2011–2012), modern medicine has, since its inception, been framed by the dramatic arts. The same might be said for the discipline of history, with historical drama found at the heart of European and American culture throughout the early modern and modern periods. That the two disciplines should overlap and inform each other in the contemporary cultural form of television should, therefore, come as no surprise. This is simply the most recent manifestation of a long and fruitful partnership that has developed on the stage, the pages of novels, and in films before emerging so extensively on the small screen. As this collection elegantly demonstrates through the wide range of periods, dramas, and topics it addresses, medical narratives form an integral part of television costume dramas across a variety of geographies and cultures.

What then, can we learn from this intersection of medicine, history, and televisual drama, particularly in this moment of global health crisis? As the chapters in this collection show, there are a number of important themes that period dramas are particularly well-placed to explore. The place of gender in historical medical practice, in relation to both patient and practitioner, for example, recurs across both topics and time periods, as well as highlighting contemporary concerns. For example, the focus on male mental health, a topic of considerable political interest in Britain in the past two decades, across dramas as diverse as *To Walk Invisible*, *Taboo*, *Peaky Blinders*, and *A Place to Call Home* raises interesting questions about how current medical concerns can be reflected in the stories we tell about the past. By contrast, considering female experiences of health and medicine as they appear in both *Harlots* and *Call the Midwife* highlights the persistence of gendered power imbalances in women's experiences of the medical encounter and the continuity of gynaecology in the construction of women as medical subjects.

This question of the balance of power between patient and practitioner is, of course, one of the central questions explored by social historians of medicine. For such historians, therefore, the consideration of medicine in period drama provides an interesting angle on the discipline. As several chapters in this collection demonstrate, such dramas allow for the representation of practitioners as both heroes and villains, and as individuals asserting their professional power within limits defined by gender, race, and class. Dramatising such struggles has the power to bring the subject to life, and to disseminate historical knowledge to a wide audience. Like all period dramas, however, they risk oversimplifying complex, messy narratives, in which many historic actors are, perforce, written out. Here the scholarship of the contributors to this volume makes an important contribution. By probing the limits and nuances of these representations, their analysis helps to bridge the divide between popular perception and scholarly understanding, providing a basis on which the two can meet in conversation.

Nor is it only from the representation of the character and role of the practitioner that such discussions emerge. Period dramas also provide important spaces in which the patient voice and patient experience can be represented and explored. Since Roy Porter first challenged historians of medicine to 'lower the historical gaze to the sufferers' (Porter, 1985: 192), the use of the patient voice has become a significant part of the methodology of the field. It has proved a particularly useful perspective in exploring mental illness, although intersections with the developing field of disability history have provided diverse avenues of investigation around physical illness and the experience of pain as well. The ability to dramatise and thereby foreground the patient voice both within and beyond the medical encounter is one of the strengths of period drama as a medium. The emergence of such voices across the programmes examined here serves to reinforce the centrality of both social relationships to medical care provision and the significance of medicine as a force for shaping such relationships.

Social relationships are, of course, the basis of all good drama, contemporary or historical, in whatever medium presented. Medicine in period drama, as noted, allows us to consider continuity and discontinuity in our understanding of mental and physical health and illness, and who has the authority to provide advice and care, across time. Is there, however, something particular about the small screen as a medium for communicating the social history of medicine as a dramatic subject? Certainly, there are advantages in comparison to filmic representations. The long-running nature of many of the dramas discussed here, covering not merely multiple episodes but often multiples seasons as well, enables developments in medical practice and social attitudes to be traced over time in ways that are harder to capture in the running time of a film. The changes in technology, demography, and social attitudes traced by *Call the Midwife*, for example, would be impossible in a feature film format. Bringing these stories of the medical past into our homes also has the potential to give them an immediacy which can, in turn, lead to identification and understanding. The contemporary relevance of the seemingly remote historical events of *La Peste* become recognisable not only through the coincidence of timing, which saw the first season released shortly before the outbreak of the current pandemic, but also through the detailed construction of the social world of the plague.

There are, of course, dangers in dramatising any aspect of the past via a form that is constrained by both the time limitation of a set number of episodes and by economic considerations of a commercial format. As with the desire to create engaging dramatic characters noted above, the need to construct a coherent narrative arc within a set time frame tends to elide the complex messiness of the past through oversimplification or the telescoping of chronologies. The elisions, omissions, and anachronisms unpicked by several contributors to this collection highlight this tendency. For the historian watching such programmes, this can be immensely frustrating, leading to a plaintive chorus of, 'But it is so much more complicated than that!', particularly when let loose on a social media platform. But when considered, as here, with scholarly seriousness, these trends and tendencies can show the ways in which historians can communicate their knowledge more widely. The choice of historical subject, character, and setting are, in the best productions, never random. In considering how medicine makes drama in the context of the past, this collection helps us navigate new ways for telling the stories about medicine *in* the past that have engaged us as researchers.

The truncation and simplification of historical narratives is an accusation that can, of course, be levelled at period dramas dealing with any subject. What then, does the form have to offer historians of medicine in particular? In conceptualising the history of the modern world, war has long been understood as one of the most powerful forces in the creation of the world as we know it today. It is, in the words of Joan W. Scott, writing about gender in particular, 'the ultimate disorder, the disruption of all previously established relationships' (Scott, 1987: 27). Yet, for all war's disruptive power and global ubiquity as a force of social and cultural change in modern history, it has nothing on health and medicine. Those of us privileged to live in the comparative stability of Western democracies are, today, unlikely to have lived experiences of warfare. As we have all become too intimately aware in this past year, however, the daily lives of all of us are shaped by our bodily health, our mental wellbeing, our ability to access appropriate and authoritative care, the politics and resilience of health care systems, and the global networks of both medical research and provision of medical supplies. Health and medicine shape our lives at all levels, from our personal subjectivities through economic and social relationships that form our communities to the diplomacy that shapes international relations, and at all points in our lives, from birth to death.

Today, in the midst of a global pandemic, the ubiquity of health and medicine feels like the very definition of the modern world as we experience it today. What period drama has the power to do, however, is to demonstrate the extent to which this was true of the past. The caregiver – whether in the form of doctor, nurse, midwife, or apothecary – has always been part of any community. Accident, illness (both physical and mental), addiction, and the frailties of old age have always had the power to disrupt previously established relationships in unexpected ways. Technological innovation and increased scientific knowledge may have made certain conditions less lethal than in the past, although only smallpox has ever been fully eradicated. But mortality rates overall remain 100 per cent. Death still comes for us all.

Engagement with health and medicine in one form or another is, in the end, a central element of the human condition because our lives are lived out within and through our bodies and minds. This is both the familiarity and the strangeness that medicine in period dramas has the power to evoke. Whatever else they have to tell us, these dramatised narratives transformed into shadows on our screens remind us that the past, like the present, was a human experience because it was an embodied one.

Note

1 See Cope (2020), White (2020), and BBC (2021).

References

BBC (2021). 'Bridgerton: Netflix Says Drama Is Its Biggest Series Ever', *BBC News*, 28 January, www.bbc.co.uk/news/entertainment-arts-55837969, accessed 31 March 2021.

Cope, R. (2020). 'Season 4 of The Crown Got More Viewers Than Prince Charles and Princess Diana's Wedding', *Tatler*, 26 November, www.tatler.com/article/the-crown-viewing-figures-tops-prince-charles-and-princess-dianas-wedding-day, accessed 31 March 2021.

Porter, R. (1985). 'The Patient's View: Doing Medical History from Below', *Theory and Society* 14:2.

White, P. (2020). '"The Queen's Gambit" Becomes Netflix's Biggest Scripted Limited Series with 62M Checking Chess Drama', *Deadline Hollywood*, November 23, https://deadline.com/2020/11/queens-gambit-62m-viewers-netflix-1234620378/, accessed 31 March 2021.

Scott, J. W. (1987). 'Rewriting History', in *Behind the Lines: Gender and the Two World Wars*, ed. M. R. Higonnet, J. Jenson, S. Michel, and M. Collins Weitz (New Haven: Yale University Press).

Index

Lightning Source UK Ltd.
Milton Keynes UK
UKHW051009091122
411853UK00043B/89

9 781526 163288